Diabetes
in Old Age

Diabetes in Old Age
SECOND EDITION

Edited by

Alan J. Sinclair

Diabetes Research Unit
Academic Department of Geriatric Medicine and Gerontology,
The University of Birmingham, UK

and

Paul Finucane

Department of Rehabilitation and Aged Care,
Flinders University, Daw Park, Australia

Supported by an unrestricted educational grant from Servier

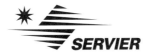

JOHN WILEY & SONS, LTD

Chichester • New York • Weinheim • Brisbane • Singapore • Toronto

First Edition published 1995
Copyright © 1995, 2001 John Wiley & Sons Ltd.,
    Baffins Lane, Chichester,
    West Sussex PO19 1UD, UK

    National   01243 779777
    International (+44) 1243 779777
    e-mail (for orders and customer service enquiries): cs-books@wiley.co.uk
    Visit our Home Page on http://www.wiley.co.uk or http://www.wiley.com

Other Wiley Editorial Offices

John Wiley & Sons, Inc., 605 Third Avenue,
New York, NY 10158-0012, USA

WILEY-VCH Verlag GmbH, Pappelallee 3,
D-69469 Weinheim, Germany

Jacaranda Wiley Ltd, 33 Park Road, Milton,
Queensland 4064, Australia

John Wiley & Sons (Asia) Pte, Ltd, 2 Clementi Loop #02-01,
Jin Xing Distripark, Singapore 129809

John Wiley & Sons (Canada), Ltd., 22 Worcester Road,
Rexdale, Ontario M9W 1L1, Canada

Library of Congress Cataloging-in-Publication Data

Diabetes in old age/edited by Alan J. Sinclair and Paul Finucane.—2nd ed.
    p. ; cm
  Finucane's name appears first on the earlier edition.
  Includes bibliographical references and index.
  ISBN 0-471-49010-5 (cased : alk paper)
  1. Diabetes in old age. I. Sinclair, Alan. II. Finucane, Paul, 1955–
  [DNLM: 1. Diabetes Mellitus—Aged. WK 810 D5375253 2000]
  RC660.75 .D4485 2000
  618.97′6462—dc21   00-043929

British Library Cataloguing in Publication Data

A catalogue record for this book is available from the British Library

ISBN 0-471-49010-5

Typeset in 10/12pt Times from the author's disks by Techset, Salisbury.
Printed and bound in Great Britain by Bookcraft (Bath) Ltd, Midsomer Norton, Somerset
This book is printed on acid-free paper responsibly manufactured from sustainable forestry,
in which at least two trees are planted for each one used for paper production.

Contents

Contributors

Susan Benbow   *Department of Medicine, Hairmyres Hospital, East Kilbride, Glasgow G75 8RG, Scotland*

E. Bonara   *Division of Endocrinology and Metabolic Diseases, Ospedale Civile Maggiore, Piazzale Stefani 1, 37126 Verona, Italy*

Andrew J. M. Boulton   *University Department of Medicine, Manchester Royal Infirmary, Oxford Road, Manchester M13 9WL, England*

E. Brun   *Division of Endocrinology and Metabolic Diseases, Ospedale Civile Maggiore, Piazzale Stefani 1, 37126 Verona, Italy*

Amanda Butcher   *Department of Medicine and Ophthalmology, Birmingham Heartlands Hospital, Birmingham, England*

Joe M. Chehade   *Division of Endocrinology, Diabetes and Metabolism, St Louis University School of Medicine, St Louis, MO 63104, USA*

Maria Crotty   *Department of Rehabilitation and Aged Care, Flinders University, Adelaide, South Australia*

Simon C. M. Croxson   *United Bristol NHS Healthcare Trust, Bristol General Hospital, Bristol BS1 6SY, England*

Paul Dodson   *Department of Medicine and Ophthalmology, Birmingham Heartlands Hospital, Birmingham, England*

Paul Finucane   *Department of Rehabilitation and Aged Care, Flinders University, General Hospital, Daws Road, Daw Park, South Australia 5041*

Brian M. Frier   *Department of Diabetes, Royal Infirmary of Edinburgh, Lauriston Place, Edinburgh EH3 9YW, Scotland*

Roger Gadsby   *Centre for Primary Healthcare Studies, Warwick University, Coventry, Warwick, England*

Geoffrey Gill   *Department of Diabetes and Endocrinology, University Hospital Aintree, Liverpool L9 1AE, England*

Tim Hendra   *Department of Geriatric Medicine, Royal Hallamshire Hospital, Sheffield, England*

P. Jean Ho   *Diabetes Centre, Royal Prince Alfred Hospital, Campertown, NSW, Australia*

Hosam K. Kamel   *Division of Geriatric Medicine, St Louis University School of Medicine, St Louis, MO 63104, USA*

Vincent McAulay   *Department of Diabetes, Royal Infirmary of Edinburgh, Lauriston Place, Edinburgh EH3 9YW, Scotland*

Graydon S. Meneilly   *Vancouver Hospital and Health Sciences Centre, UBC Site, 2211 Wesbrook Mall, Vancouver V6T 2B5, BC, Canada*

Arshag D. Mooradian   *Division of Endocrinology, Diabetes and Metabolism, St Louis University School of Medicine, St Louis, MO 63104, USA*

John E. Morley   *Division of Geriatric Medicine, St Louis University School of Medicine, St Louis, MO 63104, USA*

Michele Muggeo   *Division of Endocrinology and Metabolic Diseases, Ospedale Civile Maggiore, Piazzale Stefani 1, 37126 Verona, Italy*

Phil Popplewell   *Department of Rehabilitation and Aged Care, Flinders University, Adelaide, South Australia*

Klaas Reenders   *University of Groningen, The Netherlands*

Donald Richardson *Leonard R. Strelitz Diabetes Institute, Eastern Virginia Medical School, Norfolk, Virginia, USA*

Alan J. Sinclair *Diabetes Research Unit, Academic Department of Geriatric Medicine and Gerontology, University of Birmingham, Selly Oak Hospital, Birmingham B29 6JD, England*

Lea Sorenson *Diabetes Centre, Royal Prince Alfred Hospital, Campertown, NSW, Australia*

Christopher J. Turnbull *Arrowe Park Hospital, Upton, The Wirral, Merseyside CH49 5PE, England*

John R. Turtle *Department of Medicine, University of Sydney, NSW 2006, Australia*

G. Verlato *Division of Medical Statistics, University of Verona, Verona, Italy*

Aaron Vinik *Leonard R. Strelitz Diabetes Institute, Eastern Virginia Medical School, Norfolk, Virginia, USA*

Matthew J. Young *Department of Diabetes, Royal Infirmary of Edinburgh, Lauriston Place, Edinburgh EH3 9YW, Scotland*

Dennis K. Yue *Department of Medicine, University of Sydney, NSW 2006, Australia*

G. Zoppini *Division of Endocrinology and Metabolic Diseases, Ospedale Civile Maggiore, Piazzale Stefani 1, 37126 Verona, Italy*

Foreword

Diabetes is rapidly becoming the scourge of the modern world. Currently there are approximately 150 million people with diabetes world wide, mainly Type 2, and numbers are likely to double over the next 25 years unless drastic action is taken. Certain ethnic groups, such as people from South Asia, Amerindians and Africans, seem particularly susceptible, but even in 'low risk' groups, such as North Europeans, rates are rising alarmingly. Several factors are involved. Some are related to lifestyle, such as obesity, particularly central adiposity, and physical inactivity. A major factor is age, either acting directly or through lifestyle. From 10 to 20% of older people have Type 2 diabetes.

Overall only about half of all people with Type 2 diabetes have been diagnosed, implying a great pool of morbidity in the community, which is not being dealt with. The numbers are even higher for the elderly, particularly in nursing homes and residential care. Many of the symptoms of diabetes are attributed to ageing or other pathology.

There has long been the need for greater awareness of diabetes in the elderly. It is not a mild or trivial disease and there may be particular problems in those with multiple pathologies—a particular feature of older ill people. In the past there has been a tendency to aim for looser glycaemic control in the elderly—because they are old. This makes little sense when hyperglycaemia increases the likelihood of infections, impairs wound healing and diminishes immune function, for example.

The present book finally meets this need. It focuses on the problems of the older person with diabetes. It looks at care from several angles—including organisational aspects. It deals with previously ignored areas, such as impotence in the elderly male and also with important areas, such as drug therapy, insulin, the diabetic foot and management of the elderly diabetic patient during surgery. It will be of relevance anywhere in the world where there are older people with diabetes, in other words world wide, and, I feel, should be required reading for all those involved in the care of the older person

Sir George Alberti
Professor of Medicine
President, Royal College of Physicians of London

Preface

In our second edition we hope that we have maintained our principal goal to educate all health professionals engaged in delivering diabetes care to older citizens in society. This book should hold something for the generalist as well as the specialist with each chapter aiming to provide up-to-date knowledge in the area and practical advice to guide clinical decision making. As before, the expert authors have been recruited from the disciplines of geriatrics, diabetes and endocrinology, and primary healthcare. This creates in our view both a balance and a focus in the book that is sometimes missing in other texts. Each of the original chapter headings have been rewritten and brought up to date, and new authors have integrated their contributions accordingly.

Geriatric diabetes is now an increasing area of research interest but large clinical trials looking at interventional strategies are still infrequent. We hope that this book will stimulate interest in this challenging area and encourage research that will provide a better understanding of the benefits not only of blood glucose reduction, but also the effects of modifying other metabolic variables such as blood pressure and lipids.

Diabetes care is an exciting clinical arena at the present time with innovative developments in treatment and monitoring, organisation of care, and in prevention itself. Older people within society who develop diabetes should benefit from many of these initiatives and ensuring equity of care is an important role for the readers of this book.

Alan J. Sinclair
Paul Finucane
November 2000

Acknowledgements

This book is dedicated to my parents, Radovan and Ivy, for always being there, and to my wife, Caroline, for her endless support and encouragement. Also, to my children, Robbie, Harriet and Vicki, for their understanding when work took priority.

Alan J. Sinclair

To the many teachers and colleagues who have inspired me, especially Michael Hyland, Jacques Noel and John Pathy. To my parents, Molly and the late Frank Finucane who gave me everything and to my wife Aileen who is everything.

Paul Finucane

Section I

Epidemiology, Pathophysiology and Diagnosis

Diabetes Mellitus and Impaired Glucose Regulation in Old Age: The Scale of the Problem

Paul Finucane, Phil Popplewell

Flinders University and Flinders Medical Centre, Adelaide

INTRODUCTION

Diabetes mellitus is an important condition because it is common in developed countries, is becoming common in developing countries, and places a very great burden on individuals, healthcare systems and societies in all countries. In 1997 it was estimated that 124 million (2.1%) of the world's 5.8 billion total population had diabetes mellitus and it is projected that by 2010 this number will almost double to 221 million (Amos, McCarthy and Zimmet 1997). Of the 124 million with diabetes in 1997, 120 million (97%) had Type 2 diabetes.

In this chapter, our main purpose is to describe the incidence (i.e. the number of new cases occurring within a population over a specified period of time) and prevalence (i.e. the proportion of people in a population with that condition at a given time) rates for diabetes. We examine trends in incidence and prevalence rates for diabetes over time and in different populations. We also examine the epidemiology of impaired glucose regulation in people without overt diabetes.

DEFINITION AND CLASSIFICATION OF DIABETES AND IMPAIRED GLUCOSE REGULATION

Though definitions and classification are dealt with in detail in Chapter 3, it is necessary at this stage to explain briefly the terms used here. This is particularly important in view of some recent changes in diagnostic criteria, which impact on the interpretation of epidemiological studies. Such changes are perhaps best understood from a historical perspective.

Up until the late 1970s, epidemiological research in diabetes was bedevilled by a lack of standardization in definitions, in classification and in research methodologies. At that time, standardized diagnostic criteria were proposed (National Diabetes Data Group, 1979), were essentially adopted by the World Health Organization (WHO 1980) and were subsequently modified by that body (WHO 1985). All of these criteria placed a degree of reliance on both the fasting glucose and 2-hour post-load glucose levels to differentiate between three groups of people: those with normal glucose tolerance, those with impaired glucose tolerance (IGT) and those with diabetes.

In 1997, a modification to the 1985 WHO criteria was proposed (American Diabetes Association 1997) with the intention of moving away from reliance on the 2-hour post-load glucose level and instead basing definitions and diagnosis on fasting blood glucose levels alone. The ADA also suggested a lowering of the threshold for the diagnosis of diabetes from a fasting level of 7.8 mM (140 mg/dL) to 7.0 mM (126 mg/dL). The term 'impaired fasting glucose' (IFG) was coined to describe people whose fasting blood glucose levels were above the reference range for normality but below that required for a diagnosis of diabetes (6.1–6.9 mM). The adoption of these criteria would have led to the 2-hour post-load glucose level and to the term IGT both becoming largely obsolete.

For reasons that will be explored in Chapter 3, some limitations to the ADA criteria soon became apparent. When the WHO further revised its classifications and

Diabetes in Old Age. Second Edition. Edited by A. J. Sinclair and P. Finucane. © 2001 John Wiley & Sons Ltd.

diagnostic criteria in 1999, it adopted the ADA proposals in relation to the fasting blood glucose but retained a definition of diabetes based on the 2-hour post-load glucose level (WHO 1999). Thus the 2-hour post-load glucose level and the term IGT still have relevance. While there is significant overlap between IFG and IGT, the terms are neither synonymous nor mutually exclusive. In accordance with the new WHO guidelines, people with IFG and/or IGT can collectively be considered to have impaired glucose regulation.

EPIDEMIOLOGY

Effect of Altered Definitions and Classification of Epidemiological Data

The effect of the above changes on the interpretation of existing epidemiological studies of diabetes and impaired glucose regulation is somewhat confusing. Where data have been re-analysed using only fasting blood glucose levels and disregarding 2-hour post-load glucose levels, most studies show a fall in prevalence rates for diabetes (Davies 1999). When both the fasting blood glucose and the 2-hour post-load glucose levels are considered, prevalence rates can only increase. The impact of the new diagnostic criteria on future epidemiological studies will depend on the methodology used. This is particularly relevant to the prevalence of diabetes in older people who are more likely to be identified as having diabetes by the 2-hour post-load glucose level than by the fasting glucose level (Wahl et al 1998).

In this chapter, much of the cited epidemiological work predated the new diagnostic criteria for diabetes and this should be kept in mind when absolute incidence and prevalence rates are discussed. For example, most of the research on the epidemiology of impaired glucose regulation deals with IGT rather than with IFG. However, such 'older' studies are still relevant, particularly in their ability to examine trends in the epidemiology of diabetes and impaired glucose regulation over time. They also provide meaningful comparisons of people from different age, gender, ethnic, socioeconomic and other groups.

Limitations of Epidemiological Research

Much of the epidemiological research is of little direct relevance to elderly populations. Even studies of Type 2 diabetes have tended to focus on relatively young adult populations and some have excluded older people. However, such studies are still of value as the young adult population with diabetes of today will form a major part of tomorrow's elderly population with diabetes. Of the relatively few epidemiological studies of diabetes in elderly people, most are cross-sectional prevalence studies. Studies of disease incidence which require long-term follow-up of cohorts of patients or repeated cross-sectional analyses are relatively time-consuming and expensive and are therefore less common.

The Importance of Understanding the Scale of the Problem

Clinicians, educators, researchers and health planners alike need to appreciate the current status and future trends in the epidemiology of diabetes. This will promote:

1. Rational health planning. The magnitude of the clinical workload relevant to diabetes can be determined together with the resources required to meet it.
2. Placement of the disease in a proper perspective. Its importance relative to other disorders can be determined and this in turn can facilitate the equitable allocation of resources.
3. The identification of individuals, groups or communities who are at high risk for the development of diabetes. This offers possibilities for research into the aetiology of the disease, and for health promotion and disease prevention programs.
4. Awareness of any change in the nature of diabetes over time. Furthermore, it will facilitate the evaluation of intervention programs.

The epidemiology of IFG and IGT also needs to be considered as people with either of these disorders are at high risk of developing diabetes in the future. For example, a study involving Pima Indians from Arizona in the US followed up those with IGT for a median of 3.3 years and found that 31% developed overt diabetes, 26% continued to have IGT, while 43% reverted to normal glucose tolerance (Saad et al 1988). The cumulative incidence of overt diabetes was 25% at 5 years and 61% at 10 years.

PREVALENCE TRENDS OVER TIME

In developed and developing countries alike, prevalence rates for diabetes in the general population have been on the increase since the early 1900s. For example, Harris (1982) had drawn attention to an upward trend in US prevalence rates for diagnosed diabetes between the 1930s and 1980 (Figure 1.1). Prevalence rates rose in all age groups and in both sexes, with the number of known people with diabetes doubling between 1960 and 1980 (Bennett 1984).

In one Australian community (Glatthaar et al 1985), the prevalence rate for diabetes increased by 50% over the 15-year period 1966–1981, and in a UK population prevalence rates rose by 60% between 1983 and 1996 (Gatling et al 1998).

However, in the US at least, prevalence rates for diabetes now seem to be reaching a plateau. The annual review of 40 000 households comprising 120 000 US residents conducted by the National Health Interview Survey (NHIS) indicates that the prevalence of diabetes rose by 67% from 1959 to 1966; 41% from 1966 to 1973; 21% from 1973 to 1980; and 4% from 1980 to 1989 (Centers for Disease Control 1990a). Incidence rates also increased in the US until the early 1980s and, at least in some populations, continue to rise (Burke et al 1999).

Changes to the diagnostic criteria for diabetes and IFG/IGT hamper direct comparisons of prevalence rates between recent and earlier epidemiological studies. However, using currently accepted criteria, the prevalence rate for diabetes in older adults (i.e. aged 40–74 years) rose from 8.9% during the years 1976–1980 to 12.3% during the years 1988–1994 (Harris et al 1998).

The prevalence of any condition depends on both its incidence and its duration. At different times, these factors have made variable contributions to the increasing prevalence of diabetes, at least in Western countries. For example, in the US between 1960 and 1970, incidence rates for diabetes increased due to a greater awareness of the condition, greater surveillance and better diagnostic methods which all contributed to the earlier diagnosis of milder cases (Harris 1982). Incidence rates for Type 2 diabetes continue to rise in some populations but not in others. For example, the San Antonio Heart Study found a three-fold increase in incidence between 1987 and 1996 (Burke et al 1999) while data from the Swedish Skaraborg Diabetes Registry indicate no increase in the incidence of diabetes between 1991 and 1995 (Berger, Stenstrom and Sundkvist 1999).

Since the early 1970s, however, it is clear that much of the rise in prevalence rates for diabetes is attributable to enhanced survival in those affected. While some two-thirds of people with diabetes die from cardiovascular disease, mortality rates in diabetes are falling, though not as rapidly as mortality rates from

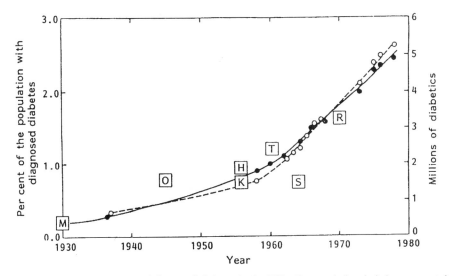

Figure 1.1 Trends in the prevalence an rate of diagnosed diabetes in the USA. Open and closed circles represent data from National Interview Surveys of the US Public Health Service. Rates from seven community-based surveys are included for comparison. M, Maryland (State); O, Oxford, Massachusetts; H, Hargerstown, Maryland; K, Kansas City, Kansas; T, Tecumseh, Michigan; S, Sudbury, Massachusetts; R, Rochester, Minnesota

cardiovascular disease in non-diabetics (Gu, Cowie and Harris 1999). Skaraborg Diabetes Registry data indicate that between 1991 and 1995, the median age of death for people with diabetes increased from 77.2 to 80.2 years (Berger et al 1999).

In developed countries in particular, the increased prevalence of diabetes and IFG/IGT over time can be further attributed to:

- aging of the population
- greater number of people from ethnic minority backgrounds who are adopting a 'transitional' lifestyle
- greater levels of overweight and obesity
- more sedentary lifestyles

The importance of these risk factors in the pathophysiology of diabetes is discussed in more detail in Chapter 2. However, from an epidemiological perspective, aging is a crucially important factor and nowadays, individuals have a longer life span during which to develop diabetes, to live with the condition and to develop its complications (Wilson, Anderson and Kannel 1986). The population with diabetes is increasingly elderly. Even twenty-five years ago, 40% of newly diagnosed people with diabetes in a US sample were aged over 65 years (Palumbo et al 1976). The NHIS survey already cited documented a greater than 100% increase in the number of people with diabetes aged over 75 years in the US between 1980 and 1987 (Centers for Disease Control 1990a).

Diabetes is fast becoming a significant problem in many developing countries where previously it was little recognized. This can be explained in part by all of the factors mentioned above: increased detection rates, improved survival rates and an aging society. More importantly, however, and as will be discussed in Chapter 2, people in many developing countries are switching from a traditional to a Western lifestyle and in the process adopting diets and exercise patterns that lead to the development of diabetes.

FACTORS INFLUENCING THE PREVALENCE OF DIABETES AND IMPAIRED GLUCOSE REGULATION

The prevalence of diabetes and IFG/IGT varies considerably in different populations and in different subgroups within populations. The most important variables (see Table 1.1) are now discussed more fully. Some factors, for example lifestyle and obesity, are

Table 1.1 Factors influencing the prevalence of diabetes and IFG/IGT

Age
Sex
Country of residence
Place of residence
Race and ethnicity
Socioeconomic status and lifestyle
Obesity

both closely interrelated and difficult to measure precisely. This makes it difficult to disentangle one from the other when analysing their relative contributions to the development of diabetes (King and Zimmet 1988).

Age

Age is the single most important variable influencing the prevalence of diabetes and IFG/IGT. Almost every epidemiological study, whether cross-sectional or longitudinal, shows that the prevalence of both diabetes and IFG/IGT initially increases with advancing aging, reaches a plateau and subsequently declines. However, the time of onset of the increase, the rate of increase, the time of peak prevalence and rate of subsequent decline differ in the various groups studied.

There is general agreement that the rise in prevalence begins in early adulthood. For example, Pima Indians aged 25–34 years are 10 times more likely to have diabetes than those aged 15–24 years (Knowler et al 1978). In Americans aged 45–55 years, diabetes is over four times more common than in those aged 20–44 years (Harris et al 1987). The subsequent rate of increase with aging is variable, being greatest in societies with the highest prevalence of glucose intolerance (King and Rewers 1993).

In Pima Indians, the prevalence of abnormal glucose tolerance peaks at 40 years for men and 50 years for women and declines in men after the age of 65 years and in women after the age of 55 years (Knowler et al 1978). In other populations, prevalence rates peak in the sixth decade and subsequently decline (King and Rewers 1993). However, in a study of elderly Finnish men, prevalence peaked in those aged 75–79, falling off in 80–84 years olds (Tuomilehto et al 1986). In some populations however, the highest prevalence rates are found in the oldest age groups (Glatthaar et al 1985; King and Rewers 1993).

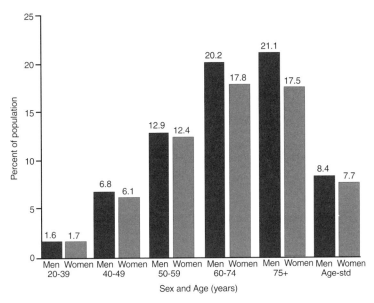

Figure 1.2 Prevalence of diabetes in men and women in the U.S. population age ≥20 years, based on NHANES III. Diabetes includes previously diagnosed and undiagnosed diabetics defined by fasting plasma glucose ≥126 mg/dl. Age-std, age-standardized. Reproduced by permission from Harris et al (1998)

Figure 1.2 shows the prevalence rates of diabetes in males and females and in different age groups, taken from the third National Health and Nutrition Examination Survey (NHANES III) carried out in the US (Harris et al 1998). This survey is the most extensive and up-to-date currently available, being conducted from 1988 to 1994 and involving some 19 000 adult Americans (i.e. aged over 20 years). Prevalence rates rise with advancing age until a plateau is reached at age 60–74 years.

Gender

There is evidence to suggest that diabetes was once more common in females than males. In recent years however, a disproportionate increase in the number of males known to have diabetes has resulted in equal prevalence rates being found in some societies while males predominate in others. Possible explanations for this change include a disproportionate increase in the incidence of diabetes in males, increased detection in males and reduced mortality in diabetic males.

Between 1980 and 1987, NHIS data showed a 33% increase in the prevalence of self-reported diabetes among white males but no increase among white fe-

males (Centers for Disease Control, 1990). Although there was a 16% increase among black males and a 24% increase among black females, this had a smaller impact as non-whites constitute only 15% of the US population. When interpreting this data, one should remember the limitations of self-reporting which the NHIS used as a measure of the prevalence of diabetes.

Recent studies involving predominantly non-elderly people have found the prevalence of Type 2 diabetes in males to exceed that in females in Australia (Glatthaar et al 1985; Welborn et al 1989) and Finland (Tuomilehto et al 1991). However, similar prevalence rates have been reported from New Zealand (Scragg et al 1991) and Japan (Sekikawa et al 1993). The NHANES III survey from the US already cited (Harris et al 1998) found no significant overall difference in the prevalence of Type 2 diabetes between the sexes (Figure 1.2). However, in that survey, prevalence rates were slightly higher in males than in females in both the 60–74 years sub-group (20.2% vs 17.8%) and in the 75 years and over sub-group (21.1% vs 17.5%). This represented a change from previous surveys in which elderly females had predominated. The prevalence of IFG was also greater in males than in females in the 60–74 years sub-group (16.2% vs 12.3%) and in the 75 years and over sub-group (17.9% vs 11.9%).

A review of the prevalence of diabetes from 75 communities in 32 countries, found the sex ratio for diabetes to vary widely (King and Rewers, 1993). Some studies found an excess of males while females predominated in others. A regional trend was apparent, whereby in Africa/Asia and the Americas there was a trend to male excess, whereas in the Pacific regions females predominated. IGT was generally found to be more common in women.

The few studies that have focussed on prevalence rates in elderly populations have either not reported a sex difference, or found either a male (Lintott et al 1992) or female (Mykkanen et al 1990) excess.

Country of residence

King and Rewers (1993) have collated data on the prevalence of abnormal glucose tolerance in over 150 000 people from 75 communities in 32 countries (Figure 1.3). As diabetes is an age-related disorder, its prevalence in individual countries varied according to

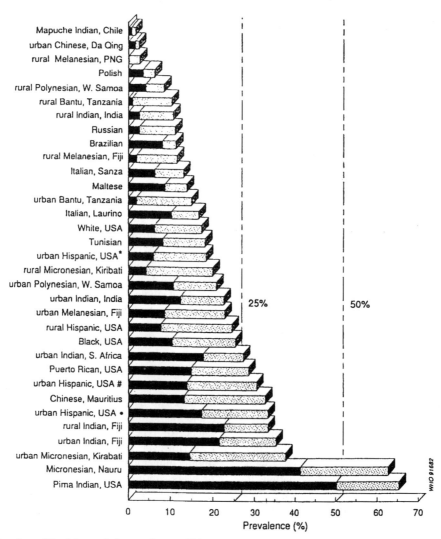

Figure 1.3 Prevalence (%) of abnormal glucose tolerance (diabetes and impaired glucose tolerance) in selected populations in the age range of 30–64 years, age standardized to the world population of Segi, sexes combined. *, Upper income; #, middle income; ●, low income; ■ diabetes mellitus; ▨ impaired glucose tolerance. Reproduced by permission from King and Rewers (1993)

the age structure of that society. Thus developed countries with a large elderly population have high prevalence rates; conversely, low rates are found in developing countries with few elderly people. Age-standardized rather than true prevalence rates are therefore used to allow valid comparisons between countries. As King & Rewers used a truncated age range of 30–64 years, their findings cannot be automatically extrapolated to elderly populations.

Diabetes was found to be absent or rare (less than 3% of people affected) in some traditional communities in developing countries. Prevalence rates in Europe were 3–10%, while some Arab, Asian Indian, Chinese and Hispanic American populations had rates of 14–20%. The highest rates were found in natives of the South Pacific island of Nauru and in Pima/Papago Indians in the USA who had prevalence rates as high as 50%.

Migrant populations are at particular risk of developing diabetes. A study of Japanese-American men who had retained their racial and cultural identity, found that 56% had abnormal glucose tolerance and that a third had diabetes (Fujimoto et al 1987). This rate is far higher than among white Americans with a similar socioeconomic profile in terms of education, occupation and income. It is also higher than the rate among the native population of Japan. Chinese and Indian migrants have a particularly high prevalence of abnormal glucose tolerance when compared with indigenous communities (King and Rewers 1993). These studies emphasize the importance of environmental factors, largely absent in the indigenous population but acquired in the migrant setting, in the development of diabetes.

ceiving hospital treatment for newly-diagnosed Type 2 diabetes (Barker, Gardner and Power 1982). Type 2 diabetes was found more frequently in towns with the poorest socioeconomic environment, irrespective of latitude. Caution must be exercised when using such 'surrogate' markers of prevalence and incidence, as illustrated by a Finnish study which found that the prevalence of known diabetes in a cohort of elderly men was 11% in the east of the country and 5% in the west. When a glucose challenge and then current WHO criteria were used to measure the true prevalence rate, it was identical at 24% in both regions (Tuomilehto et al 1986). Regional differences are not always found. For example, a study of over 6000 Tanzanian men showed that prevalence rates for diabetes, which were generally low, were similar in six villages despite having geographical, socioeconomic and dietary differences (McLarty et al 1989).

Diabetes is considered to be a disease of modernization and urbanization (Welborn 1994) and several studies have found significantly higher prevalence rates in urban than in rural environments (King and Rewers 1993). Comparisons of migrant populations living in rural and urban settings in the same country also consistently show an excess of diabetes and IGT in urban migrants.

Finally, it should be remembered that particular sub-groups of the population, such as those living in institutional care, will have a particularly high prevalence of diabetes (Grobin 1970). This is not surprising, given the advanced ages of such people and the fact that diabetic complications place them in need of residential care.

Place of Residence

The prevalence of diabetes differs between regions in the same country. In the US, for example, there is more self-reported diabetes in Hawaii and in states east of the Mississippi river (Centers for Disease Control 1990b). Even when differences in age, sex and racial/ethnic differences between states were taken into account, a greater than three-fold difference existed between the state with the highest rate and that with the lowest.

A study of people aged 18–50 years and living in nine towns in England and Wales, chosen to represent different latitude and socioeconomic status, found a greater than two-fold difference in the numbers re-

Race and Ethnicity

Studies from multicultural societies provide compelling evidence that racial background impacts greatly on the incidence and prevalence of diabetes and IFG/IGT. Here again, the NHANES III study from the US provides the best American epidemiological data. Three racial groups are identified in NHANES III: non-Hispanic whites, non-Hispanic blacks and Mexican-Americans. Compared with non-Hispanic whites, non-Hispanic blacks had a 1.6 times and Mexican-Americans a 1.9 times higher prevalence of diabetes (Harris 1998). In absolute terms, age- and sex-standardized prevalence rates for diabetes and IFG combined were 14.1% in adult non-Hispanic whites, 18.8%

in non-Hispanic blacks and 22.7% in Mexican-Americans.

Racial differences in prevalence rates of diabetes are also apparent in older people. NHANEs III reported that for people aged 60–74 years, prevalence rates for diabetes were 17.3% in non-Hispanic whites, 28.6% in non-Hispanic blacks and 29.3% in Mexican-Americans. For those aged over 75 years, corresponding figures were 17.5%, 22.4% and 29.7%.

Diabetes was found to be over twice as common in Aboriginal Australians than in non-Aboriginals living in the same community (Guest et al 1992). In the same study, both groups had similar prevalence rates for IGT. In a large multiracial New Zealand workforce the relative risk of having diabetes was 4–6 times greater in Maori, Pacific Islanders and Asians, than in people of European backgrounds (Scragg et al 1991). This increased risk remained significant after controlling for age, income and body mass index.

Attention has already been drawn to the high prevalence of abnormal glucose tolerance among the Pima Indians of Arizona in the US (Knowler 1978). For indigenous North Americans, susceptibility to Type 2 diabetes is related to the degree of racial admixing; thus Americans of mixed ethnicity have rates of diabetes intermediate between those of full native Americans and of Caucasians (Gardner 1984).

In a survey of the Southall district of London, which has a large Asian population, the overall age-adjusted prevalence of self-reported diabetes was almost four times higher in Asians than in Europeans (Mather and Keen 1985). It is also of interest that the excess prevalence of diabetes among Asians was greatest in the older age groups. However, this survey also relied on self-reporting to measure the prevalence of diabetes. Another UK study also showed that diabetes was four times higher in Asian men than white men and twice as high in Asian women as white women (Simmons, Williams and Powell 1989).

Socioeconomic Status and Lifestyle

It is difficult to disentangle the effect of socioeconomic status and lifestyle on the prevalence of diabetes from confounding factors such as country of residence, place of residence and racial origin. The evidence, suggests however, that these are independent risk factors. Certain ethnic groups are particularly susceptible to developing abnormal glucose tolerance when they forsake a traditional for an urbanzized lifestyle (Dowse et al 1990). This has been documented in

North American Indians, Mexican-Americans, Australian Aborigines, Micronesian and Polynesian Pacific Islanders and Asian Indians. For example, urban dwellers on the Pacific island of Kiribati have rates of Type 2 diabetes three times greater than those living in a rural setting; in the over 65 population, there is a four-fold urban-rural difference (King et al 1984). Large variations in the prevalence of diabetes in different Australian Aboriginal communities have been reported (Guest and O'Dea 1992) with urbanized Aboriginals having the highest rates (Cameron, Moffit and Williams 1986). Migration is a potent stimulus to lifestyle change; the higher prevalence of diabetes in migrant communities when compared with those left behind has been explained by socioeconomic advantage which migration tends to confer (King and Zimmet 1988).

Socioeconomic deprivation, which is associated with poor diet and other adverse lifestyle factors is also linked to high rates of diabetes. In the US, the 1973 National Household Interview Survey documented an inverse relationship between income and the prevalence of known diabetes (US Dept of Health, Education and Welfare 1978). A study of nine towns in England and Wales, chosen to represent different latitude and socioeconomic status, found that the detection rate for newly diagnosed Type 2 diabetes was greatest in towns with a 'poor' socioeconomic profile and least in towns with 'good' profiles (Barker et al 1982). In a survey of a large multiracial New Zealand workforce, the relative risk for glucose intolerance was inversely related to income but not to other markers of socioeconomic status (Scragg et al 1991).

A study of over 1100 Hindu Indians living in Dar-es-Salaam, Tanzania, looked at the prevalence of diabetes and IGT in seven sub-communities of different caste. The age- and sex-adjusted prevalence of diabetes differed more than five-fold (Ramaiya et al 1991). Similar differences were noted in the prevalence of IGT. These sub-communities differed in socioeconomic characteristics and lifestyle and may also have differed genetically and in their diet. Studies such as this highlight the danger of regarding people from a single geographical area or with similar racial origins as homogenous and of grouping them under a single label (e.g. 'Asians').

The effect of physical exercise on the pathogenesis of diabetes is discussed in Chapter 2; there is epidemiological evidence that exercise influences prevalence rates. For example, migrant Indians in Fiji who were physically active had half the risk of diabetes than those who were inactive (Taylor et al 1984). Physical activity was also implicated as an environmental risk factor for diabetes mellitus in a multi-racial community in Mauritius (Dowse et al 1990).

Obesity

This section outlines the epidemiological evidence for obesity as a risk factor for diabetes and IFG/IGT; its importance in the pathogenesis of Type 2 diabetes is discussed in more detail in Chapter 2. There is clear evidence that obesity is an independent risk factor for diabetes. In the NHANES II study cited earlier, obesity doubled the probability of having diabetes and was also an independent risk factor for IGT (Harris et al 1987). The Framingham study has had broadly similar findings, with people overweight by >40% having twice the prevalence of diabetes than others (Wilson et al 1986). A study of 1300 Finns aged 65–74 years found an association between diabetes and obesity and particularly between diabetes and central obesity (Mykkanen et al 1990). Central obesity, recognized by a high waist/hip girth ratio, correlates with intra-abdominal visceral fat mass. The importance of central obesity in the pathogenesis of diabetes is explained in Chapter 2. A study of elderly Hong Kong Chinese also found diabetes to be more common in overweight and obese subjects (Woo et al 1987).

In other studies, the association between obesity and diabetes has been less impressive. Among elderly New Zealanders, a positive association was found in newly diagnosed people with diabetes but not in those with known diabetes (Lintott et al 1992). Racial factors may play a part, though the evidence is somewhat confusing. For example, in a survey of a large multiracial New Zealand workforce, the increased prevalence of glucose intolerance in Maori and Pacific Islanders over people of European origin was partly attributable to obesity (Scragg et al 1991). Obesity has been implicated in the high prevalence of diabetes in Pima Indians; furthermore, in those with IGT, obesity predicted subsequent development of diabetes, though it was not an independent risk factor (Saad et al 1988). On the other hand, a study of over 6000 young Tanzanians found only a modest increase in the prevalence of diabetes with increasing body mass (McLarty et al 1989). Furthermore, obesity was not prevalent among elderly Finnish men, many of whom had diabetes (Tuomilehto et al 1986). In this study, the BMI de-

creased with age in those with diabetes, IGT and normal glucose tolerance alike.

PREVALENCE OF ABNORMAL GLUCOSE TOLERANCE IN DIFFERENT COUNTRIES

From all that has been stated above, it follows that prevalence rates for diabetes and IFG/IGT are specific to the population from which the study sample is drawn and cannot easily be extrapolated to other populations. However, it is still possible to profile a community in which the prevalence of diabetes is likely to particularly high. It will have both a large elderly and migrant population and be located in an urban setting in a 'developed' country. A high percentage of people will be at either extreme of the socioeconomic scale, many will have sedentary lifestyles and will be overweight or obese. In communities that lack these characteristics, the prevalence of glucose intolerance will be relatively low.

Amos et al (1997) estimated that in 1997 diabetes affected:

- 66 million people in Asia
- 22 million people in Europe
- 13 million people in North America
- 13 million people in Latin America
- 8 million people in Africa
- 1 million people in Oceania.

Future increases in the prevalence of diabetes are likely to affect Asia and Africa more than other regions. By 2010, its prevalence in these areas will become two to three times more common than in 1997, at which time more than 60% of all people with diabetes will live in Asia (Amos et al 1997).

The US and Canada

The key epidemiological studies of diabetes and IFG/IGT in the US in the past 25 years have been the periodic National Health and Nutrition Examination Surveys conducted by the National Center for Health Statistics of the Centers for Disease Control and Prevention. The second national survey (NHANES II) covered the period 1976–1980 (Harris et al 1987) and the third (NHANES III) covered the period 1988–1994 (Harris et al 1998). These data have been supplemented by the Hispanic Health and Nutrition Examination Survey (Hispanic HANES) which surveyed a representative sample of Mexican-Americans in the south-western US during 1982–1984 (Flegal et al 1991). All three studies used the recommended diagnostic criteria of the ADA and WHO.

In the NHANES III study, some 19 000 adult Americans aged over 20 years were questioned about having previously diagnosed diabetes. Over 6000 of this group also had measurement of fasting plasma glucose and almost 3000 of those aged 40–74 years had a formal oral glucose tolerance test. A glucose challenge was not offered to people 75 years and over. NHANES III estimated that for 1997, 15.6 million adult Americans (8.1% of the total population) had diabetes mellitus. Of these, 10.2 million (5.3%) had diagnosed diabetes and 5.4 million (2.8%) had undiagnosed diabetes.

Using ADA and the recently updated WHO criteria, a further 13.4 million (6.9%) adult Americans have IFG. It is not possible to accurately estimate the number of additional adult Americans with impaired glucose regulation (i.e. those with a normal IFG but with IGT on the basis of a 2-hour post-load glucose level). A subset of the NHANES III study population did receive a glucose challenge; these were all aged 40–74 years and 15.8% had IGT. In summary, therefore, 8.1% of adult Americans have diabetes, an additional 6.9% have IFG and some others have impaired glucose regulation, identified only by a 2-hour post-load glucose level.

With regard to elderly Americans, 18.8% of those aged 60–74 years and 18.9% of those aged over 75 years have diabetes. An additional 14% of those over 60 years have IFG and still some others have IGT but not IFG (Harris et al 1998). Some years ago it was estimated that almost 20% of white North Americans can expect to develop Type 2 diabetes if they survive into their seventh decade (King and Zimmet, 1988).

The 1991 Canadian Study of Health and Aging involved over 10 000 elderly people (aged 65–106 years) and estimated the prevalence of diabetes at 12.4% (Rockwood et al 1998). However, this estimate is at best approximate as it largely relied on self-reporting and health records and only some 700 subjects underwent random glucose estimations.

The UK

Two studies from the UK contain data that provide an estimate of the prevalence of diabetes and IGT in elderly people. Both studies predated the new ADA/WHO criteria for diabetes. In two London general practice populations, 10.3% of men and 9.5% of women aged 65–69 years had diabetes; the corresponding figures were 11.4% and 9.4% for people aged 70–75 years (Yudkin et al 1993). A further 6.5% of men and 5.6% of women aged 65–69 years had IGT as had 8.4% of men and 3.6% of women aged 70–75 years. The second study, from Melton Mowbray, estimated that 9% of people aged over 65 years had diabetes (Croxson et al 1991).

Other European Countries

The prevalence of diabetes and IGT in elderly Finns is remarkably high, with 30% of men aged 65–84 years having Type 2 diabetes and another 32% having IGT (Tuomilehto et al 1986). Less impressive rates were found in a study of 1300 younger subjects (aged 65–74 years), where 16% of men and 19% of women had diabetes and another 18% and 19% respectively had IGT (Mykkanen et al 1990). A Swedish community study estimated that 15% of people aged over 65 years had diabetes (Andersson, Svardsudd and Tibblin 1991) and similar prevalence rates have been reported from Denmark (Agner, Thorsteinsson and Eriksen 1982). In more southern parts of Europe, the prevalence rate for Type 2 diabetes has been estimated at 22.8% in Italians aged 65–84 years (Rosso et al 1998) and at 8.5% in French people aged over 65 years (Bourdel-Marchasson et al 1997). However, as the French study largely relied on self-reporting, the true prevalence rate is likely to be substantially higher.

Australia and New Zealand

National studies on the epidemiology of diabetes are lacking in both countries. What data exists are mainly derived from relatively small studies of rural or semi-rural communities. In the 1989–90 National Health Survey in Australia, the prevalence of self-reported diabetes in people aged 65–74 years was 7.8% in males and 6.5% in females (Welborn et al 1995). Prevalence rates for people aged over 75 years were 8.7% for males and 7.5% for females. Another study which relied on self-reporting and fasting blood glucose levels found that 16.4% of people aged 60–69 years, 16.7% of people aged 70–79 years and 16% of those aged 80 years or over had diabetes (Mitchell et al 1998). In a random sample of some 600 New Zealanders aged over 65, the age-adjusted prevalence of diabetes was 15% (Lintott et al 1992). However, as people living in residential care were excluded, this rate is also likely to be an underestimate.

Japan

It has been estimated that over 10% of people aged over 45 years in Japan have diabetes while another 15% have IGT (Sekikawa et al 1993). This prevalence rate is far higher than earlier estimates that used less satisfactory methodologies. Another study found that 13% of people aged 60–79 years had diabetes while an additional 25% had IGT (Ohmura et al 1993).

Other Countries

Readers with a particular interest in the world-wide prevalence of diabetes and IFG/IGT are referred to the reviews by King and Zimmett (1988) and King and Rewers (1993). An even more detailed account is provided by Amos et al (1997) who estimate 1997 prevalence rates in various counties in Asia, Europe, the Americas, Africa, and Oceania. As can be seen from Figure 1.3, some communities and countries have remarkably high prevalence rates for diabetes and IGT. The highest recorded rates are among the Pima Indians of Arizona, US, where 40% of those aged 65–74 years have diabetes (Knowler et al 1978). However, new challengers for this dubious distinction are now appearing from populations in Papua New Guinea (Dowse et al 1994) and Micronesians in Nauru (Zimmet, Humphrey and Dowse 1994).

Countries with large populations also deserve special mention even if the prevalence of diabetes is not particularly high. In Hong Kong Chinese, 10% of those aged over 60 and 17% aged over 75 have diabetes (Woo et al 1987). In Taiwan, one study showed that 26% of people aged over 60 years had diabetes and another 22% had IGT (Lu et al 1998). Demographic and socioeconomic changes in mainland China suggest that a similar prevalence rate can be expected there in time.

THE ECONOMIC COST OF ABNORMAL GLUCOSE TOLERANCE

Diabetes incurs both direct and indirect costs. Direct patient costs are the sum of what is spent on diagnosing and treating diabetes itself and on managing its acute and chronic complications; it is estimated that people with diabetes use hospital and primary health-care services two to three times as much as the general population (Damsgaard et al, 1987a,b). Lost productivity due to short term illness, disability and premature mortality accounts for the indirect costs. Estimates of the economic cost of diabetes are largely drawn from a few Western countries and cannot be extrapolated to other countries or healthcare systems.

In the US, the National Diabetes Data Group estimated the total cost of diabetes at $13.8 billion or 4% of the US health budget in 1984 (Entmacher et al 1985). The Center for Economic Studies in Medicine put the cost at $20.4 billion for 1987 (Fox and Jacobs 1988). Both figures are probable underestimates as they either failed to include the cost of diabetic complications or underestimated the prevalence of diabetes. For similar reasons, the finding that Type 2 diabetes alone cost the US economy $19.8 billion in 1986 is also an underestimate (Huse et al 1989). Even if the absolute figures are inaccurate, the breakdown of the expenditure on Type 2 diabetes in the US in 1986 is still of interest (Table 1.2). In the UK, by the late 1980s it was conservatively estimated that diabetes cost £1.2billion per annum or 5% of the NHS budget (Laing and Williams, 1989). In Australia, the direct cost of diabetes was estimated at between $0.44 billion and $1.4 billion in 1995 and this is projected to rise to between $0.9 billion and $2.3 billion by 2010 (McCarthy et al 1996).

There are age and sex differences in the economic cost of diabetes, with men aged under 65 years accounting for 35% of cost, women aged over 65 years for 30%, men aged over 65 years for 18% and women aged under 65 years for 17% (Huse et al 1989). It has been further estimated that per capita health

Table 1.2 Breakdown of estimated $19.8 billion spent on Type 2 diabetes in the US in 1986[a]

Item	Cost ($ billion)	Percentage of total cost
Total healthcare expenditure	*11.56*	*58.5*
NIDDM per se	6.83	34.6
Circulatory complications	3.85	19.5
Visual complications	0.39	2.0
Neuropathy	0.24	1.2
Skin ulcers	0.15	0.8
Nephropathy	0.10	0.5
Lost productivity	*8.2*	*41.5*
From disability	2.6	13.2
From premature death	5.6	28.3

Source: Modified from Huse et al (1989).

expenditure on people with diabetes is two to three times greater than on non-diabetics and the loss of productivity due to disability and premature death is also sizeable (Huse et al 1989).

THE HUMAN COST

In the US in 1986, Type 2 diabetes was thought to account for 144 000 deaths (6.8% of total US mortality) and the total disability of 951 000 persons (Huse et al 1989). People aged over 65 years account for 75% of these deaths (Fox and Jacobs 1988). Also in the US, coronary artery disease rates are twice in common in males with diabetes and four times as common in females (Barrett-Connor and Orchard 1985), stroke is four times more common (Kuller et al 1985), blindness five times more common (Huse et al 1989), and lower limb amputation 10–20 times more common (Palumbo and Melton 1985).

In terms of human pain and suffering, the cost of diabetes to patients, partners, children, other family members and other carers is incalculable. As well as physical costs, diabetes incurs psychological costs in terms of the major impositions that it places on lifestyle. Being relatively intangible, these costs tend to receive inadequate recognition and are too often disregarded.

DIABETES AND IFG/IGT–THE HIDDEN EPIDEMIC

Epidemiological studies consistently find that large proportions of people found to have diabetes are previously undiagnosed. For example, the NHANES III survey estimated that over one-third of the 8.1% of adult Americans with diabetes are unaware of the problem (Harris et al 1998). Other epidemiological studies from the UK (Croxson et al 1991), Japan (Sekikawa et al 1993) and Australia (McCarthy et al 1996) report that about half of all diabetes is undiagnosed. A more global picture is obtained from a comparison of the prevalence of diabetes in 32 countries which found that in most populations over 20% of people with diabetes were previously undiagnosed and in some over 50% were undiagnosed (King and Rewers 1993). There are regional differences in the prevalence of known diabetes. For example, in a study of elderly Finnish men, 45% of people in one geographical area had been aware of the diagnosis of diabetes but only 28% were aware in another region (Tuomilehto et al 1986).

FUTURE TRENDS

Worldwide, the number of people with diabetes is expected to almost double over a 13-year period, from 124 million in 1997 to 221 million in 2010 (Amos et al 1997). In most societies, demographic changes will mainly account for this, with projected large increases in the proportion of elderly people among whom diabetes is particularly prevalent. Higher prevalence rates will also result from lifestyle changes and the further adoption of habits that increase susceptibility to diabetes. These issues are discussed in more detail in Chapter 2. In some countries at least, improved surveillance and detection of diabetes, together with improved longevity for people with established diabetes, will further increase prevalence rates.

Increases in the prevalence of diabetes will be more pronounced in some countries than in others, and those countries where prevalence rates are currently low are likely to see the greatest proportional increases. For example, between 1995 and 2010, prevalence rates for Type 2 diabetes will increase by 111% in Asia, 93% in Africa, 82% in Latin America, 51% in Europe, 48% in Oceania, and 35% in North America (Amos et al 1997).

Health organizations face a major challenge in offsetting this impending pandemic of abnormal glucose tolerance. Primary prevention holds the key and success depends on promoting the maintenance of traditional lifestyles in some communities and the adoption of new lifestyles elsewhere. Many countries have now developed a national strategic plan to address the problem of diabetes (Colagiuri, Colagiuri and Ward 1998). Such plans tend to have specific goals, which aim to reduce the incidence and prevalence of diabetes as well as to reduce morbidity and improve quality of life for those with the condition.

REFERENCES

Agner E, Thorsteinsson B, Eriksen M (1982) Impaired glucose tolerance and diabetes mellitus in elderly subjects. *Diabetes Care*, **5**, 600–604.

American Diabetes Association (1997) Report of the expert committee on the diagnosis and classification of diabetes mellitus. *Diabetes Care*, **20**, 1183–1197.

Amos AF, McCarthy DJ, Zimmet P (1997) The rising global burden of diabetes and its complications: estimates and projections to the year 2010. *Diabetic Medicine*, **14**, S1–S85.

Andersson DKG, Svardsudd K, Tibblin G (1991) Prevalence and incidence of diabetes in a Swedish community 1972–1987. *Diabetic Medicine*, **8**, 428–434.

Barker DJP, Gardner MJ, Power C (1982) Incidence of diabetes amongst people aged 18–50 years in nine British towns: a collaborative study. *Diabetologia*, **22**, 421–425.

Barrett-Connor E, Orchard T (1985) Diabetes and heart disease. In: (US Department of Health and Human Services). *Diabetes in America: Diabetes data compiled 1984.* NIH Publication 85-1468, XXIX, 1–41.

Bennett PH (1984) Diabetes in the elderly: diagnosis and epidemiology. *Geriatrics*, **39**, 37–41.

Berger B, Stenstrom G, Sundkvist G (1999) Incidence, prevalence, and mortality of diabetes in a large population. *Diabetes Care*, **22**, 773–778.

Bourdel-Marchasson I, Dubroca B, Manciet G, Decamps A, Emeriau J-P, Dartigues J-F (1997) Prevalence of diabetes and effect on quality of life in older French living in the community: the PAQUID epidemiological survey. *Journal of the American Geriatrics Society*, **45**, 295–301.

Burke JP, Williams K, Gaskill SP, Hazuda HP, Haffner SM, Stern MP (1999) Rapid rise in the incidence of Type 2 diabetes from 1987 to 1996. Results from the San Antonio Heart Study. *Archives of Internal Medicine*, **159**, 1450–1456.

Cameron WI, Moffitt PS, Williams DRR (1986) Diabetes mellitus in the Australian Aborigines of Bourke, New South Wales. *Diabetes Research and Clinical Practice*, **2**, 307–314.

Centers for Disease Control (1990a) Prevalence, incidence of diabetes mellitus—United States, 1980–1987. *Journal of the American Medical Association*, **264**, 3126.

Centers for Disease Control (1990b) Regional variation in diabetes mellitus prevalence—United States, 1988 and 1989. *Journal of the American Medical Association*, **264**, 3123–3126.

Colagiuri S, Colagiuri R, Ward J. (1998) *National Diabetes Strategy and Implementation Plan.* Diabetes Australia, Canberra.

Croxson SCM, Burden AC, Bodington M, Botha JL (1991) The prevalence of diabetes in elderly people. *Diabetic Medicine*, **8**, 28–31.

Damsgaard EM, Froland A, Green A. (1987a) Use of hospital services by elderly diabetics and fasting hyperglycaemic patients aged 60–74 years. *Diabetic Medicine*, **4**, 317–322.

Damsgaard EM, Froland A, Holm N. (1987b) Ambulatory medical care for elderly diabetics: the Fredericia survey of diabetic and fasting hyperglycaemic subjects aged 60–74 years. *Diabetic Medicine*, **4**, 534–538.

Davies M (1999) New diagnostic criteria for diabetes—are they doing what they should? *Lancet*, **354**, 610–611.

Dowse GK, Gareeboo H, Zimmet PZ, Alberti KGMM, Tuomilehto J, Fareed D, Brissonnette LG, Finch CF (1990) High prevalence of NIDDM and impaired glucose tolerance in Indian, Creole, and Chinese Mauritians. *Diabetes*, **39**, 390–396.

Dowse GK, Spark RA, Mavo B, Hodge AM, Erasmus RT, Gwalimu M, Knight LT, Koki G, Zimmet PZ (1994) Extraordinary prevalence of non-insulin-dependent diabetes mellitus and bimodal plasma glucose distribution in the Wanigela people of Papua New Guinea. *Medical Journal of Australia*, **160**, 767–774.

Entmacher PS, Sinnock P, Bostic E, Harris ML (1985) The economic impact of diabetes. In: (US Department of Health and Human Services) *Diabetes in America: Diabetes data compiled 1984.* NIH Publication 85–1468, XXXII, 1–13.

Flegal KM, Ezzati TM, Harris MI, Hayes SG, Juarez RZ, Knowler WC, Perez-Stable EJ, Stern MP (1991) Prevalence of diabetes and impaired glucose tolerance in Mexican Americans, Cubans and Puerto Ricans ages 20–74 in the Hispanic Health and Nutrition Examination Survey. *Diabetes Care*, **14** (Suppl. 3), 628–638.

Fox NA, Jacobs J. (1988) Direct and Indirect Costs of Diabetes in the United States in 1987. Alexandria: American Diabetes Association.

Fujimoto WY, Leonetti DL, Kinyoun JL, Newell-Morris L, Shuman WP, Stolov WC, Wahl PW (1987) Prevalence of diabetes mellitus and impaired glucose tolerance among second-generation Japanese-American men. *Diabetes*, **36**, 721–729.

Gardner LI, Stern MP, Haffner SM, Gaskill SP, Hazuda HP, Relethford JH, Eifler CW (1984) Prevalence of diabetes in Mexican Americans: relationship to percent of gene pool derived from native American sources. *Diabetes*, **33**, 86–92.

Gatling W, Budd S, Walters D, Mullee MA, Goddard JR, Hill RD (1998) Evidence of an increasing prevalence of diagnosed diabetes mellitus in the Poole area from 1983 to 1996. *Diabetic Medicine*, **15**, 1015–1021.

Glatthaar C, Welborn TA, Stenhouse NS, Garcia-Webb P (1985) Diabetes and impaired glucose tolerance: a prevalence estimate based on the Busselton 1981 survey. *Medical Journal of Australia*, **143**, 436–440.

Grobin W (1970) Diabetes in the aged: underdiagnosis and overtreatment. *Canadian Medical Association Journal*, **103**, 915–923.

Gu K, Cowie CC, Harris MI (1999) Diabetes and decline in heart disease mortality in US adults. *Journal of the American Medical Association*, **281**, 1291–1297.

Guest CS, O'Dea K (1992) Diabetes in Aborigines and other Australian populations. *Australian Journal of Public Health*, **16**, 340–349.

Guest CS, O'Dea K, Hopper JL, Nankervis AJ, Larkins RG (1992) The prevalence of glucose intolerance in Aborigines and Europids of south-eastern Australia. *Diabetes Research and Clinical Practice*, **15**, 227–235.

Harris M (1982) The prevalence of diagnosed diabetes, undiagnosed diabetes, and impaired glucose tolerance in the United States. Proceedings of the Third Symposium on Diabetes in Asia and Oceania. *Excerpta Medica*, 70–76.

Harris MI, Hadden WC, Knowler WC, Bennett PH (1987) Prevalence of diabetes and impaired glucose tolerance and plasma glucose levels in US population aged 20–74. *Diabetes*, **36**, 523–534.

Harris MI, Flegal KM, Cowie CC, Eberhardt MS, Goldstein DE, Little RR, Wiedmeyer H-M, Byrd-Holt DD (1998) Prevalence of diabetes, impaired fasting glucose, and impaired glucose tolerance in US adults. The Third National Health and Nutrition Examination Survey, 1988–1994. *Diabetes Care*, **21**, 518–524.

Huse DM, Oster G, Killen AR, Lacey MJ, Colditz GA (1989) The economic costs of non-insulin-dependent diabetes mellitus. *Journal of the American Medical Association*, **262**, 2708–2713.

King H, Zimmet P (1988) Trends in the prevalence and incidence of diabetes: non-insulin-dependent diabetes mellitus. *World Health Statistics Quarterly*, **41**, 190–196.

King H, Rewers M (1993) Global estimates for prevalence of diabetes mellitus and impaired glucose tolerance in adults. *Diabetes Care*, **16**, 157–177.

King H, Taylor R, Zimmet, Pargeter K, Raper LR, Beriki T, Tekanene J (1984) Non-insulin-dependent diabetes (NIDDM) in a newly independent Pacific nation: the Republic of Kiribati. *Diabetes Care*, **7**, 409–415.

Knowler WC, Bennett PH, Hamman RF, Miller M (1978) Diabetes incidence and prevalence in Pima Indians: a 19-fold greater incidence than in Rochester, Minnesota. *American Journal of Epidemiology*, **108**, 497–505.

Kuller LH, Dorman JS, Wolf PA. (1985) Cerebrovascular disease and diabetes. In: (US Department of Health and Human Services). *Diabetes in America: Diabetes data compiled 1984*. NIH Publication 85-1468, XVII, 1–18.

Laing W, Williams R. (1989) *Diabetes, a Model for Healthcare Management*. London: Office of Health Economics.

Lintott CJ, Hanger HC, Scott RS, Sainsbury R, Frampton C (1992) Prevalence of diabetes mellitus in an ambulant elderly New Zealand population. *Diabetes Research and Clinical Practice*, **16**, 131–136.

Lu F-H, Yang Y-C, Wu J-S, Wu C-H, Chang C-J. (1998) A population-based study of the prevalence and associated factors of diabetes mellitus in southern Taiwan. *Diabetic Medicine*, **15**, 564–572.

Mather HM, Keen H (1985) The Southall diabetes survey: prevalence of known diabetes in Asians and Europeans. *British Medical Journal*, **291**, 1081–1084.

McCarthy DJ, Zimmet P, Dalton A, Segal L, Welborn TA (1996) *The Rise and Rise of Diabetes in Australia, 1996. A review of statistics, trends and costs*. Diabetes Australia National Action Plan, Canberra.

McLarty DG, Swai ABM, Kitange HM, Masuki G, Mtinangi BL, Kilima PM, Makene WJ, Chuwa LM, Alberti KGMM (1989) Prevalence of diabetes and impaired glucose tolerance in rural Tanzania. *Lancet*, **i**, 871–875.

Mitchell P, Smith W, Wang JJ, Cumming RG, Leeder SR, Burnett L (1998) Diabetes in an older Australian population. *Diabetes Research and Clinical Practice*, **41**, 177–194.

Mykkanen L, Laakso M, Uusitupa M, Pyorala K (1990) Prevalence of diabetes and impaired glucose tolerance in elderly subjects and their association with obesity and family history of diabetes. *Diabetes Care*, **13**, 1099–1105.

National Diabetes Data Group (1979) Classification of diabetes mellitus and other categories of glucose intolerance. *Diabetes*, **38**, 1039–1057.

Ohmura T, Ueda K, Kiyohara Y, Kato I, Iwamoto H, Nakayama K, Nomiyama K, Ohmori S, Yoshitake T, Shinkawu A, Hasuo Y, Fujishima M (1993) Prevalence of Type 2 (non-insulin dependent) diabetes mellitus and impaired glucose tolerance in the Japanese general population: the Hisayama study. *Diabetologia*, **36**, 1198–1203.

Palumbo PJ, Elveback LR, Chu C-P, Connolly DC, Kurland LT (1976) Diabetes mellitus: incidence, prevalence, survivorship, and causes of death in Rochester, Minnesota, 1945–1970. *Diabetes*, **25**, 566–573.

Palumbo PJ, Melton LJ. Peripheral vascular disease and diabetes. In: (US Department of Health and Human Services). *Diabetes in America: Diabetes data compiled 1984*. NIH Publication 85-1468, XV, 1–21.

Ramaiya KL, Swai ABM, McLarty DG, Bhopal RS, Alberti KGMM (1991) Prevalence of diabetes and cardiovascular disease risk factors in Hindu Indian subcommunities in Tanzania. *British Medical Journal*, **303**, 271–276.

Rockwood K, Tan M-H, Phillips S, McDowell I. (1998) Prevalence of diabetes mellitus in elderly people in Canada: report from the Canadian Study of Health and Aging. *Age and Aging*, **27**, 573–577.

Rosso D, Campagna S, Di Stefano F, Romano G, Maugeri D, Maggi S, Motta M, Catanzaro S, Carnazzo G (1998) Prevalence of diabetes mellitus in a sample of the elderly population of the city of Catania. *Archives of Gerontology and Geriatrics*, **27**, 223–235.

Saad MF, Knowler WC, Pettitt DJ, Nelson RG, Mott DM, Bennett PH (1988) The natural history of impaired glucose tolerance in the Pima Indians. *New England Journal of Medicine*, **319**, 1500–1506.

Scragg R, Baker J, Metcalf P, Dryson E (1991) Prevalence of diabetes mellitus and impaired glucose tolerance in a New Zealand multiracial workforce. *New Zealand Medical Journal*, **104**, 395–397.

Sekikawa A, Sugiyama K, Tominaga M, Manaka H, Takahashi K, Sasaki H, Eguchi H, Fukuyama H, Igarashi M, Miyazawa K, Ohnuma H (1993) Prevalence of diabetes and impaired glucose tolerance in Funagata area, Japan. *Diabetes Care*, **16**, 570–574.

Simmons D, Williams DRR, Powell MJ (1989) Prevalence of diabetes in a predominantly Asian community: preliminary findings of the Coventry diabetes study. *British Medical Journal*, **298**, 18–21.

Taylor R, Ram P, Zimmet P, Raper LR, Ringrose H (1984) Physical activity and prevalence of diabetes in Melanesian and Indian men in Fiji. *Diabetologia*, **27**, 578–582.

Tuomilehto J, Nissinen A, Kivela S-L, Pekkanen J, Kaarsalo E, Wolf E, Aro A, Punsar S, Karvonen MJ (1986) Prevalence of diabetes mellitus in elderly men aged 65 to 84 years in eastern and western Finland. *Diabetologia*, **29**, 611–615.

Tuomilehto J, Korhonen HJ, Kartovaara L, Salomaa V, Stengard JH, Pitkanen M, Aro A, Javela K, Uusitupa M, Pitkaniemi J (1991) Prevalence of diabetes mellitus and impaired glucose tolerance in the middle-aged population of three areas in Finland. *International Journal of Epidemiology*, **20**, 1010–1017.

US Dept of Health, Education and Welfare (1978) *Diabetes Data: Compiled 1977*, DHEW NIH Publication 78-1468. Washington: US Government Printing Office.

Wahl PW, Savage PJ, Psaty BM, Orchard TJ, Robbins JA, Tracy RP (1998) Diabetes in older adults: comparison of 1997 American Diabetes Association classification of diabetes mellitus with 1985 WHO classification. *Lancet*, **352**, 1012–1015.

Welborn TA (1994) Asia-Oceania and the global epidemic of diabetes. *Medical Journal of Australia*, **160**, 740.

Welborn TA, Glatthaar C, Whittall D, Bennett S (1989) An estimate of diabetes prevalence from a national population sample: a male excess. *Medical Journal of Australia*, **150**, 78–81.

Welborn TA, Knuiman M, Bartholomew HC, Whittall DE (1995) 1989–90 National Health Survey: prevalence of self-reported diabetes in Australia. *Medical Journal of Australia*, **163**, 129–132.

Wilson PWF, Anderson KM, Kannel WB (1986) Epidemiology of diabetes mellitus in the elderly. *American Journal of Medicine*, **80** (Suppl 5A), 3–9.

World Health Organization (1980) *Second Report of the Expert Committee on Diabetes* (Technical Report Series 646). WHO, Geneva.

World Health Organization (1985) *Study Group on Diabetes Mellitus* (Technical Report Series 727). WHO Geneva.

World Health Organization (1999) *Definition, Diagnosis and Classification of Diabetes Mellitus and its Complications*. WHO, Geneva.

Woo J, Swaminathan R, Cockram C, et al (1987) The prevalence of diabetes mellitus and an assessment of methods of detection among a community of elderly Chinese in Hong Kong. *Diabetologia*, **30**, 863–868.

Yudkin JS, Forrest RD, Jackson CA, Burnett SD, Gould MM (1993) The prevalence of diabetes and impaired glucose tolerance in a British population. *Diabetes Care*, **16**, 1530.

Zimmet P, Humphrey A, Dowse G (1994) *Report on 1994 Diabetes and Eye Disease Survey: Republic of Nauru*. Melbourne: International Diabetes Institute.

2

Pathophysiology of Diabetes in the Elderly

Graydon S. Meneilly

University of British Columbia, Vancouver.

INTRODUCTION

Numerous studies have investigated the pathogenesis of Type 2 diabetes (DeFronzo 1987), but elderly patients have been systematically excluded. Recently, a number of investigators have begun to study the pathophysiologic alterations that occur in elderly patients with diabetes. These studies, which will be reviewed below, suggest that there are many ways in which diabetes in the elderly is unique. Some of the factors that contribute to the high prevalence of diabetes in the elderly are shown in Figure 2.1.

GENETIC FACTORS

Several lines of evidence suggest that there is a strong genetic component to diabetes in the elderly, although the specific genes responsible have yet to be defined (Kahn 1984). A person with a family history of Type 2 diabetes is much more likely to develop the disease (Morris and Rimm 1991). Diabetes is also much more common in the elderly in certain ethnic groups (Lipton et al 1993). The likelihood that an elderly identical twin will develop diabetes if their sibling is affected is over 80%. Even in elderly identical twins discordant for Type 2 diabetes, the unaffected siblings clearly have evidence of abnormal glucose metabolism (Vaag et al 1995).

AGE-RELATED CHANGES IN CARBOHYDRATE METABOLISM

There are progressive alterations in glucose metabolism with age which explain why genetically susceptable older individuals may not develop diabetes until late in life. Pathogenic mechanisms which contribute to the glucose intolerance of aging include alterations in glucose-induced insulin release and resistance to insulin-mediated glucose disposal. Early investigations suggested that glucose-induced insulin release was normal in the elderly. However, more recent studies enrolling large numbers of carefully characterized healthy young and old subjects have demonstrated definable alterations in glucose-induced insulin release in the aged (Iozzo et al 1999; Muller et al 1996). Of note, the magnitude of the decrement in insulin secretion is more apparent in response to oral than to intravenous glucose (Muller et al 1996). This may be due, in part, to a decreased beta-cell response to the incretin hormones glucose-dependent insulinotropic peptide (GIP) and glucagon-like peptide (GLP-1). However, numerous studies have demonstrated that the most important pathogenic mechanism underlying the glucose intolerance of aging is resistance to insulin-mediated glucose disposal (Muller et al 1996; Ferrannini et al 1996). There is debate as to whether the insulin resistance of the elderly is intrinsic to the aging process itself or is the result of lifestyle factors commonly associated with aging. The consensus of opinion is that the aging process is the most important cause of insulin resistance, although lifestyle changes are clearly an important contributing factor (see below).

LIFESTYLE AND ENVIRONMENTAL FACTORS

Despite the strong genetic component, it is abundantly clear that various environmental and lifestyle factors can increase or decrease the likelihood that a

Diabetes in Old Age. Second Edition. Edited by A. J. Sinclair and P. Finucane. © 2001 John Wiley & Sons Ltd.

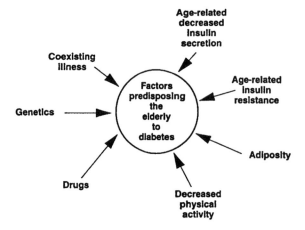

Figure 2.1 Factors contributing to the high prevalence of diabetes in the elderly. Reproduced by permission from Halter JB (1995) Carbohydrate metabolism. In Masoro EJ (ed) *Handbook of Physiology, Volume on Aging.* New York: Oxford University Press, p. 119

genetically susceptible individual will develop the disease in old age. Many older people have coexisting illnesses and take multiple drugs (such as thiazide diuretics), which can allow a latent abnormality in glucose metabolism to develop into full-blown diabetes (Pandit et al 1993). Diabetes is much more likely to occur in older individuals who are obese, especially if the fat is distributed centrally (Cassano et al 1992). Regular physical activity also appears to protect against the development of the disease (Manson et al 1992).

The above information suggests that lifestyle modifications may be of value in the prevention of Type 2 diabetes in the elderly even in patients with a strong family history of the disease.

DIET

Large epidemiologic studies have demonstrated that diabetes is more likely to develop in older patients who have a diet that is high in saturated fats and simple sugars and low in complex carbohydrates (Feskens et al 1995). It has been suggested that deficiencies of trace elements or vitamins may contribute to the development or progression of diabetes in younger subjects, and it is increasing recognized that the same may be true in the elderly. Elderly patients with diabetes have exaggerated free radical production, and administration of the antioxidant vitamins C and E to these patients improves insulin action and meta-

bolic control (Paolisso et al 1993; Paolisso et al 1994a). Many elderly patients with diabetes are deficient in magnesium and zinc, supplements of which improve their glucose metabolism (Paolisso et al 1994b; Song et al 1998). Although chromium deficiency has been shown to cause abnormalities in glucose metabolism in animals and younger patients, there is no evidence that chromium supplements improve glucose tolerance in the elderly.

In summary, there is increasing evidence to suggest that dietary abnormalities may contribute to the pathogenesis of diabetes in the elderly, and that dietary modifications may be of therapeutic benefit.

METABOLIC ALTERATIONS

The metabolic alterations occurring in middle-aged subjects with Type 2 diabetes have been characterized extensively (DeFronzo 1988). When compared with age- and weight-matched controls, both lean and obese middle-aged subjects have elevated fasting hepatic glucose production, marked resistance to insulin-mediated glucose disposal, and a profound impairment in glucose-induced pancreatic insulin release.

Recently, metabolic factors have been characterized in lean and obese elderly patients with diabetes (Arner, Pollare and Lithell 1991; Meneilly et al 1996). These studies have found some surprising differences in the metabolic profiles of middle-aged and elderly subjects. In contrast to younger subjects, fasting hepatic glucose production is normal in both lean and obese elderly subjects (Figure 2). As in younger subjects, lean elderly patients have a profound impairment in pancreatic insulin secretion, but in contrast to the young these patients have minimal resistance to insulin-mediated glucose disposal (Figures 3 and 4). In contradistinction to the young, obese elderly subjects have relatively preserved glucose-induced insulin secretion (Figure 3). Similar to the young however, these patients have a marked resistance to insulin-mediated glucose disposal (Figure 4).

In summary, the principal defect in lean elderly subjects is impaired glucose-induced insulin release, while the principal defect in obese patients is resistance to insulin-mediated glucose disposal. One of the most interesting findings of these studies was that the ability of insulin to enhance blood flow was markedly reduced in obese, insulin-resistant older patients (Figure 5) (Meneilly and Elliott 1999). Insulin-mediated vasodilation is thought to account for about 30%

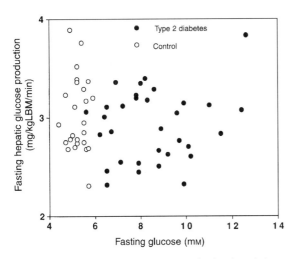

Figure 2.2 Fasting hepatic glucose production in relation to fasting glucose levels in healthy elderly controls and elderly patients with diabetes. Hepatic glucose production was measured by infusing radioactive glucose tracers

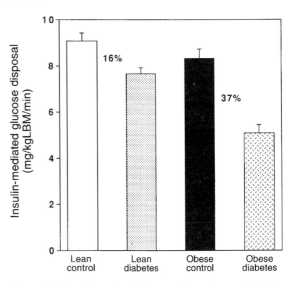

Figure 2.4 Insulin-mediated glucose disposal rates in healthy elderly controls and elderly patients with diabetes. Glucose disposal rates were measured utilizing the euglycemic clamp technique. Insulin is infused to achieve levels occurring after a meal, and glucose is infused simultaneously to prevent hypoglycemia

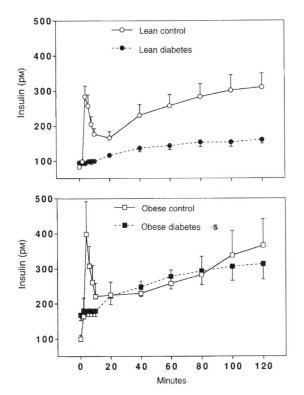

Figure 2.3 Glucose-induced insulin release in healthy elderly controls and elderly patients with diabetes. Insulin values were measured at glucose levels approximately 5 mM above fasting

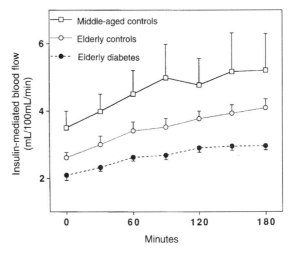

Figure 2.5 Insulin-mediated blood flow in obese middle-aged controls and obese elderly controls and patients with diabetes. Blood flow was measured in the calf during euglycemic clamp studies utilizing venous occlusion plethysmography

of normal glucose disposal, presumably because it increases the delivery of insulin and glucose to muscle tissue. Indeed, it has been demonstrated that ACE inhibitors may improve insulin sensitivity in elderly patients with diabetes and hypertension (Paolisso et al 1992). This suggests that drugs that enhance muscle blood flow may prove to be valuable adjuncts to the therapy of elderly patients with diabetes.

It has been known for a number of years that autoimmune phenomena play a pivotal role in the beta-cell failure that occurs in patients with Type 1 diabetes (Zimmet 1999). It is increasingly recognized, too, that a subset of middle-aged patients with Type 2 diabetes have a form of diabetes characterized by beta-cell failure, and these patients often have high titres of islet-cell antibodies and antibodies to GAD, similar to younger patients with Type 1 diabetes. It has been suggested that screening for anti-GAD antibodies and other autoimmune parameters should be routine in middle-aged patients, since the presence of these antibodies will predict patients destined to require insulin therapy (Zimmet 1999). Future studies may target these patients for therapies that modify the immune destruction of the beta cells, prevent islet-cell failure and reduce the need for insulin therapy, analagous to the studies currently being conducted in patients with Type 1 diabetes.

It is tempting to speculate that autoimmune phenomena contribute to the profound impairment in glucose-induced insulin secretion seen in lean older patients with Type 2 diabetes, since a substantial percentage of older patients with diabetes have islet-cell and anti-GAD antibodies. However, the clinical significance of this finding in the elderly is less certain. The author's unit has demonstrated that, although the prevalence of anti-GAD antibodies was similar in middle-aged and elderly patients with diabetes, the likelihood that a GAD-positive patient would require insulin therapy in the near future was substantially reduced in the elderly (Meneilly et al 2000). Thus, it is unclear at present whether measurement of autoimmune parameters can be used to predict future insulin requirements in the aged, or whether elderly patients with these abnormalities should be treated with therapies designed to modify autoimmune destruction of the pancreas.

It is surely appropriate, therefore, to target therapeutic interventions in the elderly based on their metabolic profile. In lean subjects, because of their profound impairment in glucose-induced insulin secretion, the principal approach should be to give sulfonylureas to stimulate insulin secretion, or to administer exogenous insulin. Obese patients should be treated with drugs that enhance insulin-mediated glucose disposal, such as metformin, rosiglitazone or athiozolidinedione.

GLUCOSE EFFECTIVENESS OR NON-INSULIN-MEDIATED GLUCOSE UPTAKE

It has been recognized for decades that insulin is an important hormone involved in the uptake of glucose into cells. Recently it has been demonstrated that glucose can stimulate its own uptake in the absence of insulin (Best et al 1996). This is known as 'glucose effectiveness' or non-insulin-mediated glucose uptake (NIMGU). Under fasting conditions, approximately 70% of glucose uptake occurs via glucose effectiveness, primarily in the central nervous system. After a meal, approximately 50% of glucose uptake in normal subjects occurs via NIMGU, the bulk of which occurs in skeletal muscle. Because many middle-aged subjects with diabetes are insulin-resistant, it has been suggested that up to 80% of postprandial glucose uptake in these patients may occur via glucose effectiveness. At this time it is uncertain whether defects contribute to elevated glucose levels in middle-aged patients with diabetes, since studies which have evaluated this parameter in middle-aged diabetics have given inconsistent results.

In healthy elderly subjects, glucose effectiveness is impaired during fasting but is normal during hypoglycemia (Meneilly et al 1989). Elderly patients with diabetes have an even greater impairment in glucose effectiveness than the healthy elderly (Figure 2.6)

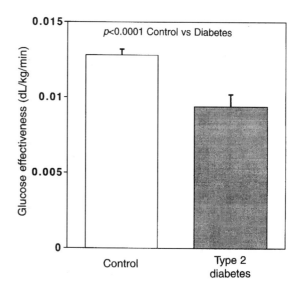

Figure 2.6 Glucose effectiveness in elderly controls and patients with diabetes. During these studies, insulin secretion was suppressed by infusing the somatostatin analogue octreotide. Glucose was then infused to assess glucose disposal in the absence of insulin

(Forbes et al 1998). Although the cause of this abnormality is uncertain, it may relate to a decreased ability of glucose to recruit glucose transporters to the cell surface in these patients.

In the future, this metabolic abnormality may prove to be of great therapeutic relevance to the elderly. In younger patients, exercise, anabolic steroids and a reduction of free fatty acid levels have been shown to enhance glucose effectiveness (Best et al 1996). In preliminary experiments, the author's unit has shown that the incretin hormone glucagon-like-peptide-1 (GLP-1) may enhance NIMGU in elderly patients with diabetes. Thus, it is possible that future therapies for the elderly may be directed not only at increasing insulin secretion and reversing insulin resistance, but also at enhancing glucose effectiveness.

MOLECULAR BIOLOGY STUDIES

There is little information available regarding molecular biologic abnormalities that may be present in elderly patients with diabetes. The glucokinase gene controls the glucose sensor for the beta cell. Defects in this gene could lead to the impairment in glucose-induced insulin secretion which is present in lean elderly patients with diabetes. Evidence for mutations in this gene in elderly patients is conflicting (Laakso et al 1995; McCarthy et al 1993).

In skeletal muscle, insulin binds to its receptor, resulting in activation of the insulin receptor tyrosine kinase. Activation of this enzyme sets in motion a cascade of intracellular events—at present incompletely understood—that results in the translocation of glucose transporters to the cell surface. Theoretically, a defect in any of these pathways could lead to insulin resistance. To date, these intracellular processes are incompletely studied in elderly patients with diabetes. Preliminary information suggests that insulin receptor number and affinity are normal, but insulin receptor kinase activity may be defective (Obermaier-Kusser et al 1989). Clearly further studies are required to elucidate the subcellular defects that cause abnormal glucose metabolism in the elderly patient with diabetes.

GLUCOSE COUNTER-REGULATION

Numerous studies have found that elderly patients with diabetes, when compared with younger patients, have an increased frequency of severe or fatal hypoglycemia (Stepka, Rogala and Czyzyk 1993). A number of studies have evaluated glucose counter-regulation in elderly subjects to try to determine the cause of the increased frequency of hypoglycemia, and some important observations have emerged. Many elderly patients with diabetes have not been educated about the warning symptoms of hypoglycemia and as a consequence do not know how to interpret the symptoms when they occur (Thomson et al 1991). The most important hormone in the defence against hypoglycemia in normal subjects is glucagon. If glucagon responses are deficient, epinephrine becomes important, and growth hormone and cortisol come into play if hypoglycemia is prolonged for several hours. Glucagon and growth hormone responses to hypoglycemia are impaired in healthy elderly subjects and to an even greater extent in older patients with diabetes (Figure 2.7) (Meneilly et al 1994). Even when they are educated about the symptoms of hypoglycemia, the elderly

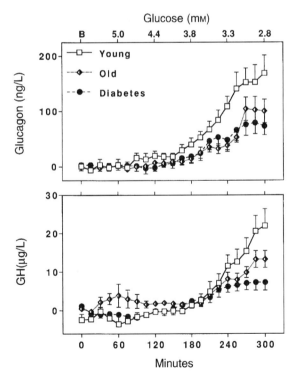

Figure 2.7 Glucagon and growth hormone (GH) responses to hypoglycemia in healthy young, healthy old and elderly patients with diabetes. Controlled hypoglycemia was induced using the glucose clamp technique. Glucose values at which hormone levels were measured are shown on the top horizontal axis

have reduced awareness of the autonomic warning symptoms (sweating, palpitations, etc.) at glucose levels that would elicit a marked response in younger subjects. Finally, elderly patients have impaired psychomotor performance during hypoglycemia, which would prevent them from taking steps to return the blood glucose value to normal even if they were aware that it was low. Thus the increased frequency of hypoglycemia in the elderly is due to a constellation of abnormalities, including reduced knowledge and awareness of warning symptoms, decreased counter-regulatory hormone secretion and altered psychomotor performance.

The levels of pancreatic polypeptide (PP) is elevated during hypoglycemia, and this response is mediated by the vagus nerve. The role of PP in normal glucose counter-regulation is uncertain, but in younger patients with diabetes reduced PP responses to hypoglycemia are an early marker of autonomic insufficiency. Although elderly patients with diabetes often have evidence of autonomic dysfunction, their PP responses to hypoglycemia are normal (Meneilly 1996). Thus PP responses to hypoglycemia cannot be used to predict autonomic function in elderly patients.

It has been suggested that some younger patients with diabetes, when switched to human from animal insulins, develop hypoglycemic unawareness and an increased frequency of hypoglycemic events. It has been demonstrated that animal insulin results in a greater awareness of the warning symptoms of hypoglycemia than human insulin in elderly patients with diabetes, although a small clinical trial found no difference in the frequency of hypoglycemic events in elderly patients treated with animal or human insulin (Meneilly, Milberg and Tuokko 1995; Berger 1987). It has been the author's clinical experience that elderly patients treated with human insulin who develop hypoglycemic unawareness and frequent hypoglycemic events on human insulin do better with beef–pork insulin. Pending the results of further studies, animal insulins should continue to be made available for use in the elderly.

Based on the above information, there are a number of interventions that can be proposed to prevent hypoglycemic events in the elderly. First, it would seem prudent to educate elderly patients about the warning symptoms of hypoglycemia so that they can appreciate them when they occur. Second, consideration should be given to the use of oral agents or insulin preparations that are associated with a lower frequency of hypoglycemic events in the elderly.

CONCLUSIONS

Diabetes in the elderly is caused by a combination of genetic and environmental factors superimposed on the normal age-related changes in carbohydrate metabolism. The metabolic alterations occurring in elderly patients with diabetes appear to be distinct from those occurring in younger patients. As we gain a greater appreciation of the pathophysiologic abnormalities that occur in the elderly, we can develop more focused approaches to therapy in this age group. It is only in this way that we will be able to better cope with the epidemic of diabetes in the elderly which will befall us in the coming decades.

ACKNOWLEDGMENTS

The author's work described was supported by grants from the Medical Research Council of Canada, the Canadian Diabetes Association, the British Columbia Health Research Foundation, and the Pacific Command-Royal Canadian Legion. I gratefully acknowledge the support of the Allan McGavin Geriatric Endowment at the University of British Columbia, and the Jack Bell Geriatric Endowment Fund at Vancouver Hospital and Health Science Centre. I am especially indebted to my longstanding collaborators in this work, particularly Dr Dariush Elahi at Harvard University and Dr Daniel Tessier at the University of Sherbrooke. I thank Rosemarie Torressani, Eugene Mar, Gail Chin and Christine Lockhart for technical assistance in conducting these studies.

REFERENCES

Arner P, Pollare T, Lithell H (1991) Different Aetiologies of Type 2 (non-insulin-dependent) diabetes mellitus in obese and non-obese subjects. *Diabetologia*, **34**, 483–487.

Best JD, Kahn SE, Ader M, Watanabe RM, Ni TC, Bergman RN (1996) Role of glucose effectiveness in the determination of glucose tolerance. *Diabetes Care*, **19**, 1018–1030.

Berger M (1987) Human insulin: much ado about hypoglycaemia (un)awareness. *Diabetologia*, **30**, 829–833.

Cassano PA, Rosner B, Vokonas PS, Weiss ST (1992) Obesity and body fat distribution in relation to the incidence of non-insulin-dependent diabetes mellitus. *American Journal of Epidemiology*, **136**, 1474–1486.

DeFronzo RA (1988) Lilly Lecture 1987. The triumvirate: (β-cell, muscle, liver. A collusion responsible for NIDDM. *Diabetes*, **37**, 667–687.

Ferrannini E, and the European Group for the Study of Insulin Resistance (1996) Insulin action and age. *Diabetes*, **45**, 949.

Feskens EJM, Virtanen SM, Rasanen L, Tuomilehto J, Stengard J, Pekkanen J, Nissinen A, Kromhout D (1995) Dietary factors determining diabetes and impaired glucose tolerance. *Diabetes Care*, **18**, 1104–1112.

Forbes, Elliott T, Tildesley H, Finegood D, Meneilly GS (1998) Alterations in non-insulin-mediated glucose uptake in the elderly patient with diabetes. *Diabetes*, **47**, 1915–1919.

Iozzo P, Beck-Nielsen J, Laakso M, Smith U, Yki-Jarvinen H, Ferrannini E (1999) Independent influence of age on basal insulin secretion in non-diabetic humans. European group for the study of insulin resistance. *Journal of Clinical Endocrinology and Metabolism*, **84**, 863–868.

Kahn CR (1984) Banting Lecture. Insulin acton, diabetogenes, and the cause of Type 2 Diabetes. *Diabetes*, **43**, 1066–1084.

Laakso M, Malkki M, Kekalainen P, Kuusisto J, Mykkanen L, Deeb SS (1995) Glucokinase gene variants in subjects with late-onset NIDDM and impaired glucose tolerance. *Diabetes Care*, **18**, 398–400.

Lipton RB, Liao Y, Cao G, Cooper RS, McGee D (1993) Determinants of incident non-insulin-dependent diabetes mellitus among blacks and whites in a national sample. The NHANES 1 epidemiologic follow-up study. *American Journal of Epidemiology*, **138**, 826–964.

Manson JE, Nathan DM, Krolewski AS, Stampter MJ, Willett HWC, Hennekens CH (1992) A prospective study of exercise and incidence of diabetes among US male physicians. *JAMA*, **268**, 63–67.

McCarthy MI, Hitman GA, Hitchins M, Riikonen A, Stengard J, Nissinen A, et al (1993) Glucokinase gene polymorphisms: A genetic marker for glucose intolerance in cohort of elderly Finnish men. *Diabetic Medicine*, **10**, 198–204.

Meneilly GS, Elahi D, Minaker KL, Sclater AL, Rowe JW (1989) Impairment of noninsulin-mediated glucose disposal in the elderly. *Journal of Clinical Endocrinology and Metabolism*, **63**, 566–571.

Meneilly GS, Cheung E, Tuokko H (1994) Counter-regulatory hormone responses to hypoglycemia in the elderly patient with diabetes. *Diabetes*, **43**, 403–410.

Meneilly GS, Milberg WP, Tuokko H (1995) Differential effects of human and animal insulin on the responses to hypoglycemia in elderly patients with NIDDM. *Diabetes*, **44**, 272–277.

Meneilly GS, Hards L, Tessier D, Elliott T, Tildesley H (1996) NIDDM in the elderly. *Diabetes Care*, **19**, 1320–1375.

Meneilly GS (1996) Pancreatic polypeptide responses to hypoglycemia in aging and diabetes. *Diabetes Care*, **19**, 544–546.

Meneilly GS, Elliott T (1999) Metabolic alterations in middle-aged and elderly obese patients with Type 2 diabetes. *Diabetes Care*, **22**, 112–18.

Meneilly GS, Tildesley H, Elliott T, Palmer JP, Juneja R (2000) Significiance of GAD positivity in elderly patients with diabetes. *Diabetic Medicine*, **17**, 247–248.

Morris RD, Rimm AA (1991) Association of waist to hip ratio and family history with the prevalence of NIDDM among 25,272 adult, white females. *American Journal of Public Health*, **81**, 507–509.

Muller DC Elahi D, Tobin JD, Andres R (1996) The effect of age on insulin resistance and secretion: a review. *Seminars in Nephrology*, **16**, 289–298.

Obermaier-Kusser B, White MF, Pongratz DE, Su L, Ermel B, Muhlbacher C, et al (1989) A defective intramolecular auto-activation cascade may cause the reduced kinase activity of the skeletal muscle insulin receptor from patients with non-insulin-dependent diabetes mellitus. *Journal of Biological Chemistry*, **264**, 9497–9504.

Pandit MK, Burke J, Gustafson AB, Minocha A, Peiris AN (1993) Drug-induced disorders of glucose tolerance. *Annals of Internal Medicine*, **118**, 529–539.

Paolisso G, Gambardella A, Verza M, D'Amora A, Sgambato S, Varrichio M (1992) ACE-inhibition improves insulin-sensitivity in age insulin-resistant hypertensive patients. *Journal of Human Hypertension*, **6**, 175–179.

Paolisso G, D'Amore A, Galzerano D, Balbi V, Giugliano D, Varricchio M, D'Onofrio F (1993) Daily vitamin E supplements improve metabolic control but not insulin secretion in elderly Type 2 diabetic patients. *Diabetes Care*, **16**, 1433–1437.

Paolisso G, D'Amore A, Balbi V, Volpe C, Galzerano D, Giugliano D, Sgambato S, Varricchio M, and D'Onofrio F (1994a) Plasma vitamin C affects glucose homeostasis in healthy subjects and in non-insulin-dependent diabetics. *American Journal of Physiology*, **266**, E261–E268.

Paolisso G, Scheen A, Cozzolino D, De Maro G, Varricchio M, D'Onofrio F, et al (1994b) Changes in glucose turnover parameters and improvement of glucose oxidation after 4-week magnesium administration in elderly non-insulin-dependent (Type 2) diabetic patients. *J Clin Endocrinol Metab*, **78**, 1510–1515.

Song MK, Rosenthal MJ, Naliboff BD, Phanumas L, Kang KW (1998) Effects of bovine prostate powder on zinc, glucose and insulin metabolism in old patients with non-insulin-dependent diabetes mellitus. *Metabolism*, **47**, 39–43.

Stepka M, Rogala H, Czyzyk A (1993) Hypoglycemia: a major problem in the management of diabetes in the elderly. *Aging*, **5**, 117–121.

Thomson FJ, Masson EA, Leeming JT, Boulton AJ (1991) Lack of knowledge of symptoms of hypoglycaemia by elderly diabetic patients. *Age and Aging*, **20**, 404–406.

Vaag A, Henriksen JE, Madsbad S, Holm N., Beck-Nielsen H (1995) Insulin secretion, insulin action, and hepatic glucose production in identical twins discordant for non-insulin-dependent diabetes mellitus. *Journal of Clinical Investigations*, **95**, 690–698.

Zimmet PZ (1999) Diabetes epidemiology as a tool to trigger diabetes research and care. *Diabetologia*, **42**, 499–518.

.

3

Establishing the Diagnosis

P. Jean Ho and John R. Turtle
Royal Prince Alfred Hospital and the University of Sydney

WHY DIABETES IS A PROBLEM IN ELDERLY PEOPLE

Diabetes is one of the most common chronic diseases which can lead to complications that seriously affect quality of life and life span. It has an incidence and prevalence which increase greatly with age (Harris 1990; King and Rewers 1993) and is therefore particularly relevant to the elderly age group, defined here as persons who are 65 years or older. Diagnosed diabetes is present in 7–10% of the elderly population, making up approximately 40% of persons with known diabetes in the general population. In addition, approximately 10% of elderly persons have undiagnosed diabetes, are untreated and at an even higher risk from the morbidity and mortality of diabetes. Another 20% of elderly persons have impaired glucose tolerance (IGT) and are at increased risk of developing macrovascular disease and diabetes. Thus nearly one in five of the elderly population have diabetes, diagnosed or undiagnosed. When IGT is included, 40% of the elderly population have some degree of impaired glucose homeostasis.

With increasing longevity, this age group, which currently represents 11% of the population, will increase to approximately 20% by the year 2021 (Lipson 1986). Globally, obesity and sedentary lifestyle are resulting in more people developing diabetes and vascular disease, and this is affecting the developing countries, minority groups and disadvantaged communities within industrialized countries particularly rapidly (Harris et al 1998; IDF Asian-Pacific Type 2 Diabetes Policy Group 1999; King and Rewers 1993). Thus demands on healthcare resources will continue to rise among diabetic persons who are 65 years and over.

Morbidity from Diabetes

The main argument in favour of detection of diabetes in its early stages is to reduce or prevent its complications, which otherwise would lead to further morbidity (Samos and Roos 1998). Elderly diabetic persons have much higher use of ambulatory services than those without diabetes. Poor vision and blindness due to diabetic eye disease, lower limb amputation due to peripheral vascular disease, neuropathy and infection, ischaemic heart disease, cerebrovascular accidents and chronic renal failure can all severely limit an elderly person's mobility, independence and quality of life.

Chronic complications are often present in elderly people with newly diagnosed diabetes; at diagnosis, 10–20% have established retinopathy or nephropathy and 10% have cardiovascular disease and neuropathy (Harris et al 1992; Muggeo 1998). Hypertension and Q-wave myocardial infarction are more prevalent, and the subsequent risk of developing retinopathy, peripheral vascular insufficiency and peripheral neuropathy is increased with age at diagnosis of diabetes (Davis et al 1997; Scheen 1997). Chronic diabetic complications can be more devastating to the patient's well-being when they first occur at an elderly age. By diagnosing diabetes early, complications may be prevented or even reversed. The current life expectancy for Australians is 76 years for men and 81 years for women and increasing yearly, so prevention of long-term diabetic complications is important even in this age group.

The elderly diabetic person is prone to certain acute complications of the disease. Hyperglycaemia leads to osmotic diuresis. With the decreased sense of thirst, the

Diabetes in Old Age. Second Edition. Edited by A. J. Sinclair and P. Finucane. © 2001 John Wiley & Sons Ltd.

elderly diabetic person is less able to ingest sufficient fluids and therefore is at risk of sodium and water depletion, hypotension, hyperosmolality, hypokalaemia (especially if the patient is taking diuretics), reduction in insulin secretion, and thrombotic events. Following myocardial infarction or septicaemia, elderly patients are more likely to develop shock, which may lead to lactic acidosis particularly in patients with poorly controlled diabetes. Such acute complications can become life-threatening but many can also be prevented by early diagnosis of diabetes and appropriate management.

Mortality from Diabetes

The majority (86–92%) of elderly people with diabetes have Type 2. Patients with Type 2 diabetes have an overall 10-year mortality rate as high as 44%. The diagnosis of diabetes at the age of 65 years reduces a person's life expectancy by approximately 4–5 years. In one study, elderly diabetic subjects were 4.5 times more likely to die than their non-diabetic controls over a 5-year period (Croxson et al 1994). With advancing age of onset of Type 2 diabetes, overall mortality increases, although it has been suggested that the increment from diabetes falls, and there may be no further increase in mortality due to diabetes when the diagnosis is made after the age of 75 years (Morley et al 1987). However, a recent systematic review of this area indicates a continuing high mortality rate for older subjects with diabetes even when the diagnosis is made above the age of 65 years (Sinclair, Robert and Croxson 1997).

Cardiovascular disease is the most common complication of hyperglycaemia and the major cause of death in elderly people with diabetes, and ischaemic heart disease may account for up to half the number of deaths in this group (Vilbergsson et al 1998; Waugh et al 1989). Persons with diabetes have 1.5 times the in-hospital mortality rate after acute myocardial infarction and 1.4 times the post-discharge mortality rate compared with non-diabetic persons (Sprafka et al 1991). It is imperative, therefore, that diabetes be diagnosed early to reduce, delay or prevent its morbidity, mortality and cost in this age group.

With increasing life span, the opinion that people who get diabetes in the older age group do not live long enough to develop complications—and so do not need treatment for mild to moderate hyperglycaemia—is no longer valid. Early detection of diabetes may be of benefit in other ways. A physician may consider the possibility of diabetes-related problems more promptly in an emergency. The offspring of a person with diabetes can be induced into screening and preventative measures themselves.

WHEN DIABETES SHOULD BE SUSPECTED

Early diagnosis of diabetes requires a high degree of vigilance on the part of the physician. Many people with diabetes, especially the elderly, are asymptomatic. At the time of diagnosis of diabetes, long-term complications are often present but the patient may be asymptomatic. Elderly patients may present with nonspecific symptoms only, which may be dismissed as 'normal aging' by themselves and their physicians. Elderly patients are generally more likely to present at a later stage of illness; this leads to underreporting of illness, confusion as to the cause of the illness, and atypical presentation. Multiple pathology is usually present and may further complicate the diagnosis.

Even a typical mode of presentation of diabetes may be missed. Mild to moderate weight loss and fatigue may be unnoticed, unreported or dismissed. Even the classical symptoms of hyperglycaemia—namely polyuria, thirst, polydipsia and polyphagia—may be absent. Polyuria may be misinterpreted as dribbling, as incontinence from mechanical bladder problems, or as urinary tract infection. Polydipsia is often mild or absent owing to the increased renal threshold for glucose and reduced thirst mechanism with aging (Samos and Roos 1998). Polyphagia is difficult to elicit, as the elderly usually present with anorexia when ill. Infection, usually of mild severity, is often present but may be asymptomatic until a very late stage.

Several diabetic-related conditions are more common in elderly patients, and may be the presenting illness in previously undiagnosed diabetic patients. These conditions include painful shoulder periarthrosis, diabetic amyotrophy, diabetic neuropathic cachexia and diabetic dermopathy with intraepidermal bullae (Samos and Roos 1998).

Some clinical manifestations of hyperglycaemia which should lead a physician to suspect diabetes are presented in Table 3.1. However it must be emphasized that diabetes often mimics, coexists with and complicates other diseases.

Some elderly patients may present with symptoms of chronic complications of diabetes such as visual

Table 3.1 Clinical features of hyperglycaemia in elderly people

Primary effect	Secondary effect
Osmotic diuresis	Increased urination, nocturia, poor sleep, nocturnal falls, incontinence, dehydration, excessive thirst, polydipsia, weakness
Fluctuating refraction	Poor vision, decreased mobility, falls, impaired ability to drive
Poor red cell deformability and platelet adhesiveness	Intermittent claudication, thrombotic stroke, myocardial infarction
Recurrent infections	
Poor wound healing	
Nonspecific complaints (e.g. weight loss, fatigue)	
Alteration in mentation	Poor memory, poor compliance
Depression	
Decreased pain threshold	Increased painful symptoms
Impaired recovery from stroke	
Hyperosmolar non-ketotic hyperglycaemia	Severe dehydration, decreased consciousness, coma, hyperglycaemia visual disturbances, seizures, cerebral thrombosis
Diabetic ketoacidosis	

Source: Adapted from Rosenthal MJ, Morley JE (1992) Diabetes and its complications in older people. In: Morley JE, Korenman SG (eds) *Endocrinology and Metabolism in the Elderly.* Boston: Blackwell Scientific.

loss, peripheral nerve abnormalities, ischaemic heart disease, congestive cardiac failure, peripheral vascular or cerebrovascular disease. Even when there are no symptoms suggestive of hyperglycaemia, a survey for risk factors for diabetes mellitus in every elderly patient is warranted (Table 3.2) because of the high prevalence of undiagnosed diabetes in this age group, and the large proportion of diabetic elderly who are asymptomatic. Such a survey is simple to perform and highlights the relevance of various aspects of routine primary care of the elderly patient.

Table 3.2 Risk factors for diabetes mellitus in elderly people

1. Obesity: body mass index >25 (weight in kg/height in m^2) or percentage ideal weight ≥115%
2. Abdominal obesity: waist circumference ≥95 cm in women and >100 cm in men
3. Positive family history of Type 2 diabetes in direct relatives
4. Ischaemic heart disease
5. Hypertension
6. Cerebrovascular disease
7. Peripheral vascular disease
8. Dyslipidaemia
9. Positive history of glucose intolerance
10. Morbid obstetrical history or a history of babies over 4 kg at birth
11. Certain racial groups; e.g. Arab, Asian migrant, Hispanic American (King et al 1993)
12. Use of diabetogenic drugs; e.g. corticosteroids, oestrogens, thiazides, beta-blockers, phenytoin

Most elderly persons who develop diabetes have Type 2. Obesity may be one of the most important factors related to Type 2 diabetes (Harris et al 1998). Body mass index, and in particular abdominal obesity and weight gain after age 18–20 years predict increased mortality and risk of diabetes (Bray 1998). Adiposity reduces the number of insulin receptors and increases the production of free fatty acids, both leading to decreased effectiveness of insulin (Hansen 1999). Major genes for Type 2 diabetes have not been identified. Yet unknown autosomal dominant gene(s) and environmental factors are thought to interact to result in Type 2 diabetes. It occurs in identical twins with high concordance (Barnett et al 1991) and its high prevalence in certain racial groups is decreased by foreign genetic admixture (Zimmet et al 1986). In comparison with the general population, the risk of Type 2 diabetes is four times higher in the siblings of cases and eight times higher in the offspring of two parents with Type 2 diabetes (Krolewski and Warran 1990). Hypertension, diastolic blood pressure, triglycerides, lower HDL cholesterol have all been associated with increased risk of subsequent diagnosis of diabetes in persons over 65 years (Mykkanen et al 1993).

Considering the morbidity associated with diabetes and its high prevalence in the elderly, all elderly persons should be screened for diabetes. Elderly persons with one or more risk factors (other than advanced age) should have the diagnosis of diabetes ruled out definitively.

ESTABLISHING THE DIAGNOSIS OF DIABETES MELLITUS IN ELDERLY PEOPLE

Prior to 1997, the widely accepted criteria for the diagnosis of diabetes mellitus had been those recommended by the National Diabetes Data Group (NDDG 1979), which were later slightly modified by the World Health Organization (WHO 1985). Fasting hyperglycaemia was defined as plasma glucose ≥ 7.8 mM, while normality and diabetes for the 2-hour value in the standard 75 g oral glucose tolerance test (OGTT) were < 7.8 mM and ≥ 11.1 mM respectively. In patients without unequivocal glucose elevation in two instances, either in the fasting or random state, the OGTT was required for diagnosis.

Much knowledge on the pathophysiology of diabetes has accumulated since the above criteria were established. In 1997, a new classification and diagnostic criteria for diabetes were established by the American Diabetes Association (ADA 1997); and in 1998, recommendations were presented provisionally by WHO (Alberti et al 1998). The purpose of revising the diagnostic criteria was to more accurately predict those persons who are at risk of diabetic complications so that preventive measures can be started earlier. The essential change in the new diagnostic criteria that is relevant to persons aged over 65 years is the lowering of the diagnostic fasting plasma glucose level for diabetes to ≥ 7.0 mM. This is based on equivalence to the 2-hour level of ≥ 11.1 mM in the 75 g 2-hour OGTT, and on the predictive power of the fasting level for microvascular complications found in cross-sectional studies (Engelgau et al 1997; Finch, Zimmet and Alberti 1990; McCance et al 1994).

To accommodate the new diagnostic fasting level, a new category of impaired fasting glycaemia (IFG, fasting plasma glucose 6.1–6.9 mM) was created to replace the former category of glucose intolerance. In addition to the above changes, ADA also recommends the use of the fasting level alone, and the abolishment of the OGTT for routine clinical diagnosis. In contrast, WHO recommends that, for clinical purposes, the OGTT be used in cases where random glucose levels are in the uncertain range (venous plasma glucose between 5.5 mM and 11.1 mM; see below), while the fasting level be used alone only when the OGTT is not practicable.

A number of studies have examined the implications of using the fasting glucose level without the OGTT on prevalence, disease phenotype and mortality. It appears that the new criteria are not identifying the same population as did the old criteria. In older adults, variable changes in the prevalence of diabetes have been reported using the 1997 ADA fasting criteria alone compared with the 1985 WHO fasting and 2-hour criteria in different populations (Balkau 1999; Davies et al 1999; DECODE Study Group 1998; Unwin et al 1998; Wahl et al 1998). Substantial numbers of people diagnosed by one set of criteria were missed by the other, and vice versa.

There is also substantial discordance between patients classified as IFG by the 1997 ADA criteria and those classified as IGT by the earlier criteria (Wiener and Roberts 1999b). Our knowledge about the prognosis of IGT is much greater than that of IFG. Elevated fasting glucose may not have as high a risk of progression to diabetes compared with impaired post-load glucose (Charles et al 1991). Isolated post-load hyperglycaemia with normal fasting glycaemia (<7.0 mM) is associated with increased fatal cardiovascular disease and heart disease in elderly women (Barrett-Connor and Ferrara et al 1998). In another study, high 2-hour post-load blood glucose was associated with a higher risk of death independently of fasting glucose level, whereas mortality was associated with increasing fasting glucose only in the subjects with normal glucose tolerance. Overall, mortality was higher in people diagnosed by the old 2-hour glucose than the new fasting criteria alone (DECODE Study Group 1999). These studies suggest that the OGTT is more useful prognostically than the use of fasting glucose alone.

Thus it appears that the ADA criteria, though simplifying diagnostic procedures, are likely to change the diagnostic category of a substantial number of individuals. It is not yet established whether this change will be more effective in identifying those with increased risk of morbidity and mortality associated with abnormal glucose metabolism. The more moderate change of lowering the diagnostic fasting glucose level while retaining the OGTT for less clear-cut cases as proposed by WHO is adopted in this chapter.

If a patient has unequivocal elevation of plasma glucose level (random level ≥ 11.1 mM or fasting level ≥ 7.0 mM) with obvious symptoms of hyperglycaemia (polyuria, polydipsia and weight loss) or acute metabolic decompensation, the diagnosis of diabetes mellitus is established. No further biochemical confirmation is required. This is the recommendation of the 1998 WHO consultation report (Alberti and Zimmet 1998). The 1997 ADA criteria differ slightly: when there is no acute metabolic decompensation, confirmation by either another elevated glucose level with symptoms, or elevated fasting glucose, or an elevated 2-hour post-OGTT glucose level on a separate day is required.

Screening of Asymptomatic Elderly Patients Who Have No Risk Factors for Diabetes Other Than Age

What is the justification for screening for diabetes in the population who are 65 years or older? The prevalence of diabetes is increased in these individuals. It has a significant impact on quality of life and life span. There is an asymptomatic period, during which effective treatment reduces morbidity, mortality and financial cost due to the disease. Tests are available at reasonable cost to detect diabetes in the asymptomatic period.

In one study, yearly screening of venous plasma glucose levels post-prandially or after oral glucose loading in elderly nursing-home residents (average age 82 years) revealed progressive deterioration in glucose tolerance (Grobin 1970). Almost one-half of those subjects with abnormal screening levels were diabetic in the OGTT, suggesting how easily diabetes can be missed in this group without screening, noting that the disease is present in 14.5% of nursing-home residents (Morley et al 1987). The National Health and Medical Research Council of Australia recommends that elderly people 65 years of age or older be screened annually for diabetes during their routine visits to general practitioners (NHMRC of Australia 1992). This should be done in all in this age group whether or not there are symptoms of hyperglycaemia, or any other high risk factors for diabetes mellitus.

Screening Procedure

The primary purpose of screening is to identify those who have a high probability of meeting the diagnostic criteria of diabetes. Screening is simply done by measuring a random venous plasma glucose level. The fasting plasma glucose level or the OGTT have higher sensitivity, specificity and positive predictive value for diagnosing diabetes (Harris 1993) but require more organization. Glycosylated haemoglobin is not recommended by the WHO or the ADA as a diagnostic criterion although it is an invaluable guide to therapy, and may have a role in identifying cases with relatively poor glycaemic control (Peters et al 1996). HbA_{1c}

shows large interindividual differences in non-diabetic persons (Kilpatrick, Maylor and Keevil 1998) and is insufficiently sensitive as a diagnostic test (Wiener and Roberts 1998). Thus even if analytical methods were improved and standardized, HbA_{1c} may still have a poor sensitivity as a screening test for diabetes. In older persons, several factors other than plasma glucose concentration commonly present may alter the glycosylated haemoglobin level (Bunn 1981).

Interpreting the Result of Screening and Follow-up

A random venous plasma glucose of <11.1 mM, is non-diagnostic of diabetes. If it is 5.6–11.0 mM, the diagnosis of diabetes is uncertain (WHO 1985), so a fasting venous plasma glucose should be measured as discussed below. If it is ≤ 5.5 mM, diabetes is unlikely (WHO 1985), but a repeat screen is indicated a year later provided that no high risk factors emerge in the interim. Should risk factors emerge, the patient should have a fasting venous plasma glucose measured.

If the random venous plasma glucose is ≥ 11.1 mM, a fasting venous plasma glucose level should be measured (see below). However, if two random levels ≥ 11.1 mM have already been documented, the diagnosis of diabetes is established without further testing.

Establishing the Diagnosis

Unless there are unequivocal symptoms of hyperglycaemia, the diagnosis of diabetes requires two diagnostic test results obtained on separate days. This includes individuals in the following groups:

1. Those who are asymptomatic of hyperglycaemia and do not have any high risk factors for diabetes other than age, but have a single random venous plasma glucose concentration of 11.1 mM or greater during routine screening.
2. Those who are asymptomatic of hyperglycaemia but have one or more high risk factors for diabetes other than age.
3. Those who have mild symptoms suggestive of hyperglycaemia, with or without high risk factors for diabetes other than age.

A fasting venous plasma glucose level is measured. If it is <7.0 mM, an OGTT is indicated (see below). If the level is ≥ 7.0 mM, and a random level ≥ 11.1 mM has already been documented, the diagnosis of diabetes is established. If the level is ≥ 7.0 mM, but the random level is < 11.1 mM, the fasting level should be measured again. Then if both fasting levels are ≥ 7.0 mM, the diagnosis of diabetes mellitus is established (ADA 1997; Alberti and Zimmet 1998); an OGTT is not required. If only one fasting level is ≥ 7.0 mM, and the random level is < 11.1 mM, an OGTT is required to rule out the diagnosis of diabetes.

The WHO has not yet finalized its recommendations about alterations to the classification and diagnostic criteria for diabetes. Epidemiological studies have shown that a significant proportion of people have an abnormal glucose level in either the fasting or post-load state but not both. The diagnosis of diabetes would be missed in the latter group if the OGTT were omitted. Thus the authors continue to support the use of the OGTT if fasting glucose is in the high normal range (6.1–6.9 mM), or if there is any other suspicion or risk factor suggesting glucose intolerance. This is in agreement with the position statement of the Australian Diabetes Society and the New Zealand Society for the Study of Diabetes (Colman et al 1999).

In situations of acute illness, stress or immobilization in a hospital bed, elevated fasting blood glucose levels indicate defective mechanisms to deal with glucose under stress. It is incorrect to interpret such elevated blood sugar levels as falsely positive. A provisional diagnosis of glucose intolerance or possible diabetes should be made. Blood sugar levels should be monitored and treated as indicated by the degree of hyperglycaemia. On recovery from acute illness, the diagnosis of diabetes should be ruled out by fasting plasma glucose levels or by OGTT if the fasting plasma glucose is non-diagnostic.

Oral Glucose Tolerance Test (OGTT)

Test Procedure

The OGTT is indicated only when repeated fasting glucose levels are borderline or inconsistent. It is performed in the following way (Alberti and Zimmet 1998). Prior to the test, the patient should be ambulant and without any restriction on usual physical activity. An unrestricted diet (more than 150 g of carbohydrate per day) is taken for 3 days before the test. If possible, medications should be discontinued for 3 days before the test. The test is administered in the morning after a fast (except for water) of 8–14 hours. During the test, the patient should remain seated and not smoke. A

loading dose of 75 g glucose solution is administered orally over 5 minutes. Venous plasma glucose is measured immediately before and at 2 hours after the patient begins to drink the solution.

Contraindications to the Test

The test should *not* be performed in the following circumstances:

1. If the diagnosis of diabetes has already been established by an unequivocal elevation of plasma venous glucose level and classic symptoms of hyperglycaemia, or by two fasting venous plasma glucose levels of ≥ 7.0 mM. Performance of the OGTT may cause a harmful degree of hyperglycaemia and would not give any further information.
2. In patients who are experiencing acute medical or surgical stress, as it may lead to a false positive result. The OGTT should be delayed until several months after recovery.
3. In persons who are chronically malnourished.
4. In persons who have been confined to bed for 3 days or more.

Interpretation of the Test Results

The method of interpretation shown in Table 3.3 is based on the diagnostic criteria recommended by the 1998 WHO consultation (Alberti and Zimmet 1998) and those reported by the 1997 ADA Expert Committee (ADA 1997). In contrast to the older 1979 NDDG criteria, the OGTT is simplified by not using a mid-test level.

Table 3.3 Interpretation of fasting and 2-hour post-75 g OGTT glucose levels[a]

Classification	Fasting	OGTT
Normal	≤ 6.0	< 7.8
IFG[b]	6.1–6.9	< 7.8
IGT[c]	< 7.0	7.8–11.0
Diabetes	< 7.0	≥ 11.1
Diabetes	≥ 7.0	—[d]

[a]Venous plasma glucose concentration in mM.
[b]IFG – impaired fasting glycaemia.
[c]IGT – impaired glucose tolerance.
[d]OGTT not indicated.

Current Opinion on Glucose Tolerance Testing in the Elderly

The usefulness of the OGTT in the elderly has been questioned. Most patients (about 75%) diagnosed with IGT never develop diabetes. Many people diagnosed with diabetes by the OGTT never develop fasting hyperglycaemia or symptomatic diabetes (Foster 1991). Repeat OGTTs done in the same individual under standard conditions may give different results (Mooy et al 1996). Social, employment and insurance ramifications of the label of diabetes can be economically and psychologically stressful for the elderly diabetic person. Consequently, the OGTT is rarely indicated in clinical practice (Foster 1991). The ADA's recommendation for the use of the fasting hyperglycaemia without performing the OGTT in clinical diagnosis is particularly relevant in the elderly group.

Another reason for limiting use of the OGTT in the clinical setting is that some studies suggest that glucose intolerance appears to be almost physiological in the elderly. Decline in glucose tolerance starts in the third decade and continues throughout life. This is characterized by the moderate increase in 1-hour and 2-hour post-prandial plasma glucose concentrations. After a 100 g oral glucose challenge, there is a rise in arterialized venous plasma glucose concentration from 60 to 180 minutes of 0.7–0.8 mM per decade. A small increase in fasting plasma glucose concentration has also been demonstrated in some but not all studies (Jackson and Jaspan 1992). The pathogenesis of glucose intolerance in the elderly is multifactorial, involving impaired glucose-induced insulin secretion, delayed and prolonged insulin-mediated suppression of hepatic glucose output, as well as delayed insulin-stimulated peripheral glucose uptake which appears to be the major disturbance, with skeletal muscle being the primary site of the defect (Jackson and Jaspan 1992). The relative importance of factors such as decreased physical activity, diet changes, reduced muscle mass and obesity is not fully understood. A comparison of metabolic abnormalities in aging, obesity and Type 2 diabetes suggested that Type 2 diabetes and glucose intolerance of aging were distinct entities (Jackson and Jaspan et al 1992).

However, other lines of evidence suggest that the hyperglycaemia of aging may indeed be pathological. In many though not all studies, the percentage of glycosylated haemoglobin increases with aging in non-diabetic persons (Kilpatrick, Maylor and Keevil 1996; Ko et al 1998; Wiener and Roberts 1999a) even when

no rise is fasting plasma glucose is detected (Kilpatrick et al 1996), suggesting that at least there is increased glycosylation of haemoglobin in these persons. The findings that glucose may mediate cross-linkage of proteins and that advanced glycosylation end-products accumulate in some tissues with age and in diabetes may help explain how glucose intolerance of aging also leads to atherosclerotic macrovascular complications of diabetes (Monnier et al 1999).

In conclusion, most cases of diabetes in the elderly are readily diagnosed without the OGTT. In the individual patient, when less intensive testing for diabetes is non-diagnostic, the OGTT may be the only way of obtaining a definitive diagnosis so that effective management can be commenced to improve glycaemic control and prevent complications of the disease.

The risks of an individual with IFG or IGT developing diabetes or macrovascular disease are increased, substantially unrelated to age (Bennett 1984). Diagnosis of IFG or IGT in the elderly therefore demands active intervention to improve the risks. Currently, there are no generally accepted age-adjusted criteria for the diagnosis of diabetes, IGT or IFG in the elderly. The diagnostic criteria described above are intended for use in any non-pregnant adult.

Should Annual Screening for Diabetes Mellitus in the Elderly be Limited?

Grobin's (1970) early study of nursing-home residents reported that blood sugar levels after a 50 g oral glucose load and the percentage of subjects with abnormal screening levels did not rise after the age of 80 years. Both parameters showed a consistent drop after the age of 90 years. Age-specific prevalence of diagnosed diabetes appears to plateau at about 10% after the age of 74 years (Harris 1990). In contrast, the prevalence of diabetes diagnosed or undiagnosed in individuals over the age of 80 has been estimated to be as high as 40% (Morley et al 1987). Thus there is probably a large number of elderly persons with undiagnosed diabetes in whom the diagnosis of diabetes may reduce morbidity and probably mortality. There is no clear age above which persons with consistently normal annual screening plasma glucose levels may not benefit from further yearly screening. However, the decision should be made on an individual patient basis, taking into account coexisting diseases, general well-being and life expectancy.

EVALUATION OF THE ELDERLY PATIENT WITH DIABETES, IGT OR IFG

The vast majority of newly diagnosed diabetic persons who are 65 years of age or older have Type 2 diabetes. Some of them may require insulin for glycaemic control after a short trial of treatment with diet, exercise and oral hypoglycaemic agents, but they are not dependent on insulin to prevent ketoacidosis or to sustain life. However, some elderly patients with long-standing Type 2 diabetes may lose the ability to secrete insulin and thus become insulin-dependent and may be diagnosed at this late stage. Before starting treatment for IFG, IGT or diabetes, a comprehensive evaluation should be carried out, focusing on factors which may influence the management plan (Table 3.4).

At the time of diagnosis of IFG, IGT or diabetes, the contribution of medication or other illness (especially infection, cancer, hyperthyroidism) which may affect glucose tolerance must be considered. Patients with diabetes, IGT or IFG are at increased risk of macro-vascular disease. Therefore, risk factors for athero-sclerosis should be sought: obesity, dyslipidaemia, smoking, hypertension, and lack of exercise. Elevated serum triglycerides and reduced HDL cholesterol are commonly found in patients with Type 2 diabetes. Clinical evidence of existing macrovascular disease should be sought; i.e. ischaemic heart disease, cerebrovascular disease and peripheral vascular disease. Patients with diabetes should have a baseline glycosylated haemoglobin or fructosamine measured to give an integrated measure of recent glycaemic control and for monitoring progress.

MANAGEMENT OF THE ELDERLY PATIENT WITH IGT OR IFG

Management Goals

These patients should be informed that they have an increased chance of developing diabetes and the macrovascular complications of diabetes, but it is not predictable in the individual patient. The management goals for these patients are to normalize blood glucose levels and decrease risk-factors for macrovascular disease. When risk-factor modifications regarding obesity, diet and exercise are undertaken, the glucose tolerance of many of these individuals often returns to normal.

Management Strategies

The following guidelines apply to patients with IFG, IGT or diabetes. Additional issues concerning patients with diabetes are discussed later.

Weight, diet and exercise. Obese patients should aim to achieve some weight reduction by adopting a healthy lifestyle with a combination of correct diet and regular exercise. Weight reduction should be gradual and need not reach ideal body weight to improve glycaemic control. Patients should be encouraged to take a balanced, nutritionally correct diet and reduce their intake of simple sugars and fat. Unsaturated fat should be substituted by monounsaturated or poly-unsaturated types. Although the optimal dietary composition is unknown, a diet composed of 15–20% of total energy intake as protein, 25–30% as fat, 50–60% as complex carbohydrate and less than 10% as simple sugars is a generally accepted recommendation (European Diabetes Policy Group 1999; IDF Asian-Pacific Type 2 Diabetes Policy Group 1999; National Health and Medical Research Council of Australia 1992).

Table 3.4   Evaluation of the elderly patient diagnosed with IFG, IGT or diabetes

---

Routine history
Relevant past medical history
Risk factors for diabetes (Table 3.2)
Family history of vascular disease, hypertension, dyslipidaemia,
    other endocrine disorders
Eating habits
Weight history, especially recent changes
Level of physical activity
Socioeconomic status
Smoking and alcohol usage
Drug history
Symptoms of diabetic complications

Routine physical examination
Including determination of BMI and waist circumference

Laboratory tests in those diagnosed with diabetes, IGT or IFG
Urine microscopy and culture
Fasting serum total cholesterol, HDL cholesterol and triglycerides
Estimation of LDL cholesterol
Serum uric acid
Thyroid function tests

Other laboratory tests in those with diabetes
Urinalysis for protein, glucose and ketones
Glycosylated haemoglobin or fructosamine
Liver function tests
Serum urea and creatinine
Electrocardiogram

Sodium should be restricted in patients with hypertension. Alcohol restriction is recommended, especially for those with obesity, hypertriglyceridaemia or hypertension. Meal plans should be simple, flexible, and adaptable to the elderly patient's way of life and food preferences. Patients should be referred to a dietitian to facilitate successful dietary management.

Regular exercise improves bodyweight, plasma lipids, blood pressure, insulin sensitivity and glucose tolerance. It also maintains general fitness, balance, mobility and sense of well-being. Prior to starting regular exercise, the patient should be assessed with respect to cardiovascular, respiratory and musculoskeletal systems by the physician. A stress electrocardiogram is indicated in those with suspected ischaemic heart disease. Ideally, moderate exercise should be done for at least 20 minutes each time, three or four times a week, but the actual duration, frequency and progression of exercise should be individualized. Avoidance of injury during exercise should be taught.

Macrovascular disease. Treatment of hypertension, dyslipidaemia and cessation of smoking are essential in the prevention or management of macrovascular disease. Low-dose aspirin should be considered in these patients, especially in those with known coronary artery disease, unless contraindications are present (Harpaz et al 1998).

The severity of symptomatic peripheral vascular disease should be documented noninvasively by Doppler ultrasonography. Mild disease may improve with exercise and cessation of smoking. Severe disease may benefit from referral to a vascular surgeon. Those with an asymptomatic carotid bruit should be managed conservatively, with attention to risk factors for atherosclerosis. Those with active lesions causing recurrent cerebral ischaemia will benefit from neurological referral. A baseline electrocardiogram should be obtained in patients with suspected or known cardiovascular disease. Ischaemic heart disease should be treated vigorously as it is a major cause of death in patients with macrovascular disease. In spite of their adverse effects on lipid profiles, glycaemic control, and symptoms of hypoglycaemia, beta-blockers have a definite role in reducing post-infarct mortality (Herlitz and Malmberg 1999).

Hypertension. Hypertension is a risk factor for macrovascular disease. Most hypertension in patients with IFG, IGT or diabetes is essential hypertension. Treatment of essential hypertension in the elderly, including diastolic or isolated systolic hypertension, has been shown to reduce stroke and cardiovascular mortality (Dahlof et al 1991; SHEP Cooperative Research Group 1991), and the benefits can be expected to extend to the elderly with IFG, IGT or diabetes. Pharmacological treatment should be considered if blood pressure remains 140/90 mmHg or higher. Maximal non-drug management—diet, exercise, weight reduction, cessation of smoking, limited alcohol intake and moderate sodium restriction—should be pursued before drugs are introduced.

Elderly persons are prone to postural hypotension. No particular antihypertensive drug is contraindicated in the patient with IFG or IGT. However, side-effects of different antihypertensive drugs—such as hypokalaemia with diuretics, unfavourable lipid profiles with thiazides and beta-blockers, postural hypotension with alpha-adrenergic blockers, central adrenergic inhibitors and vasodilators—should always be considered when choosing an antihypertensive drug.

Dyslipidaemia. Dyslipidaemia is a major risk factor for macrovascular disease. Dietary saturated fatty acid restriction and substitution with monosaturated or polyunsaturated fatty acids under a dietitian's supervision is the first-line treatment for reduction of serum cholesterol and triglyceride levels. This can be effective even in the absence of weight reduction. Regular exercise in all patients and weight reduction for those who are overweight will also improve serum lipid levels. If non-pharmacological therapy is inadequate, lipid-lowering drugs should be considered. Gemfibrozil and the 3-hydroxy-3-methylglutaryl (HMG)-coenzyme A (HMG-CoA) reductase inhibitors are useful first-line agents in patients with IFG, IGT or diabetes (IDF Asian-Pacific Type 2 Diabetes Policy Group 1999). The former predominantly lowers fasting triglyceride and raises HDL cholesterol levels, while the latter predominantly lowers low-density lipoprotein (LDL) cholesterol levels. The increased risk of drug toxicity and non-compliance with multiple drug use in the elderly must be considered before adding drugs to an existing regimen.

Diabetogenic drugs. If the patient is taking diabetogenic drugs, they should be continued only if essential. Substitution with non-diabetogenic drugs should be tried.

MANAGEMENT OF THE ELDERLY PATIENT WITH DIABETES

Management Goals

The vast majority of these patients have Type 2 diabetes. The goals of management are to control the degree and symptoms of hyperglycaemia without precipitating large swings in glucose levels or hypoglycaemia, to prevent or delay complications, and to maintain the patient's general well-being and independence.

Management Strategies

Target glucose levels. Hypoglycaemia is more frequent and can be more deleterious in older diabetic patients. The WHO criteria for ideal glycaemic control for diabetic people in general (venous plasma glucose <5.5 mM fasting and <7.8 mM two hours post-prandial) are too strict for many elderly people. A fasting venous plasma glucose of <7.8 mM fasting and <11.1 mM two hours post-prandial is more appropriate for the majority in this age group. In patients taking insulin, higher post-prandial levels are acceptable (e.g. up to 15 mM).

Weight, diet and exercise. Much has been written on glycaemic control in the elderly diabetic (Mooradian 1992). The first line and cornerstone of treatment to control glycaemia is diet. Many elderly people with Type 2 diabetes respond well to diet and exercise alone without pharmacological intervention for glycaemic control. Gradual and moderate weight reduction is desirable in the obese diabetic. The general principles of a suitable diet are the same as described earlier for the person with glucose intolerance. In addition, attention should be directed to even distribution of carbohydrate through the day and in relation to exercise, particularly if oral hypoglycaemic agents or insulin are taken.

All patients with diabetes should follow a regular exercise program appropriate for their mobility and fitness. Guidelines for people with glucose intolerance also apply to people diagnosed with diabetes. Any ischaemic heart disease or proliferative retinopathy must be assessed when planning an exercise program. Glycaemic stability should be achieved prior to starting the program. Attention should be paid to the presence and prevention of foot problems related to neuropathy, vasculopathy or skeletal deformities. Suit-able footwear must be used. A podiatrist's advice can be invaluable.

Oral hypoglycaemic agents (see Chapter 10). If symptomatic hyperglycaemia and high blood glucose levels persist despite adherence to diet and an exercise program, pharmacological treatment should be considered. Sulphonylureas are the first-line drugs in non-obese patients. Short-acting sulphonylureas (e.g. glicazide) are preferred because elderly patients are more prone to hypoglycaemia and its deleterious effects. Significant renal or hepatic impairment further increases the risk of hypoglycaemia. Only one sulphonylurea should be used at any time. It should be introduced at a low dose taken with the morning meal before gradual increase to twice a day dosage if necessary. Metformin is often useful as a first-line oral hypoglycaemic agent, or in addition to a sulphonylurea in obese patients to assist in weight loss. However, metformin is contraindicated in the presence of cardiac, renal or hepatic impairment because of the risk of lactic acidosis. Alpha-glucosidase inhibitors have a good safety profile; they can be used as first-line drugs, alone or in combination with sulphonylureas or metformin. In order to minimize their gastrointestinal side-effects, metformin and alpha-glucosidase inhibitors need to be commenced at low dosage and increased gradually.

Several newer agents have recently been introduced into clinical use. Some carry less risk of hypoglycaemia, and may in time prove to be especially useful in elderly patients. Insulin secretors such as rapaglinide may be more suitable than sulphonylureas for elderly patients because of their rapid onset and shorter duration of action, thereby decreasing the risk of hypoglycaemic episodes. Thiazolidinediones increase insulin sensitivity. Troglitazone, the first thiazolidinedione on the market, was withdrawn recently owing to its hepatotoxicity. Other thiazolidinediones with less severe adverse effects may become useful agents in elderly diabetic patients in the future.

Insulin (see Chapter 12). If diet, exercise and maximal dosage of oral hypoglycaemic agents in combination are still inadequate in controlling hyperglycaemia and its symptoms, insulin will have to be considered in addition, to or instead of, hypoglycaemic agents. However, insulin carries with it further risk of hypoglycaemia, and should be used only when absolutely required and at the lowest dose that is effective to keep the blood glucose levels in an acceptable range. The choice of insulin regimen depends on the individual patient's requirements and resources and will be considered elsewhere in this text. Community nursing care services are often useful in implementing and maintaining the correct insulin prescribed, and in home blood glucose monitoring.

Home monitoring of glycaemic control and ketonuria. Home blood glucose monitoring is essential in any patient who takes insulin, and is helpful in those using oral hypoglycaemic agents. This may be done using a home glucose meter or by visual colour comparison with standard charts. The frequency of monitoring depends on the stability of glycaemic control and the frequency of insulin injections. Home blood glucose monitoring can be difficult for the elderly patient with limited visual acuity, dexterity or financial resources. Community nursing services are often required for these patients.

Urine dipstick testing for glycosuria is not useful because it is affected by the renal threshold for glucose which may be elevated. Testing for ketonuria should be done when blood glucose is persistently elevated above 20 mM and during intercurrent illness.

Macrovascular disease. Cardiovascular disease accounts for the majority of deaths in patients with diabetes. Reduction of all risk factors for atherosclerosis is a vital part of management of the diabetic patient. Principles of management of coexistent dyslipidaemia, hypertension, ischaemic heart disease, cerebral and peripheral vascular disease outlined in the previous section for patients with IFG or IGT should be applied with equal vigour to those with diabetes.

Hypertension. Hypertension is a risk factor for macrovascular disease and nephropathy in patients with diabetes. Weight reduction, regular physical activity, reduction in alcohol and salt intake are important parts of hypertension management, whether drugs are used or not. Angiotensin-converting enzyme (ACE) inhibitors and calcium-channel blockers are considered to be the first-line drugs for treating hypertension in diabetic patients. ACE inhibitors have an important role in delaying any deterioration in renal function in diabetes. If side-effects are severe, angiotensin receptor antagonists can be used. Thiazide diuretics and beta-adrenergic blockers are also effective in lowering blood pressure and cardiovascular risk. Concern regarding the effects of thiazides and beta-adrenergic blockers on blood glucose levels and lipid profiles are insignificant when the drugs are used individually, but they may have larger effects if used in combination. Beta-adrenergic blockers can blunt the adrenergic symptoms of hypoglycaemia as well as delay recovery from hypoglycaemia, which is particularly dangerous in insulin-treated patients. In patients with diabetic nephropathy, diuretics are often required for adequate antihypertensive control, and elderly patients should be monitored closely for electrolyte disturbances. Protective cardiovascular reflexes are attenuated with aging, and so extra caution is needed to avoid over-reduction in blood pressure when initiating treatment in patients in this age group. The target blood pressure of 130/85 mmHg generally used for diabetic patients (WHO–ISH Guidelines Subcommittee 1999) may need to be modified to avoid postural hypotension.

Dyslipidaemia. The prevalence of dyslipidaemia is increased by at least two-fold in persons with Type 2 diabetes, and involves all classes of lipoprotein. The most common lipid disorder seen in diabetic patients is hypertriglyceridaemia and reduced HDL cholesterol. Diet, exercise, weight reduction and improvement of glycaemic control improve but rarely correct the dyslipidaemia in patients with Type 2 diabetes completely. If after 2–3 months of such therapy, total serum cholesterol and LDL cholesterol are still above 4.5 and 2.5 mM respectively, pharmacological intervention should be considered, although it is seldom used unless the total cholesterol is above 5.0 mM. As with patients with IFG or IGT, HMG-CoA reductase inhibitors and gemfibrozil are the drugs of choice.

Ischaemic heart disease. Ischaemic heart disease is the major cause of death in diabetes. Atherosclerosis progresses at a more rapid rate and is more extensive in older diabetic patients than in their non-diabetic fellows. Myocardial ischaemia or infarction may be painless and myocardial infarction atypical in presentation in these patients (Vokonas and Kannel et al 1996). Post-infarct cardiac failure is more common and survival is lower in diabetics (Sprafka et al 1991). Thus treatment of ischaemic heart disease and risk factor modification in diabetic patients should have a high priority.

Patient education. Education is a fundamental part of management of the elderly person with diabetes. Programs have been shown to improve knowledge, metabolic control, desirable lifestyle changes and psychological functioning (Gilden et al 1989). The content of diabetes education programs needs to be adapted to the elderly with different degrees of independence and comorbidity. Involvement of the patient's family or carer should be encouraged to maximize the benefits.

General management. Management of the elderly diabetic patient poses a special challenge. He or she is likely to have multiple comorbid conditions which must be identified and prioritized for effective management. Limited financial and psychosocial resources, cognitive dysfunction and depression often create barriers to effective management (Scheen 1997). Directions for all medications should be in writing and education programs may need to be repeated to maximize compliance. The patient's drug regimen should be reviewed regularly. Polypharmacy should be minimized to prevent drug toxicity and to improve compliance. Potentially diabetogenic drugs should be used only if essential. Home care and nursing services or residential care facilities can often facilitate effective management.

SCREENING FOR DIABETIC COMPLICATIONS

Currently, many elderly people already have chronic complications of diabetes which may be asymptomatic at diagnosis. These should be screened systematically by history, examination and appropriate laboratory investigations. Table 3.5 presents some guidelines for initial examination and appropriate laboratory investigations for chronic diabetic complications.

Symptoms of sensory, motor and autonomic neuropathy should be documented at the time of diagnosis of diabetes and reassessed at least every 6 months. Other neurological conditions must be ruled out before a diagnosis of diabetic neuropathy is made. The patient should be informed that symptoms of diabetic neuropathy may improve slowly with improved glycaemic control.

All elderly people with diabetes should be reviewed at least 6-monthly for refraction, and at least yearly for ophthalmoscopic examination with pupil dilatation. Detection of any retinopathy, cataract or other ocular abnormality warrants referral to an ophthalmologist. Early retinopathy can be reversed by improved metabolic control or halted by laser therapy.

Table 3.5 Initial screening for chronic diabetic complications

Atherosclerotic disease
Cardiovascular examination
Electrocardiogram
Serum total cholesterol, HDL cholesterol and triglycerides

Neuropathy
Neurologic examination, with particular attention to peripheral sensation and autonomic nervous system (valsalva manoeuvre, postural hypotension, sinus arrhythmia)

Eye disease
Visual acuity
Fundoscopy with pupils dilated

Nephropathy
Dipstick urinalysis for protein
Microalbuminuria if negative dipstick proteinuria
Quantification of proteinuria and creatinine clearance if dipstick for proteinuria is positive
Serum creatinine and urea
Blood pressure

Foot problems
Vascular, neurologic, musculoskeletal and cutaneous and soft tissue examination of the feet
Examination and improvement of footwear

Renal function should be monitored at least annually by measurement of microalbuminuria and plasma creatinine. Urinalysis should be checked regularly to detect occult urinary tract infection. Strict control of hypertension is important for preventing or reversing early diabetic nephropathy.

The feet should be examined at every visit to the physician. Ulcers and infection must be treated promptly. A podiatrist should be involved in the education and management of footcare (see Chapter 6).

SUMMARY

In developed countries, people aged 65 years or over with diabetes account for a growing majority among people with diabetes (King, Aubert and Herwan 1998). Globally, the number of diabetic people in this age group is increasing progressively. Early diagnosis is important to improve glycaemia, correct hyperglycaemic symptoms, prevent medical complications, and maintain quality of life and independence. Routine screening for diabetes by primary physicians is recommended for all persons 65 years of age or older. Those with multiple high risk factors require definitive exclusion of the diagnosis of diabetes. The diagnostic criteria for diabetes in the elderly are identical to those for non-pregnant adults in general. With the introduction of the lower diagnostic plasma glucose level, it may be expected that a larger proportion of elderly people might be diagnosed with diabetes, as diagnosis in this age group in particular has always relied much more on fasting rather than on 2-hour post-load glucose measurements. Patients diagnosed with IFG or IGT are at increased risk of diabetes and macrovascular disease. Non-pharmacological measures are often successful in improving glucose tolerance in these patients, and lowering their atherosclerotic risks. For those with diabetes, diet is the cornerstone of treatment. Oral hypoglycaemic agents and insulin are valuable drugs which must be used with caution in the elderly because of the increased risk of hypoglycaemia and drug toxicity. Regular screening for diabetic complications and risk factors for atherosclerosis should be performed on all persons with diabetes. Management of diabetes in the elderly should involve education and take into account the patient's level of independent living, intercurrent illness, life expectancy and lifestyle.

REFERENCES

ADA Expert Committee on the Diagnosis and Classification of Diabetes Mellitus (1997) Report of the Expert Committee on the diagnosis and classification of diabetes mellitus. *Diabetes Care*, **20**, 1183–1197.

Alberti KGMM, Zimmet PZ (1998) Definition, diagnosis and classification of diabetes mellitus and its complications; 1. Diagnosis and classification of diabetes mellitus. Provisional report of a WHO consultation. *Diabetic Medicine*, **15**, 539–553.

Balkau B (1999) New diagnostic criteria for diabetes and mortality in older adults. *Lancet*, **353**, 68–69.

Barnett AH, Eff C, Leslie RDG, Pyke DA (1991) Diabetes in identical twins: a study of 200 pairs. *Diabetologia*, **20**, 87–93.

Barrett-Connor E, Ferrara A (1998) Isolated postchallenge hyperglycaemia and the risk of fatal cardiovascular disease in older women and men. The Rancho Bernardo study. *Diabetes Care*, **21**, 1236–1239.

Bennett PH (1984) Diabetes in the elderly: diagnosis and epidemiology. *Geriatrics*, **39**, 37–41.

Bray GA (1998) Obesity: a time bomb to be defused. *Lancet*, **352**, 160–161.

Bunn HF (1981) Evaluation of glycosylated hemoglobin in diabetic patients. *Diabetes*, **30**, 613–617.

Charles MA, Fontbonne A, Thibult N, Warnet J-M, Rosselin GE and Eschwege E (1991) Risk factors for NIDDM in the white population: Paris prospective study. *Diabetes*, **40**, 796–799.

Colman PG, Thomas DW, Zimmet PZ, Welborn TA, Garcia-Webb P, Moore MP (1999) New classification and criteria for the diagnosis of diabetes mellitus. Position statement from the Australian Diabetes Society, New Zealand Society for the Study of Diabetes, Royal College of Pathologists of Australasia,

and Australasian Association of Clinical Biochemists. *Medical Journal of Australia*, **170**, 375–378.

Croxson SC, Price DE, Burden M, Jagger C, Burden AC (1994) The mortality of elderly people with diabetes. *Diabetic Medicine*, **11**, 250–252.

Dahlof B, Lindholm LH, Hansson L, Schersten B, Ekbom T, Wester P-O (1991) Morbidity and mortality in the Swedish trial in old patients with hypertension (STOP-hypertension). *Lancet*, **388**, 1281–1285.

Davies MJ, Muehlbayer S, Garrick P, McNally PG (1999) Potential impact of a change in the diagnostic criteria for diabetes mellitus on the prevalence of abnormal glucose tolerance in a local community at risk of diabetes: impact of new diagnostic criteria for diabetes mellitus. *Diabetic Medicine*, **16**, 343–346.

Davis TM, Stratton IM, Fox CJ, Holman RR, Turner RC (1997) UK prospective study 22: effect of age at diagnosis on diabetic tissue damage during the first 6 years of NIDDM. *Diabetes Care*, **20**, 1435–1441.

DECODE Study Group on behalf of the European Diabetes Epidemiology Study Group (1998) Will new diagnostic criteria for diabetes change phenotype of patients with diabetes? Reanalysis of European epidemiological data. *British Medical Journal*, **317**, 371–375.

DECODE Study Group on behalf of the European Diabetes Epidemiology Group (1999) Glucose tolerance and mortality: comparison of WHO and American Diabetes Association diagnostic criteria. *Lancet*, **354**, 617–621.

Engelgau MM, Thompson TJ, Herman WH, Boyle JP, Aubert RE, Kenny SJ, Badran A, Sous ES, Ali MA (1997) Comparison of fasting and 2-hour glucose and HbA1c levels for diagnosing diabetes: diagnostic criteria and performance revisited. *Diabetes Care*, **20**, 785–791.

European Diabetes Policy Group (1999) A desktop guide to Type 2 diabetes mellitus. *Diabetic Med*, **16**, 716–730.

Finch CF, Zimmet PZ, Alberti KGMM (1990) Determining diabetes prevalence: a rational basis for the use of fasting plasma glucose measurements? *Diabetic Medicine*, **7**, 603–610.

Foster DW (1991) Diabetes Mellitus. In: Wilson JD, Braunwald E, Isselbacher KJ, Petersdorf RG, Martin JB, Fauci AS, Root RK (eds), *Harrison's Principles of Internal Medicine*, New York, McGraw-Hill, 1739–1759.

Gilden JL, Hendryx M, Casia C, Singh SP (1989) The effectiveness of diabetes education programs for older patients and their spouses. *Journal of the American Geriatric Society*, **37**, 1023–1030.

Grobin W (1970) Diabetes in the aged: underdiagnosis and overtreatment. *Canadian Medical Association Journal*, **103**, 915–923.

Hansen BC (1999) Obesity and diabetes: the natural history. In: Turtle JR, Kaneko T, Osato S (eds), *Diabetes in the New Millennium*. Sydney: Endocrinology and Diabetes Research Foundation of the University of Sydney, 151–160.

Harpaz D, Gottlieb S, Graff E, Boyko V, Kishon Y, Behar S (1998) Effects of aspirin treatment on survival in non-insulin-dependent diabetic patients with coronary artery disease. *American Journal of Medicine*, **105**, 494–499.

Harris MI (1990) Epidemiology of diabetes mellitus among the elderly in the United States. *Clinics in Geriatric Medicine*, **6**, 703–719.

Harris MI (1993) Undiagnosed NIDDM: clinical and public health issues. *Diabetes Care*, **16**, 642–652.

Harris MI, Klein R, Welborn TA, Knuiman MW (1992) Onset of NIDDM occurs at least 4–7 yr before clinical diagnosis. *Diabetes Care*, **15**, 815–819.

Harris MI, Flegal KM, Cowie CC, Eberhardt MS, Goldstein DE, Little RR, Wiedmeyer H-M, Byrd-Holt DD (1998) Prevalence of diabetes, impaired fasting glucose, and impaired glucose tolerance in US adults. The Third National Health and Nutrition Examination Survey, 1988–1994. *Diabetes Care*, **21**, 518–524.

Herlitz J, Malmberg K (1999) How to improve the cardiac prognosis for diabetes. *Diabetes Care*, **22**(Suppl 2), B89–96.

IDF Asian-Pacific Type 2 Diabetes Policy Group (1999) *Type 2 Diabetes. Practical Targets and Treatments*. Sydney: Health Communications Australia.

Jackson RA, Jaspan JB (1992) Glucose intolerance and aging. In: Morley JE (ed) *Endocrinology and Metabolism in the Elderly*, Boston: Blackwell Scientific, 353–372.

Kilpatrick ES, Dominiczak MH, Small M (1996) The effects of aging on glycation and the interpretation of glycaemic control in Type 2 diabetes. *Quarterly Journal of Medicine*, **89**, 307–312.

Kilpatrick ES, Maylor PW, Keevil BG (1998) Biological variation of glycated hemoglobin: implications for diabetes screening and monitoring. *Diabetes Care*, **21**, 261–264.

King H, Rewers M (1993) Global estimates for prevalence of diabetes mellitus and impaired glucose tolerance in adults. WHO Ad Hoc Diabetes Reporting Group. *Diabetes Care*, **16**, 157–177.

King H, Aubert RE, Herman WH (1998) Global burden of diabetes, 1995–2025: prevalence, numerical estimates, and projections. *Diabetes Care*, **21**, 1414–1431.

Ko GT, Chan JC, Woo J, Lau E, Yeung VT, Chow CC, Li JK, So WY, Chan WB, Cockram CS (1998) Glycated haemoglobin and cardiovascular risk factors in Chinese subjects with normal glucose tolerance. *Diabetic Medicine*, **15**, 573–578.

Krolewski AS, Warran JH (1990) Natural history of diabetes. In: Becker KL (ed.) *Principles and Practice of Endocrinology and Metabolism*, Philadelphia, JB Lippincott, 1084–1087.

Lipson LG (1986) Diabetes in the elderly: diagnosis, pathogenesis, and therapy. *American Journal of Medicine*, **80**(Suppl 5A), 10–21.

McCance DR, Hanson RL, Charles MA, Jacobsson LTH, Pettitt DJ, Bennett PH, Knowler WC (1994) Comparison of tests for glycated haemoglobin and fasting and two-hour plasma glucose concentrations as diagnostic methods for diabetes. *British Medical Journal*, **308**, 1323–1328.

Monnier VM, Bautista O, Kenny D, Sell DR, Fogarty J, Dahms W, Cleary PA, Lachin J, Genuth S (1999) Skin collagen glycation, glycoxidation, and cross-linking are lower in subjects with long-term intensive versus conventional therapy of Type 1 diabetes: relevance of glycated collagen products versus HbA1c as markers of diabetic complications. DCCT Skin Collagen Ancillary Study Group. Diabetes Control and Complication Trial. *Diabetes*, **48**, 870–880.

Mooradian AD (1992) Management of diabetes in the elderly. In: Morley JE, Korenman (eds) *Endocrinology and Metabolism in the Elderly*. Boston: Blackwell Scientific, 388–405.

Mooy JM, Grootenhuis PA, deVries H, Kostense PJ , Popp-Snijders C, Bouter LM and Heine RJ (1996) Intra-individual variation of glucose, specific insulin and proinsulin concentrations measured by two oral glucose tolerance tests in a general Caucasian population: the Hoorn Study. *Diabetologia*, **39**, 298–305.

Morley JE, Mooradian AD, Rosenthal MJ, Kaiser FE (1987) Diabetes mellitus in elderly patients. Is it different? *American Journal of Medicine*, **83**, 533–544.

Muggeo M (1998) Accelerated complications in Type 2 diabetes mellitus: the need for greater awareness and earlier detection. *Diabetic Medicine*, **15**(Suppl 4), S60–S62.

Mykkanen L, Kuusisto J, Pyorala K, Laakso M (1993) Cardiovascular disease risk factors as predictors of Type 2 (non-insulin-dependent) diabetes mellitus in elderly subjects. *Diabetologia*, **36**, 553–559.

National Diabetes Data Group (1979) Classification and diagnosis of diabetes mellitus and other categories of glucose intolerance. *Diabetes*, **28**, 1039–1057.

National Health and Medical Research Council of Australia (1992) *Diabetes in Older People*. Canberra: Australian Government Publishing Service.

Peters AL, Davidson MB, Schriger DL, Hasselbald V (1996) A clinical approach for the diagnosis of diabetes mellitus: an analysis using glycosylated hemoglobin levels. *Journal of the American Medical Association*, **276**, 1246–1252.

Samos LF, Roos BA (1998) Diabetes mellitus in older persons. *Medical Clinics of North America*, **82**, 791–803.

Scheen AJ (1997) Non-insulin-dependent diabetes mellitus in the elderly. *Bailliére's Clinical Endocrinology and Metabolism*, **11**, 389–406.

SHEP Cooperative Research Group (1991) Prevention of stroke by antihypertensive drug treatment in older persons with isolated systolic hypertension: final results of the systolic hypertension in the elderly program (SHEP). *Journal of the American Medical Association*, **265**, 3255–3264.

Sinclair AJ, Robert IE, Croxson SCM (1997) Mortality in older people with diabetes mellitus. *Diabetic Medicine*, **14**, 639–647.

Sprafka JM, Burke GL, Folsom AR, McGovern PG, Hahn LP (1991) Trends in prevalence of diabetes mellitus in patients with myocardial infarction and effect of diabetes on survival: the Minnesota heart survey. *Diabetes Care*, **14**, 537–543.

Unwin N, Alberti KGMM, Bhopal R, Harland J, Watson W, White M (1998) Comparison of the current WHO and new ADA criteria for the diagnosis of diabetes mellitus in three ethnic groups in the UK. *Diabetic Medicine*, **15**, 554–557.

Vilbergsson S, Sigurdsson G, Sigvaldason H, Sigfusson N (1998) Coronary heart disease mortality amongst non-insulin-dependent diabetic subjects in Iceland: the independent effect of diabetes. The Reykjavik Study 17-year follow-up. *Journal of Internal Medicine*, **244**, 309–316.

Vokonas PS, Kannel WB (1996) Diabetes mellitus and coronary heart disease in the elderly. *Clinics in Geriatric Medicine*, **12**, 69–78.

Wahl PW, Savage PJ, Psaty BM, Orchard TJ, Robbins JA, Tracy RP (1998) Diabetes in older adults: comparison of 1997 American Diabetes Association classification of diabetes mellitus with 1985 WHO classification. *Lancet*, **352**, 1012–1015.

Waugh NR, Dallas JH, Jung RT, Newton RW (1989) Mortality in a cohort of diabetic patients: causes and relative risks. *Diabetologia*, **32**, 103–104.

WHO (1985) *Diabetes mellitus: Report of a WHO Study Group*. (WHO Technical Report Series 7), Geneva: WHO.

WHO–ISH Guidelines Subcommittee (1999) Guidelines for the management of hypertension. *Journal of Hypertension*, **17**, 151–183.

Wiener K, Roberts NB (1998) The relative merits of haemoglobin A1c and fasting plasma glucose as first-line diagnostic tests for diabetes mellitus in non-pregnant subjects. *Diabetic Medicine*, **15**, 558–563.

Wiener K, Roberts NB (1999a) Age does not influence levels of HbA1c in normal subject. *Quarterly Journal of Medicine*, **92**, 169–173.

Wiener K, Roberts NB (1999b) New diagnostic criteria for diabetes: a way of identifying all those at risk of long-term complications of diabetes is still needed. *British Medical Journal*, **318**, 532.

Zimmet P, Serjeantson S, King H, Kirk R (1986) The genetics of diabetes mellitus. *Australian and New Zealand Journal of Medicine*, **16**, 419–424.

4

Screening and Treatment Strategies for Diabetes Complications in the Elderly

Lea Sorensen, Dennis K. Yue
Royal Prince Alfred Hospital, and the University of Sydney

INTRODUCTION

Diabetic complications are the major causes of morbidity and mortality for people with diabetes. They can be grouped into those specific to diabetes (e.g. retinopathy, nephropathy or neuropathy) and macrovascular diseases which are shared with non-diabetic individuals but occur earlier and in more severe forms in diabetes (e.g. coronary heart disease, cerebrovascular disease and peripheral vascular disease). A few pertinent facts serve to illustrate the medical, social and economic importance of diabetic complications. Diabetic retinopathy is the commonest cause of blindness in young people. Diabetic nephropathy is now the commonest cause of end-stage renal disease in the world. Diabetic neuropathy and peripheral vascular disease account for 60 000 amputations in the USA each year. Diabetes is the most important condition underlying macrovascular diseases such as myocardial infarction and stroke.

Our approach to diabetic treatment is therefore profoundly affected by the endeavour to maintain good glycaemic control and so reduce the development of diabetic complications. An attempt to ensure adherence with everything prescribed in various treatment guidelines is responsible for the multiple tests and visits to doctors that the patient is asked to undergo. Our anxiety to achieve early detection of diabetic complications is often transferred to patients and their family. These problems become accentuated with the greatly increased prevalence of diabetes, which is reaching epidemic proportion in many countries and imposing serious economic burdens. Diabetes increases with age, and by the seventh decade as many as

one in ten individuals will be affected. Thus, the clinician is often faced with an older patient either with newly diagnosed or existing diabetes. Our approach to the prevention, screening and management of diabetes complications in this group of older patients will have great impact not only on individuals, but also on healthcare spending.

In this chapter, we first discuss the importance of glycaemic control in the prevention and treatment of diabetic complications. Subsequently, we discuss each of the major diabetic complications with respect to how aging affects its clinical manifestation, detection and treatment. Naturally, this topic is more relevant to those with Type 2 diabetes; but where appropriate, matters pertinent to people with Type 1 diabetes will also be addressed.

GLYCAEMIC CONTROL AND DIABETIC COMPLICATIONS

Much objective information concerning the benefits of good glycaemic control for older people with diabetes is now available through the results of the United Kingdom Prospective Diabetes Study (UKPDS 1998a). In this study of newly diagnosed Type 2 diabetic subjects, patients were randomly assigned to treatment with diet, a sulphonylurea, metformin or insulin. There was a stepwise approach to the introduction of additional treatment (e.g. metformin was used as a second agent if a sulphonylurea alone did not sufficiently maintain a predetermined level of glycaemic control). Though a progressive inability of beta-cells to secrete enough insulin meant that most

Diabetes in Old Age. Second Edition. Edited by A. J. Sinclair and P. Finucane. © 2001 John Wiley & Sons Ltd.

patients eventually required two oral agents or insulin therapy, analysis was performed according to the treatment group to which patients had originally been assigned. Overall, the pharmacologically treated groups achieved a mean HbA_{1c} level of 7.0% compared with the dietary treated group of 7.9%. The mean age of the approximately 4000 patients at the onset of diabetes was 52 years. After a median of 15 years of follow-up, the groups assigned to pharmacological treatment had a significant reduction of microvascular complications of about 25%, almost entirely due to a reduction in retinopathy. There were no significant effects on overall mortality or the development of diabetic nephropathy or neuropathy. Results for macrovascular disease were disappointing. There was no effect of improved glycaemic control on cerebrovascular disease, although reduction of myocardial infarction was tantalisingly close to significance at $P = 0.052$.

The results and clinical implications of the UKPDS are still being debated. In the context of our discussion, the most important aspect to emphasize is that it takes more than 10 years for the benefits of good glycaemic control to emerge. Therefore, if an elderly person with diabetes has a life expectancy of less than this, it seems reasonable to assume that good glycaemic control would make little difference to the emergence of microvascular complications and would make no difference to the development of macrovascular disease. With an elderly diabetic patient, therefore, the prime objective is to control blood glucose to a degree that alleviates symptoms of hyperglycaemia rather than aim for a complication-free assessment 10–15 years later. At a practical level, this could make a difference when considering the introduction of insulin treatment for an elderly person whose quality of life might be adversely affected by the resulting need for additional dietary restriction and glucose monitoring. Deciding against insulin could also spare many elderly patients from unnecessary hypoglycaemic episodes due to overzealous treatment. There are no firm guidelines about how to manage an older Type 2 diabetic patient who perhaps has had diabetes for many years and has already developed some complications. Clinicians need to take a holistic approach, considering the relevant clinical, social and psychological factors, to help the patient and family to adopt a treatment strategy of appropriate intensity. By contrast, as will be discussed later, the UKPDS found that, at least with the treatment then available, reductions in blood pressure brought benefits much sooner and for elderly people

are clearly of greater importance than improved glycaemic control.

It has now also been established beyond doubt that good glycaemic control plays an important role in the prevention of microvascular and neuropathic complications in Type 1 diabetic subjects. The Diabetes Control and Complications Trial (DCCT Research Group 1993) showed that intensive insulin therapy could maintain diabetic control at an average HbA_{1c} level of about 7.2%, compared with 8.9% achieved with conventional insulin therapy. With such improved control, it was possible to reduce the development of diabetic retinopathy, neuropathy and microalbuminuria. Unfortunately, the price associated with the favourable outcome of improved glycaemic control was a three-fold increase in hypoglycaemic episodes in the intensive-treatment group. In real life, this factor alone would preclude many individuals from undertaking such therapy. The DCCT only included people with Type 1 diabetes and these were mainly young and with minimal or no diabetic complications on entry to the study. The applicability of these findings to older age groups has not been formally tested.

In older Type 1 diabetic subjects, as a result of the longer duration of the disease, diabetic complications are likely to be already present at a more advanced stage although they may be completely asymptomatic. Good glycaemic control is less effective in reversing or preventing deterioration of established diabetic complications. This is true for diabetic retinopathy, overt diabetic nephropathy and neuropathy. Even near-normal glycaemic control conferred by pancreatic transplantation takes 5–10 years to make any worthwhile changes to renal morphology. Older Type 1 diabetic patients with a history of more than 20–30 year history of diabetes are also likely to have impaired counter-regulatory secretion of glucagon and adrenaline in response to hypoglycaemia. They are therefore much more prone to develop severe hypoglycaemia during intensive insulin treatment. These considerations suggest that the risk/benefit ratio of good glycaemic control in older Type 1 diabetic patients is likely to be less favourable than that reported for the DCCT cohort. In the case of diabetic nephropathy at least, it is probable that someone with a 20–30 years history of diabetes, and who has avoided devastating complications to date, is unlikely to develop such severe complications thereafter. It is therefore prudent to relax glycaemic control in the elderly Type 1 diabetic patient to minimize the risk of severe hypoglycaemia.

EYE DISEASE

Diabetic retinopathy can be divided broadly into two types: non-proliferative diabetic retinopathy (NPDR) and proliferative retinopathy (PDR). In NPDR, the major manifestations are microaneurysms, dot and blot haemorrhages and exudates in the retina. The cardinal feature of PDR is the proliferation of abnormal capillaries (also called new vessels) growing forward from the retina and into the vitreous. In addition, both types of retinopathy can be affected by macular oedema, caused by swelling and thickening of the fovea, the region of retina responsible for central vision. In NPDR, macular oedema is the principal cause of visual loss and this occurs gradually. In PDR, bleeding of the fragile new vessels leads to visual loss that is more severe and abrupt in nature. Although there is overlap, NPDR is the predominant type of retinopathy that occurs in older individuals.

Retinopathy is best detected clinically by examining the retina with an ophthalmoscope through dilated pupils. In older individuals, chronic open-angle glaucoma is often a coincidental condition. By itself, glaucoma is not a contraindication to the use of mydriatics to dilate the pupil although this task is less easy when a patient is using pupil-constricting eye-drops. On the other hand, the presence of cataract makes visualization of the fundi much more difficult. Quite often, retinal examination has to be deferred until after cataract extraction. In older diabetic patients, NPDR with macular oedema is the main cause of vision loss. The clinical presentation is less dramatic than that seen with the sudden bleeding of proliferative retinopathy. Instead, vision just becomes less with each successive year. As elderly patients are often much less complaining than their younger counterparts and may have a concurrent cause of visual impairment, such retinopathy is easily missed. Once vision declines to 6/24 or less, it is much less amenable to treatment. Therefore a routine yearly check of visual acuity and fundal examination through dilated pupils is essential in elderly diabetic subjects. Once significant abnormalities are detected, further investigations such as fluorescein angiography and more regular monitoring will need to be arranged.

There are more hurdles in the treatment of diabetic retinopathy in the elderly. In addition to the difficulty of assessment referred to above, cataract may need to be extracted before laser photocoagulation can be delivered. Cataract surgery itself may aggravate retinopathy. Laser treatment for macular oedema is technically more demanding because it has to be directed near to the macula without getting so close to it as to damage or distort central vision (Early Treatment Diabetic Retinopathy Study Group 1987). The UKPDS (1998b) has clearly shown the importance of good blood pressure control on preventing deterioration of retinopathy. However, many clinicians still fail to treat hypertension vigorously enough in the elderly population.

Despite its many difficulties, it is essential to ensure early diagnosis and optimal treatment of diabetic retinopathy in older people. This often allows them adequate vision to administer insulin injections, to remain ambulatory outdoors and to maintain social contacts.

PAINFUL AND PAINLESS NEUROPATHY

Diabetic neuropathy can affect both the peripheral and autonomic nervous systems resulting in such devastating sequelae as foot ulceration and infection, lower limb amputation, sexual dysfunction and cardiac arrhythmias. Of the neuropathies, peripheral sensory neuropathy is most widely seen in clinical practice and is primarily responsible for diabetic foot disease. This type of neuropathy is typically bilateral and symmetrical. This helps to distinguish it from other conditions commonly found in elderly people, such as arthritis and peripheral vascular disease, which are more often asymmetrical.

Peripheral sensory neuropathy essentially presents in two overlapping forms: the type with pain or that without pain but with loss of sensation. The pathogenesis of this duality in clinical presentation is not clear, although there are many theories based on involvement or regeneration of different types of nerve fibres. Those with painful neuropathy are naturally more inclined to seek medical attention. On the other hand, people with painless neuropathy often remain undiagnosed because testing of sensation is cumbersome, imprecise and often not routinely conducted. The estimated prevalence of peripheral neuropathy in the literature therefore varies from 10 to 90%, according to whether the diagnosis is based on symptoms alone, reduced sensation on testing or both. Estimates of the true prevalence rate are further confounded by the use of diagnostic tests of varying sensitivity. For example, nerve conduction studies would detect many more patients with diabetic neuropathy than clinical examination. This section deals with our clinical approach of focusing on those with significant symptoms, or sufficient objective sensory loss to be at risk of neuropathic ulceration.

Approximately 6% of people with diabetes have painful neuropathy. The symptoms are generally described as burning, or short, sharp stabbing pains in the feet. Some patients will complain of pins and needles, numbness or hot and tight feet. The precise relationship of these symptoms to pain is not clear, but the current definition of pain by the International Association for the Study of Pain (IASP) includes these moieties if the patient considers them distressing (IASP Task Force 1994). Other common findings are:

- hyperalgesia (an increased response to a stimulus that is normally painful), and
- allodynia (feeling a painful sensation from non-painful stimuli, such as bedclothes covering the feet).

While painful symptoms can be quite mild, at their worst, even walking or trying to cope with daily activities may become unbearable, preventing satisfactory sleep and diminishing quality of life.

Painless neuropathy is more common than painful neuropathy. Despite its name, it is not an innocuous condition, as the loss of sensation is fundamental to the development of painless neuropathic ulcer that often leads to amputation. The common methods of assessing sensation are by testing with a pin, cotton wool or a tuning fork. These procedures are difficult to standardize and quantify, resulting in poor interexaminer and interpatient reproducibility. To overcome some of these problems, a commonly used instrument is the 'biothesiometer' which is in essence a tuning fork calibrated to vibrate progressively more strongly when the stimulus is increased from 0 to 50 volts. Studies show that a patient who cannot feel the biothesiometer at 30 volts or greater is at high risk of developing neuropathic ulceration. The biothesiometer costs about US$1000 and this limits its availability in most clinical settings. Instead, the Semmes–Weinstein 10 g monofilament (Figure 4.1) can be used and costs only a few dollars. This filament is applied to the foot until it buckles, at which point it exerts a force of 10 g. If the patient cannot feel the filament, it again signifies a dangerous loss of sensation.

It is important to recognize that from the age of around 60 years even non-diabetic individuals progressively lose some peripheral sensation. Thus, it is not uncommon to see a normal elderly person with a biothesiometer reading of 40 volts and who cannot feel

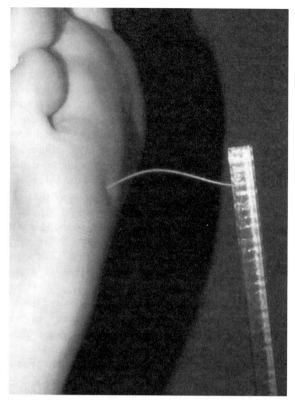

Figure 4.1. The Semmes–Weinstein 10 g monofilament (photo courtesy of The Diabetes Centre, Royal Prince Alfred Hospital, Sydney)

the Semmes–Weinstein 10 g monofilament. Failure to appreciate this can be a 'normal' aging phenomenon will lead to the overdiagnosis of insensate neuropathy in the elderly. When faced with an elderly patient with abnormal biothesiometer or monofilament findings, the clinician should take account of other factors when making a diagnosis of neuropathy. These might include the duration of diabetes, the presence of dry skin on the feet (due to anhidrosis from coexisting autonomic neuropathy) and clawed toes (due to subtle muscular imbalance as a result of neuropathy).

The treatment of painful neuropathy depends on the clinical situation. Patients often perceive pain as the first step towards possible amputation. However, once rest pain due to ischaemia can be confidently excluded, neuropathic pain without associated severe sensory loss is not usually a prelude to amputation. Reassurance of patients in this regard is sometimes all that is required. When pain has been present only for a short time (e.g. a few weeks to a few months) and sensation is normal, it often spontaneously resolves within a few months. In this acute situation, improving glycaemic control often helps to reduce the pain. On the other hand, when pain has already been present for a long time (e.g. for more than one year) and is associated with some loss of sensation, it is much more likely to persist. In this chronic situation, improving glycaemic control does not reduce pain as readily. With older people in particular, it is important not to strive over-zealously for normoglycaemia for this purpose, thus exposing the patient to a high risk of severe hypo-glycaemia.

With chronic pain, depression is common and older people in particular need support, explanation and in some cases pharmacological help. It is prudent to first determine if the patient does have pain severe enough to warrant treatment. There is also an element of trial and error in drug selection. In milder cases, simple analgesics may give some relief. When patients' life-style or sleep pattern is adversely affected, more potent agents should be considered. Tricyclic antidepressants are useful but their side-effects of dry mouth, tachy-cardia and tiredness are common and in elderly males may aggravate urinary symptoms from prostatic dis-ease. It is therefore necessary to start with low doses and titrate upward. This is important, as typically high doses are ultimately required. Anecdotal evidence suggests that tricyclic drugs act best in patients who are depressed and whose pain is described as deep and aching. The antiarrhythmic agent, mexiletine, may also be useful, particularly for those with burning or stabbing pain. It can cause bradycardia and this often precludes its use in older patients with coexisting heart diseases. Other agents that have been used include antiepileptic drugs such as phenytoin, carbamazepine and gabapentin.

For patients with more superficial and localized burning pain but no severe sensory loss, it is our practice to first try a topical cream containing capsicin. It is preferable to use a higher strength preparation of at least 0.075%. It works by stimulating the pain-conducting nerve fibres to deplete the neurotrans-mitter, substance P. To achieve this, it needs to be applied to the area of pain four times a day. This will in itself cause a local burning sensation in the first week, so patients should be advised to persevere with it for several weeks. If patients cannot tolerate or fail to re-spond to any of these pharmacological agents, then acupuncture or transcutaneous electrical nerve stimu-lation (TENS) can be tried.

There is no specific treatment for the insensate type of diabetic neuropathy. Despite many clinical trials, the aldose reductase inhibitors have not been shown to be effective. Similarly, two large but as yet unpublished studies on the use of nerve growth factor in this con-dition did not demonstrate favourable outcomes. Peo-ple with this type of neuropathy are those at high risk of neuropathic ulceration, particularly at sites of ex-cessive pressure such as on the plantar surface of the foot. Management of patients with insensate neuro-pathy revolves around the provision of good footcare education so that they appreciate the danger of ul-ceration and can take measures to prevent it. Important measures include daily inspection of the feet, appli-cation of moisturising cream to maintain skin integrity, regular removal of callus by a podiatrist, and wearing appropriate footwear. Elderly diabetic people are often disadvantaged in this regard, being limited by poor eyesight, immobility and financial constraints. If a neuropathic ulcer occurs, patients need much more intensive supervision by a number of health profes-sionals who are often scattered in several locations and this further magnifies the difficulties that arise. More-over, peripheral vascular disease is more common with advancing age and this results in a much worse prog-nosis for healing.

Apart from the problems discussed above, elderly diabetic patients occasionally suffer from other mani-festations of neuropathy. Postural hypotension is more common with age and may be aggravated by auto-nomic neuropathy. This can be a particular problem in the treatment of hypertension. Instability of gait can be a manifestation of diabetic peripheral neuropathy, aggravating unsteadiness in older people. Diabetic radiculopathy with its associated weight loss in older patients is often confused with occult malignancy. Erectile dysfunction is common in older males with or without diabetes. Although diabetic autonomic neu-ropathy is often quoted as an underlying cause, it is probably seldom important in this age group. If erectile dysfunction is a problem for the patient, they should be referred for appropriate counselling and assessed as to their suitability for conventional treatments.

NEPHROPATHY

On a worldwide basis, there are equal numbers of Type 1 and Type 2 diabetic patients with end-stage renal disease (ESRD) requiring dialysis or transplantation. As survival improves for people with Type 2 diabetes, more and more survive to the stage where they develop renal failure. This is a particular problem in many ethnic groups who develop Type 2 diabetes at an earlier age, often as early as the third decade. They live long enough to develop renal failure before the high prevalence of cardiovascular disease and cancer begin to take their toll. This consideration underlies the importance of controlling diabetes as soon as it is diagnosed, particularly when one takes into account that oral hypoglycaemic agents are much more effective early in the natural history of diabetes.

Diabetic nephropathy is essentially a symptom-free condition until it is moderately advanced (e.g. serum creatinine of about 400–500 μM) when associated conditions such as anaemia, fluid retention and cardiac failure become problems. Therefore routine screening is required to detect diabetic nephropathy and findings of proteinuria (>0.5 g/day or 2+ on a dipstick) or microalbuminuria (20–200 μg/min or 30–300 mg/day) are the main warning signs of overt and early diabetic nephropathy respectively. Their presence in any individual is an indication of an increased risk of developing ESRD and, interestingly, a much higher risk of macrovascular disease (Mogensen 1999; Deckert et al 1989).

In the management of a patient with proteinuria or microalbuminuria, the clinician needs to take into consideration the patient's age and serum creatinine. For the majority of older individuals, the presence of coincidental macrovascular disease is a greater concern. This is an important clinical point. In treating elderly patients who have proteinuria or microalbuminuria but still have a normal serum creatinine, too much emphasis is often placed on preventing renal failure which they are unlikely to live long enough to develop. By contrast, not enough is done to minimize their vascular risk factors such as treating hypertension and dyslipidaemia. On the other hand, patients with proteinuria or microalbuminuria and significantly elevated creatinine are at risk of ESRD if they survive long enough from macrovascular disease or cancer. These individuals need to have hypertension, hyperglycaemia and dyslipidaemia treated appropriately to retard the deterioration of renal filtration (Table 4.1). In the context of their treatment in older people, these issues will be discussed elsewhere in this chapter. The evidence that treatment with an angiotensin converting enzyme (ACE) inhibitor has beneficial effects on diabetic nephropathy above and beyond its anti-hypertensive action is not as strong in Type 2 as in Type 1 diabetic subjects. It is difficult to design a clinical trial to test this when the majority of Type 2 diabetic subjects with proteinuria or microalbuminuria die from macrovascular disease before they develop overt renal failure.

In the management of older diabetic patients with renal disease, particularly when serum creatinine is elevated, several precautions need to be taken. From a drug treatment perspective, glibenclamide should be used very cautiously because of its tendency to cause profound and prolonged hypoglycaemia in this group of patients. Other sulphonylureas are preferred in this

Table 4.1 Management of diabetic renal disease in the elderly

Microalbuminuria Normal serum creatinine	Proteinuria Normal serum creatinine	Elevated Serum Creatinine
Aim for good BP control	Aim for tight BP control	Aim for very tight BP control
Use of ACE Inhibitor to protect vasculature and kidney	Use of ACE Inhibitor to protect vasculature and kidney	Use ACE Inhibitor to protect vasculature and kidney but monitor serum creatinine and potassium regularly
Treat dyslipidaemia	Aggressive treatment of dyslipidaemia to reduce macrovascular risk	Aggressive treatment of dyslipidaemia to reduce macrovascular risk
Aim for appropriate glycaemic target for age and prognosis of patients	Aim for appropriate glycaemic target for age and prognosis of patients	Aim for appropriate glycaemic target for age and prognosis of patients
Check albumin excretion and serum creatinine each year	Check albumin excretion and serum creatinine each year	Check creatinine clearance at regular intervals
		Arrange for dietary advice to minimise phosphate retention
		Use caution with radiographic contrast

situation, even if one has to accept a slightly worse degree of diabetic control. Theoretically, metformin should also be avoided in the presence of an elevated creatinine. However, on many occasions patients will not accept insulin treatment and metformin is required to keep the patient symptom free and to prevent the development of a hyperglycaemic crisis. In this situation, metformin should be used in as small a dosage as possible. In patients with renal disease, special precaution also needs to be exercised when undertaking any investigation involving injection of radiographic contrast agents as this can lead to a sudden deterioration in renal function. Adequate hydration and the use of high-quality, non-ionic contrast materials have reduced the development of this complication in elderly diabetic subjects.

Increasingly, many elderly diabetic patients are being treated by peritoneal or haemodialysis when their renal function is no longer adequate to sustain life. This often imposes considerable hardship, not only for the individuals and their families, but also for the governments which in many nations are expected to provide the necessary resource. Overall, the long-term survival of these patients is not good, with many succumbing to vascular diseases. In many registries, diabetes is one of the diseases associated with the worst prognosis when life is sustained by dialysis. However, it is difficult to turn the tide of community expectation for patients to receive this form of treatment.

HYPERTENSION

The relationship between hypertension and cerebrovascular and cardiovascular disease is indisputable. This is particularly important when one considers the high prevalence of hypertension in diabetes, in those with Type 1 diabetes as a manifestation of their renal disease and in those with Type 2 diabetes as part of their insulin-resistance syndrome. However, patients with diabetes were often excluded from earlier studies conducted to examine the benefits of blood pressure reduction. Thus the value of blood pressure control in diabetic subjects was widely accepted but not rigorously tested. However, more recently, diabetic subjects have been included in many pivotal studies comparing either various antihypertensive regimens or differing levels of blood pressure control (Mogensen 1999; Curb et al 1996; Hansson et al 1998). Fortunately, patients

with diabetes seem to derive as much, if not more, benefit from blood pressure reduction in comparison with their non-diabetic counterparts. In addition, the UKPDS, which studied only subjects with Type 2 diabetes, also clearly demonstrated that blood pressure treatment reduced not only macrovascular events but also retinopathy (UKPDS 1998b). The benefit of blood pressure treatment in diabetes is therefore no longer in doubt.

In older people, isolated systolic hypertension becomes a common, under-recognized and under-treated clinical problem. The pathophysiological basis of isolated systolic hypertension is interesting (O'Rourke 1990). With aging our arteries become progressively stiffer, a phenomenon referred to as arteriosclerosis (which should not be confused from the much more commonly known atherosclerosis). Normally with each heartbeat, a pressure wave is transmitted along the arterial wall from the heart to the periphery, from where it is reflected back. In young people the reflected wave arrives back centrally in diastole. In older people with stiffer arteries, the wave transmission along the arterial wall is faster and arrives back centrally in systole. This adds to the systolic pressure, a phenomenon known as 'augmentation' and explains the emergence of isolated systolic hypertension in the elderly. Recent studies have shown that in both Type 1 and Type 2 diabetes, augmentation of systolic blood pressure with aging is exaggerated (Brooks, Molyneux and Yue 1999). For generations, medical students were taught that systolic hypertension is unimportant and does not require treatment. Recent clinical trials have shown this concept to be anything but the truth. Even in elderly people, a reduction in systolic blood pressure results in less cardiovascular morbidity and mortality (Tuomilehto et al 1998). As elderly diabetic subjects have accentuated augmentation of their systolic blood pressure, treatment of systolic hypertension is even more important. Certainly, even in older individuals systolic blood pressure should be kept as near to 130 mmHg as possible.

Polypharmacy is an almost inevitable consequence of aggressive blood pressure reduction. In the UKPDS, nearly one-third of patients required three or more antihypertensive agents to achieve a blood pressure level that would be considered unacceptable by modern standards. Elderly people are often confused by the numerous medications they are prescribed, and it is therefore important to ensure that proper supervision is provided as required.

MACROVASCULAR DISEASE

Macrovascular disease is a leading cause of morbidity and mortality in people with or without diabetes, and in both groups elderly people have more disease than their younger counterparts. However, people with diabetes develop more macrovascular disease from an earlier age and even premenopausal women are often affected. This needs to be taken into consideration in determining what is the 'older' population. People with diabetes also have a worse prognosis following a macrovascular event than those without diabetes, even after adjusting for the severity of disease, such as the size of a myocardial infarct (Fisher 1999).

There are a few points worth noting from a clinical point of view. The coexistence of autonomic neuropathy can reduce chest pain as a symptom of angina or myocardial infarction. Thus, the more subtle symptoms of breathlessness, tachycardia, fatigue or a general feeling of being unwell are often the only indicators of cardiac ischaemia. In the elderly, these may be attributed erroneously to the aging process. Cardiac failure and atrial fibrillation are common cardiovascular problems in elderly people and are even more prevalent in those with diabetes. Apart from that due to ischaemic heart disease and hypertension, a form of diabetic cardiomyopathy seems to exist and is characterized by diastolic dysfunction with impaired relaxation of the ventricles. Atrial fibrillation has been shown by the UKPDS to be common in diabetes and is associated with an eight-fold increase in cerebrovascular events.

Transient ischaemic attacks can be difficult to distinguish from hypoglycaemia in elderly people, and sometimes the diagnostic confusion can be clarified only by assessing the response to reducing the dosage of insulin or oral hypoglycaemic agents. Peripheral vascular disease in people with diabetes also differs slightly from those without diabetes. The damage is more extensive, typically involving the arteries between the knee and the ankle, rather than being limited to those above the knee. This makes surgical revascularization more difficult. Calcification of arteries is common in diabetes, especially in older people with a long history of diabetes, making the ankle brachial index less reliable as an index of perfusion pressure. In taking a history, it is worth noting that peripheral vascular disease may not be obvious in those elderly patients whose limited physical activity does not provoke claudication. In older people, rest pain due to ischaemia can be confused with arthritis or neuropathy.

Even without causing distressing symptoms, peripheral vascular disease is problematic in elderly people when it is associated with a neuropathic ulcer (i.e. the so-called neuro-ischaemic ulcer), increasing the risk of infection and impeding healing.

Evaluation of macrovascular status should be an integral part of the assessment of adult diabetic patients. Apart from routine measurement of blood pressure, pulse rate, biochemistry and plasma lipids, in older patients baseline electrocardiography is worthwhile. On physical examination, we find it most useful to listen for carotid bruits to identify carotid stenosis and to palpate the pedal pulses to help identify peripheral vascular disease. These simple clinical procedures can identify people at high risk of developing macrovascular events. Where myocardial ischaemia is suspected, a radioisotope scan may be necessary to assess myocardial perfusion, as an exercise stress test can be difficult for older age groups.

With increasing healthcare standards, elderly people with macrovascular disease are now commonly treated with procedures such as arterial bypass grafting, angioplasty and anticoagulant therapy. Diabetic patients are over-represented in this cohort and they also do not fare as well. This should strengthen our resolve to treat risk factors aggressively. Issues relating to control of hypertension and hyperglycaemia have been addressed earlier in this chapter. From a dyslipidaemia point of view, it has been shown that cholesterol reduction with statins reduces mortality in patients with established coronary heart disease. In a sub-group analysis of the Scandinavian Simvastatin Survival Study (4S Study), people with diabetes did as well as those without diabetes with regard to reducing the chance of a subsequent cardiovascular event (Pyorala et al 1997). Similar results were demonstrated in the cholesterol and recurrent events (CARE) study (Plehn et al 1999).

A number of these trials included patients up to the age of 75 years, so there is relatively little argument with the value of lipid-lowering treatment in this age group. In elderly patients with diabetes but with no history of macrovascular events, the benefit of treatment is less well defined, although data are emerging. The AFCAP/TexCAP study targeted middle-aged and older men and women aged up to 73 years, with no macrovascular history and with average lipid profiles, and showed a 33–40% reduction in coronary and cardiovascular event rates for those taking lovastatin compared with those taking placebo (Downs et al 1998). Based on our experience that lipid-lowering agents are generally well-tolerated, we tend to initiate treatment, particularly in the presence of other risk factors such as a history of smoking, long duration of diabetes and the presence of albuminuria. However, with every treatment strategy, health professionals must consider its potential impact on the patients' quality of life and the likelihood of making a worthwhile reduction to the risk of macrovascular events.

REFERENCES

Brooks B, Molyneux L, Yue DK (1999) Augmentation of central arterial pressure in Type 1 diabetes. *Diabetes Care*, **22**, 1722–1727.

Curb JD, Pressel SL, Cutler JA, Savage PJ, Applegate WB, Black H, Camel G, Davis, BR, Frost PH, Gonzalez N, Guthrie G, Oberman A, Ruton GH, Stamler J (1996) Effect of diuretic-based antihypertensive treatment on cardiovascular disease risk in older diabetic patients with isolated systolic hypertension. Systolic Hypertension in the Elderly Program Cooperative Research Group. *Journal of the American Medical Association*, **276**, 1886–1892.

Deckert T, Feldt-Rasmussen B, Borch-Johnsen K, Jensen T, Kofoed-Enevoldsen A (1989) Albuminuria reflects widespread vascular damage: the Steno hypothesis. *Diabetologia*, **32**, 219–226.

Diabetes Control and Complications Trial Research Group (1993) The effect of intensive treatment of diabetes on the development and progression of long-term complications in insulin-dependent diabetes mellitus. *New England Journal of Medicine*, **329**, 977–986.

Downs JR, Clearfield M, Weis S, Whitney E, Shapiro D, Beere P, Langendorfer A, Stein E, Kruyer W, Gotto A (1998) Primary prevention of acute coronary events with lovastatin in men and women with average cholesterol levels: results of AFCAPS/TexCAPS. *Journal of the American Medical Association*, **279**, 1615–1622.

Early Treatment Diabetic Retinopathy Study Research Group (1987) Treatment techniques and clinical guidelines for photocoagulation of diabetic macular edema. Early Treatment Diabetic Retinopathy Study Report Number 2. *Ophthalmology*, **94**, 761–774.

Fisher BM (1999) Diabetes and myocardial infarction *International Diabetes Reviews*, **3**, 15–19.

Hansson L, Zanchetti A, Carruthers SG, Dahlof B, Elmfeldt D, Julius S, Menard J, Rahn KH, Wedel H, Westerling S (1998) Effects of intensive blood-pressure lowering and low-dose aspirin in patients with hypertension: principal results of the Hypertension Optimal Treatment (HOT) randomised trial. *Lancet*, **351**, 1755–1762.

International Association for the Study of Pain (IASP) Task Force on Taxonomy (1994) *Classification of Chronic Pain*, 209–214.

Mogensen CE (1999) Microalbuminuria, blood pressure and diabetic renal disease: origin and development of ideas. *Diabetologia*, **42**, 263–285.

O'Rourke M (1990) Arterial stiffness, systolic blood pressure and logical treatment of arterial hypertension. *Hypertension*, **15**, 339–346.

Plehn JF, Davis BR, Sacks FM, Rouleau JL, Pfeffer M, Bernstein V, Cuddy TE, Moye LA, Piller LB, Rutherford J, Simpson L, Braunwald E (1999) Reduction of stroke incidence after myocardial infarction with pravastatin: the cholesterol and recurrent event events (CARE) study. *Circulation*, **99**, 216–223.

Pyorala K, Pedersen TR, Kjekshus J, Faergeman O, Anders GO, Thorgeirsson G (1997) Cholesterol lowering with simvastatin improves prognosis of diabetes patients with coronary heart disease: a subgroup analysis of the Scandinavian Simvastatin Survival Study (4S). *Diabetes Care*, **20**, 614–619.

Tuomilehto J, Rastenyte D, Thisj L, Staessen J (1998) Reduction of mortality and cardiovascular events in older diabetic patients with isolated systolic hypertension in Europe treated with nitrendipine-based antihypertensive therapy (Syst-Eur-Trial). *Diabetes*, **47**, A54.

United Kingdom Prospective Diabetes Study Group (1998a) Intensive blood glucose control with sulphonylureas or insulin compared with conventional treatment and risk of complications in patients with Type 2 diabetes (UKPDS 33). *Lancet*, **352**, 837–853.

United Kingdom Prospective Diabetes Study Group (1998b) Tight blood pressure control and risk of macrovascular and microvascular complications in Type 2 diabetes (UKPDS 38). *British Medical Journal*, **317**, 703–713.

Section II

Complications

5

Metabolic Decompensation

Simon C. M. Croxson
Bristol General Hospital, Bristol

INTRODUCTION

This chapter covers the major metabolic disturbances affecting the elderly diabetic person. It considers the special characteristics in the elderly, their precipitating factors and their management. Many of these problems can be avoided by careful use of hypoglycaemic medication, patient education (e.g. with 'sick day rules') and diabetes specialist nurses to educate patients and intervene early when problems start to occur. It must be remembered that a diabetic person could be unconscious for a reason other than metabolic decompensation; however, it is often likely to be an abnormal glucose level that is missed (due to un-diagnosed diabetes or poor attention to the diabetes) rather than another cause of altered consciousness. The main message is that the majority of these problems can be avoided, and all ill elderly people need their plasma glucose measured whether or not diabetes has been diagnosed. Indeed, the omission of venous plasma glucose measurement in an elderly person ill enough to require hospitalization is ill-advised given the high frequency of diabetes (both diagnosed and undiagnosed) in the elderly, and the nonspecific presentation of hyperglycaemia and hypoglycaemia.

HYPERGLYCAEMIC CONDITIONS

There are three hyperglycaemic problems occurring in the elderly:

- diabetic keto-acidosis (DKA)
- hyper-osmolar non-ketotic (HONK) coma
- Normo-osmolar, non-ketotic, hyponatraemic hyperglycaemia associated with impaired renal function.

The key to management is to recognize the problem, so all sick elderly subjects must have plasma glucose estimation. Elderly subjects with DKA or HONK coma are often not known to have diabetes, and care home residence is a risk factor for HONK coma and death.

Both diabetic ketoacidosis and hyper-osmolar comas occur in the elderly. Although there are criteria for their diagnosis, these can vary slightly (Page and Hall 1999; Krentz and Nattrass 1997; Alberti 1989; Berger and Keller 1992; Wachtel et al 1991; Wachtel 1990; Kitabchi and Murphy 1988). A synthesis that fits with most criteria is given in Table 5.1 In practice, some patients will seem to be half way between the two ends of the spectrum (Wachtel et al 1991). The definition of coma is variable (Alberti 1989), but one would accept any, even minor, disturbance of consciousness. The plasma osmolality can be either measured directly or calculated from the sum of urea + glucose + $2 \times (Na^+ + K^+)$ (all concentrations in mM).

DKA or HONK coma can be precipitated by similar events. Examples are any infarction (e.g. myocardial infarction, cerebrovascular accident), any infection (e.g. pneumonia or urinary tract infection), inadequate hypoglycaemic treatment (e.g. if undiagnosed diabetes or unrecognized Type 1 diabetes), and use of diabetogenic drugs, particularly oral glucocorticosteroids.

What factors determine whether a patient develops DKA or HONK coma? This issue has been reviewed by Kitabchi and Murphy (1988). It is thought that the elderly person with DKA has just enough insulin to suppress lipolysis, but not enough to suppress hepatic gluconeogenesis or stimulate peripheral glucose utilization. However, one study showed similar insulin levels in subjects with DKA or HONK coma, but

Diabetes in Old Age. Second Edition. Edited by A. J. Sinclair and P. Finucane. © 2001 John Wiley & Sons Ltd.

Table 5.1 Diagnostic criteria

Diagnostic criteria for DKA
Hyperglycaemia (venous plasma glucose >15.0 mM)
Ketosis (either urinary ketones >++ on dipstick testing or
  plasma ketones+)
 Acidosis (plasma bicarbonate less than 15 mM or arterial pH less
  than 7.3)

Diagnostic criteria for HONK coma
Hyperglycaemia (venous plasma glucose >15.0 mM, although
  usually much higher)
No significant ketosis (urinary ketones 0 to++ on dipstick)
No significant acidosis (plasma bicarbonate >15 mM or arterial
  pH >7.3)
Hyper-osmolar state (plasma osmolality >350 mOsmol/L)

subjects with the latter had lower counter-regulatory hormones leading to less lipid breakdown with less hepatic ketogenesis (Gerich, Martin and Recant 1971). Finally, it may be that the hyper-osmolar state suppresses lipolysis and hence ketogenesis.

Compared with younger subjects, older subjects with hyperglycaemic comas exhibit a much higher mortality, are less likely to have had their diabetes previously diagnosed or insulin treated, spend longer in hospital, are more likely to have renal impairment, and need a greater amount of insulin, presumably owing to a higher proportion with Type 2 diabetes and insulin resistance. (Gale, Dornam and Tattersall 1981; Barnett, Wilcox and Marble 1962; Malone, Gennis and Goodwin 1992).

People dying from DKA or HONK coma often have three things in common (Basu et al 1993; Hamblin et al 1989). They are elderly, they have previously not been diagnosed as being diabetic, and they have previously seen their general practitioner or family physician within the preceding two weeks. Symptoms of un-diagnosed diabetes in the elderly can be vague or absent (Croxson and Burden 1998). Thus the main message is that, in an ill elderly person who is deteriorating and not known to be diabetic, at the bare minimum a finger prick blood glucose measurement should be taken.

DKA Risk Factors and Management

Type 1 diabetes does occur in elderly people (Sturrock et al 1995) and the age-specific incidence is the same from 30 to 80 years of age (Mølbak et al 1994). It is relatively uncommon as a *de novo* presentation, and can catch the physician out. It may present as DKA,

but may also present as an outpatient appearing very similar to a subject with Type 2 diabetes in whom the plasma glucose levels never really lower in response to rapidly escalating doses of oral agents.

DKA does occur in Type 2 diabetic subjects and they may well be able to avoid ongoing insulin treatment when recovered (Leutscher and Svendsen 1991; Alberti 1989).

Risk factors for DKA in the elderly include un-diagnosed or recently diagnosed diabetes, and social isolation (Gale et al 1981; Barnett et al 1962). Precipitants are generally infection (Wachtel et al 1991), predominantly of chest or urinary tract (Berger and Keller 1992). In one report, 65% of deaths occurred within the first 2 days and two-thirds of these deaths seemed to be purely from the diabetic coma (Gale et al 1981).

The main step in management is to consider the possibility of DKA in an ill elderly person. The patient may have osmotic symptoms particularly if questioned closely, and may well present with general deterioration and confusion, and possibly have nausea and vomiting (Alberti 1989). Thorough clinical assessment and investigations to confirm the diagnosis, elicit a cause and define the baseline are essential. One can define acidosis by a plasma bicarbonate level less than 15 mM; thus arterial blood gases for pH are not routinely necessary unless there are concerns about respiratory function, and arterial puncture is not without pain and risk. If the patient is not passing urine, plasma can be tested for ketones with a urine dipstick; leave a lithium heparin tube to stand for 15 minutes before testing.

Intravenous fluid should be normal saline, but how rapid the infusion should be to correct the usual 6 L deficit has been debated. Adrogué et al (1989) randomized subjects who were not shocked, had at least 30 mL/h urine output initially and who did not have severe renal impairment to either a high rate (1 L/h for 4 h and then $\frac{1}{2}$ L/h for 4 h) or a low rate ($\frac{1}{2}$ L/h for 4 h and then $\frac{1}{4}$ L/h for 4 h); the low rate group corrected their bicarbonate levels more quickly, but otherwise there was no difference between the groups. However, this study excluded shocked subjects in whom one would give rapid infusions of normal saline, or possibly colloid. Thus it would appear that correction of the subjects' shocked state is paramount initially, and then use the above low-rate fluid replacement. Once the plasma glucose reaches 15 mM, change to 5% dextrose as the infusion fluid so that the insulin plus carbohydrate can continue to metabolize the ketone bodies. In practice, patients are often able to eat and drink by this stage, so that it is easier to start a basal/bolus insulin regime and feed them. A central line can be invaluable if the patient's state of hydration is uncertain, if there is coexistent cardiac failure, or if venous access is difficult.

An insulin infusion should be set up using soluble insulin (e.g. 50 units of Actrapid in 50 mL normal saline), and the rate of infusion adjusted on the basis of hourly fingerprick plasma glucose determinations and a sliding-scale infusion (see Table 5.2). Sliding-scale designs vary depending on the reference source. The major differences is whether or not the insulin infusion is stopped for very low plasma glucose values (e.g. Page and Hall 1999). In a Type 1 diabetic subject, DKA would rapidly occur if their insulin treatment was withdrawn, so that perhaps a low (0.5 unit per hour) infusion would be appropriate for the lowest plasma glucose levels. However, in this situation one would worry about patients having insulin without carbohydrate; hence the advice to switch to either a glucose–insulin–potassium (GIK) regime or a food plus subcutaneous insulin regime once the glucose readings are under 15 mM. Most well, insulin-treated patients need about 30 units of insulin per day; but if they are normally taking much more insulin than this (some patients are on 200 units per day), then there could be a need to proportionately increase the variable insulin infusion. If they are very obese or very catabolic, then again they will have increased insulin requirements. Another method used in some units is to run an infusion at 6 units per hour, watch the fingerprick plasma glucose fall gently to 15 mM, and then convert to a glucose–potassium–insulin regime (Krentz Nattrass 1997). The prescription of the sliding-scale insulin infusion does not magically fix the problem; the patient needs frequent, experienced medical review.

Potassium levels will initially be high normal, but will fall due to the effect of insulin. This will need monitoring every 4 hours over the first 12 hours; this is also an opportunity to check the accuracy of the bed-side plasma glucose monitoring. Suggested potassium replacement is 20 mmol per litre of normal saline if the potassium level is normal (3.5 to 5.5 mM), no added potassium if the level is high, and 40 mmol per litre of normal saline if the potassium level is low; Page and Hall have a simple table of this in their book (1999). Severe DKA is associated with marked loss of potassium which should be replaced using an additional 7-day course of Sando-K 2 g per day once the patient is well.

Care of the unconscious elderly diabetic person with a hyperglycaemic coma must include attention to pressure areas. In a prolonged unconscious state, consider also passing a nasogastric tube to avoid the risk of aspiration secondary to gastric stasis.

Should bicarbonate be given in severe acidosis? Several small trials have randomized subjects of all ages with DKA and arterial blood pH of 6.8–7.19 to bicarbonate or no bicarbonate, showing that the bicarbonate did not improve outcome (Hale, Crase and Nattrass 1984; Lever and Jaspan 1983; Morris, Murphy and Kitabchi 1986), which suggests that its use may be limited. However, acidosis can impair cardiac function. If there is severe acidosis (pH <6.9) and the patient is still hypotensive despite adequate treatment otherwise, bicarbonate (e.g. 500 mL of isotonic bicarbonate 1.4%) may be tried (Page and Hall 1999).

Cerebral oedema is a risk in young subjects with DKA, but does not seem to be a problem in the elderly. It presents as sudden neurological deterioration 2–24 hours after starting treatment, and is treated by intravenous mannitol (Hammond and Wallis 1992).

HONK Coma Risk Factors and Management

As with DKA, undiagnosed diabetes is a major risk factor for HONK coma, and infection is a common precipitant. In one series, 68% of subjects with HONK coma had undiagnosed diabetes, and infection was the precipitant in 55% (Small, Alzaid and MacCuish 1988). Residents of care homes are also at increased risk of HONK coma (Wachtel et al 1991), with a greater risk of fatal outcome. Often a patient (a resident) is not known to be diabetic and seems to have had a UTI recently; whether they have had a UTI precipitating the coma or they have urinary symptoms due to glycosuria is unknown. HONK coma can also be precipitated by diuretic therapy (Fonseca and Phear 1982).

Table 5.2 A typical sliding-scale insulin infusion

Plasma glucose (mM)	Insulin infusion rate (units per hour)
0.0–4.0	0.0
4.1–7.0	1.0
7.1–11.0	2.0
11.1–17.0	4.0
>17.1	6.0

As per DKA, the clinical features of HONK coma include osmotic symptoms, general deterioration etc., but in particular can include neurological symptoms such as fits and focal neurological deficits (Lorber 1995). Again, the first step in management is to recognize that a problem exists and to perform the tests to look for HONK coma, establish baseline biochemical variables and look for an underlying cause.

The main difference from DKA is in the type of fluid replacement. Use half-normal (0.45 mM) saline if serum sodium is 150 mM or more; but if the patient is hypotensive, use normal saline or colloid in similar rates to DKA until the hypotension is corrected, when the hypernatraemia needs attention. The insulin infusion used is the same as for DKA, but these patients may be quite insulin-sensitive. Otherwise the management is very similar to that for DKA. After the illness, the patient may (or may not) be controlled on diet alone.

Anticoagulation in Hyperglycaemic Coma

There is a major threat of acute thrombotic events in HONK coma, and full anticoagulation has been employed. However, unless the indications are strong— pulmonary embolism, large deep vein thrombosis, unstable angina—the author would not fully anti-coagulate the subject, since many with HONK have haemorrhagic gastritis, the vascular event may already have happened prior to medical attention, and there are no studies to guide us on this decision. Other authors (Krentz and Nattrass 1997; Alberti 1989; Small et al 1988) also do not support the need for full anti-coagulation. Given the subject's immobility, always consider deep venous thrombosis prophylaxis in subjects with hyperglycaemic coma.

Traps for the Unwary in Subjects with Hyperglycaemic Coma

- Ketone bodies can interfere with the creatinine assay, so that an elevated creatinine may be due to ketosis rather than to impaired renal function (Page and Hall 1999; Kitabchi and Murphy 1988).
- Ketosis can also cause a falsely elevated amylase level (Page and Hall 1999; Kitabchi and Murphy 1988).
- Dehydration can cause an elevated leucocytosis (Page and Hall 1999; Kitabchi and Murphy 1988).
- Ensure that the patient's heels are regularly inspected to prevent pressure sores.

- The plasma glucose level should halve every 4–6 hours. If it does not fall, either the syringe pump is not working, or the variable-dose infusion is set too low.
- Finger prick determination of plasma glucose can be falsely low in the shocked state (Atkin et al 1991).
- When an insulin infusion is halted, the patient's exogenous insulin level will be zero after 10 minutes. Switch the pump off 30 minutes after the first dose of regular treatment, (Page and Hall 1999).
- Subjects with HONK coma often will manage on diet alone. If stabilized on hypoglycaemic medication, they need careful review initially to avoid hypoglycaemia.

Normo-osmolar, Non-ketotic, Hyponatraemic Hyperglycaemia Associated with Impaired Renal Function

There are several case reports (Ryder and Hayes 1983; Popli et al 1990) of subjects with hyperglycaemia who are relatively well with mild dehydration only, and hyponatraemia. The subjects are known to have pre-existing renal impairment, and it is thought that the renal impairment protects the subject from osmotic diuresis. Because the plasma glucose is extracellular, it acts to draw water from the intracellular space and dilutes the plasma sodium. It is possible to adjust for the effect of hyperglycaemia on plasma sodium (1.6 mM plasma sodium is equivalent to 5.56 mM plasma glucose). The treatment is to recognize the syndrome initially, because the main risk is over-generous fluid replacement. In case reports most subjects recovered having received approximately 2 L of normal saline per day. Insulin can be given as an insulin infusion as per DKA, although early conversion to a basal bolus regimen may be feasible. Stabilize them and look towards their long-term treatment; many of these subjects can later be controlled on diet alone.

Well-tolerated marked hyperglycaemia does occur in subjects not known to be diabetic; the patient has some osmotic symptoms or general malaise, the general practitioner sensibly checks the venous plasma glucose, and is then surprised by a rather high level (e.g. 30–50 mM). The author has had several patients like this in recent years. These subjects have no evidence of an acute illness, normal mental function, no clinical or biochemical evidence of dehydration, and no evidence of hyper-osmolar state or keto-acidosis. Again their sodium level is generally low.

A two-stage treatment strategy can be adopted. First stabilize the patient on a basal/bolus regime. Second, obtain a dietitian's assessment, decide on long-term glycaemic management (see below), and try it after a few days of good glycaemic control. The justification for this initially aggressive approach in relatively asymptomatic subjects comes from one study showing that intermittent good glycaemic control by insulin treatment caused persistent acceptable glycaemic control on diet alone, presumably by improved beta-cell function and insulin sensitivity (Ilkova et al 1997). Also, it would be unwise to leave a frail elderly person alone with marked hyperglycaemia, since it would be so difficult to monitor for decompensation. Where excellent back-up facilities with frequent blood glucose monitoring and assessments of the patient's well-being have been present, the author has managed newly diagnosed Type 2 diabetic subjects with plasma glucoses in the low 30s at home with diet, sulphonylurea, careful instruction, and frequent review.

Management after the Hyperglycaemic Coma

The aim is to select a treatment regimen which will achieve plasma glucose levels as normal as possible with low risk of side-effects, such as hypoglycaemia or weight gain. To do this it is necessary to separate out the subjects with Type 1 diabetes. The guidelines for an outpatient in the author's unit state that diabetes is Type 1 if either there is significant ketosis, or the individual has two of the features suggesting Type 1 diabetes (Gale and Tattersall 1990a) in Table 5.3.

Having identified the subjects with Type 1 diabetes, and given them insulin, it is then necessary to decide on the best regime for the Type 2 diabetic subjects by considering four questions:

1. Was the patient's previous diet satisfactory regarding management of diabetes and obesity? Beware

Table 5.3 Features suggesting Type 1 diabetes

Short history
Marked symptoms
Marked weight loss, regardless of initial weight
First-degree relative with Type 1 diabetes
Personal history of autoimmune disease

of patients consuming large amounts of glucose-containing drinks when thirsty.
2. Was the patient's glycaemic control previously satisfactory (e.g. from their own monitoring or from a recent glycosylated haemoglobin)?
3. Has the patient had an acute illness to precipitate the hyperglycaemia?
4. Has the patient had an adequate trial of appropriate oral agents?

If the patient has Type 1 diabetes then insulin is required. If the patient was previously insulin-requiring, then insulin is probably the treatment of choice. Considering those with Type 2 diabetes, if the patient's diet was previously inadequate, then a trial of diet looking for improvement in glycaemic control or weight (or both) is appropriate. A subject may be given metformin, acarbose or a thiozoledinedione (where licensed) at an early stage since these drugs do not cause hypoglycaemia or weight gain. In the absence of an acute illness, and if the subject's diet was previously acceptable, then oral agents may be required from the start since they have had their trial of diet and the choice would depend on what agents were contra-indicated. If the patient is underweight, an agent to raise insulin levels is required, such as a sulphonyl-urea or insulin.

Finally, if the patient does need to continue high-dose oral steroids (e.g. 20 mg per day or more), then often insulin is required and a basal/bolus regimen is needed (plasma glucose seems to rise over the afternoon despite splitting the dose of prednisolone).

The patient must be reviewed after discharge to ensure that glycaemic control is acceptable. It is vitally important to allocate to both patient and carer where appropriate (and to the primary and secondary care teams) responsibility and targets for the main areas of importance such as glycaemic control, blood pressure control, attention to other risk factors for large vessel disease, care of feet, eyes and kidneys.

HYPOGLYCAEMIC CONDITIONS

Clinical Features, and Risk Factors

Hypoglycaemia can have neuroglycopenic, autonomic or nonspecific features in the elderly, and these individuals often have poor hypoglycaemia awareness. There are multiple risk factors (see also Chapter 10). Careful prescription of sulphonylureas and insulin and ensuring regular diet are mandatory. The key to management is to recognize the problem; all sick elderly subjects must have a plasma glucose estimation.

Hypoglycaemia is defined clinically by Whipple's triad of clinical symptoms of hypoglycaemia, low plasma glucose level, and recovery with glucose administration (Hall et al 1990). Although for many endocrine purposes hypoglycaemia is defined as less than 2 mM, for clinical purposes hypoglycaemia is less than 4 mM.

As the blood glucose level falls, the patient characteristically displays sympathetic effects such as sweating, tachycardia, anxiety, etc. If the plasma glucose continues to fall, neuroglycopenia ensues with decreased consciousness level, confusion and possibly fits. Jaap et al (1998) reviewed 132 subjects with Type 2 diabetes aged 70 or more, of whom 102 had had hypoglycaemia in the preceding 2 months. Patients seemed to have three different clusterings of symptoms, autonomic (e.g. sweating and trembling), general neuroglycopenic (e.g. weakness and confusion) and specific neuroglycopenic with poor coordination and articulation (e.g. unsteadiness, incoordination, light-headedness, and slurred speech). Importantly, all clusterings were just as common, but the third specific neuroglycopenic group of symptoms are obviously liable to diagnostic confusion in the elderly. Indeed, an important problem in the elderly is that hypoglycaemic episodes ('hypos') will be misdiagnosed as stroke, transient ischaemic attack, unexplained confusion, 'gone off legs' (? cause) or a fit due to cerebrovascular disease.

Many studies have demonstrated that the elderly person has difficulty appreciating the sympathetic features of hypoglycaemia and may mount a diminished counter-regulatory hormone response (Ortiz-Alonso et al 1994; Meneilly, Cheung and Tuokko 1994a; Meneilly, Cheung and Tuokko 1994b; Marker, Cryer and Clutter, 1992; Brierley et al 1995). This may lead to a delay in recovery from hypoglycaemia. Using hyperinsulinaemic hypoglycaemic clamps in young and old men, Matyka et al (1997) showed that, in young men, the threshold for appreciating hypoglycaemic symptoms was 1 mM higher than the threshold for delayed reaction times, whereas in old men these two thresholds were similar. Thus by the time an older person suspects that they are becoming hypoglycaemic, they may be unable to correct the situation. They are also unlikely to have been educated about hypoglycaemia (Thomson et al 1991). In younger subjects with Type 1 diabetes, an intensive education program led to less hypoglycaemia, with improved glycaemic control (Schiel, Ulbrich and Muller 1998), but there are no similar trials in the elderly.

Hypos are generally due to specific treatments raising the level of circulating insulin, such as insulin administration or insulin-secretagogues such as sulphonylureas or meglitinides. Other agents which improve insulin sensitivity or retard carbohydrate digestion do not cause hypoglycaemia on their own; if these patients' plasma glucose levels fall excessively, then their pancreatic islet cells merely produce less insulin and the patients do not become hypoglycaemic.

Several studies have looked at subjects who have become hypoglycaemic and have identified various risk factors (see especially Shorr et al 1976; also Asplund Wilholm and Lithner 1983; Stahl and Berger 1999; Jennings, Wilson and Ward 1989; Shorr et al 1996; Harrower 1994; Clarke and Campbell 1975; Tessier et al 1994; Diabetes Control and Complications Trial Research Group 1993. Table 5.4 summarizes the main risks).

Impaired hepatic function appears to be a risk factor for sulphonylurea-induced hypoglycaemia, given that most sulphonylureas are initially metabolized by the liver. The hypoglycaemic episode is likely to have a more serious outcome if the patient has cerebrovascular disease or ischaemic heart disease (Asplund et al 1983).

Shorter-acting sulphonylureas such as tolbutamide and gliclazide are less likely to cause episodes than longer-acting agents such as glibenclamide or chlorpropamide (Asplund et al 1983; Stahl and Berger 1999; Jennings et al 1989; Shorr et al 1996; Harrower 1994; Clarke and Campbell 1975; Tessier D et al 1994). However, the short-acting agent glipizide may not be safe in the elderly (Asplund, Wiholm and Lundman 1991). Although naturally more expensive owing to their recent invention, there is a role for the meglitinides such as repaglinide in subjects who may miss meals (Tronier et al 1995).

Table 5.4 Risk factors for hypoglycaemia

Choice of sulphonylurea/insulin
Tight glycaemic control
Increasing age
Male gender
Recent discharge from hospital
Polypharmacy
New hypoglycaemic treatment
Impaired renal function
Excess alcohol

Insulin therapy has a greater risk of hypoglycaemia than treatment with oral hypoglycaemic agents (UKPDS Group 1998a; Shorr et al 1997b). This risk is increased by the use of long-acting zinc-based insulin preparations (Taylor et al 1999) or short-acting soluble insulin (Taylor et al 1994) compared with isophane insulin. The insulin analogues may be less prone to cause hypoglycaemia than the traditional soluble insulins (Garg et al 1996; Home et al 1998), and there is some evidence that the elderly are more aware of hypoglycaemia due to animal than human insulins (Meneilly, Milberg and Tuokko 1995).

For various reasons, elderly men may be more likely to be unable to organise regular meals than elderly women, which would partly explain their increased risk of hypoglycaemia. It is important to ensure that the patient has a reliable supply of food. Meals may be delivered by home care services during the week, but not at the weekend when the patient's intake declines substantially. During intercurrent illnesses patients may also not get enough carbohydrate, and they must be given 'sick day rules'. A further change of diet can occur on transfer to a care home when hypoglycaemia can ensue due to sudden compliance with a diabetic diet.

There are many possible drug interactions with sulphonylureas (Krentz, Ferner and Bailey 1994), and thus polypharmacy is a risk factor for hypoglycaemia. Hypoglycaemia also occurs when diabetogenic treatment (particularly oral steroids) is reduced without a concomitant decrease in hypoglycaemic medication. There is a possibility of hypoglycaemia with the introduction of ACE inhibitors since they decrease insulin resistance (Herings et al 1995; Morris et al 1997; Shorr et al 1997a).

Improved glycaemic control leads to improved (beta-cell function and insulin sensitivity (Ilkova et al 1997); hence hypoglycaemia can occur after improvement in glycaemic control due to introduction of a new agent, rather than purely due to overdosing the patient with the new agent. Similarly, if the diabetic patient losses weight, they will require less hypoglycaemic treatment.

Elderly subjects who are cognitively impaired sometimes become hypoglycaemic either because they forget to eat or because they repeat their dose of insulin having failed to remember their previous dose has already been given.

Finally, although it is appreciated that an episode of hypoglycaemia is due to either inappropriate medication, excess exercise, or inadequate food supply, often the cause of the hypoglycaemia may not be apparent (Potter et al 1982).

Management of Hypoglycaemia

The key to management is realizing that there is a problem. If a diabetic subject on insulin, sulphonylurea or meglitinide starts to feel unwell, then the plasma glucose must be measured, preferably using a venous specimen. It is surprising that many ill diabetic subjects are admitted without documented evidence of their plasma glucose level. Having discovered that someone is hypoglycaemic, management can be divided into immediate, short-term and long-term approaches.

Immediate management (Page and Hall 1999) consists of 25 g of quick-acting carbohydrate to increase the alertness of the subject. This could be oral glucose (remember long-chain polysaccharides will have a decreased effect in the presence of acarbose) given as 50 mL of 50% dextrose solution intravenously, or approximately 100 mL of sugary fizzy drink such as Lucozade, Coke Cola given orally, or a sugary gel such as Hypostop or real fruit jam being fed to the patient (if they are alert enough) or smeared on their gums.

Glucagon can also be used as IM/subcutaneous injection if the above methods are impracticable. In Type 1 diabetes, glucagon works nearly as well as intravenous dextrose (Collier et al 1987). However, glucagon is contraindicated if there is still beta-cell function since glucagon stimulates further insulin release with possibly disastrous consequences (Marri, Cozzolino and Palumbo 1968). Thus glucagon should be used with caution in Type 2 diabetic subjects. Glucagon is also ineffective if liver glycogen stores are decreased, such as during prolonged hypoglycaemia or recent use of glucagon. After recovery, the patient then takes approximately 25 g complex carbohydrate (e.g. two slices of bread) to prevent them becoming hypoglycaemic again.

Medium-term management involves avoiding a repetition of the hypoglycaemic episode. If the patient was on short-acting insulins or sulphonylureas, then they can probably be allowed home in the care of a family member. If a patient on intermediate-acting insulins or sulphonylureas has had a severe hypoglycaemic event needing medical assistance, they require admission. A 5% dextrose infusion running at one litre over 24 hours would be a wise precaution, with close observation of the patient for clinical and biochemical evidence of hypoglycaemia (4-hourly capillary blood glucose monitoring) for 24 hours. The blood glucose will be higher after a hypoglycaemic episode and one must expect this rather than increase hypoglycaemic medication.

The long-term management entails working out why the patient became hypoglycaemic and preventing its recurrence.

Three a.m. hypoglycaemia is not uncommon, and the Somogyi effect whereby the body naturally over-compensates can cause early morning hyperglycaemia—which can trick the patient and professionals concerned into increasing the hypoglycaemic medication. It is not known how common this is.

Intentional poisoning of patients with hypoglycaemic medication is not unknown and this should be borne in mind, particularly where someone other than the patient is dispensing the medication. There are also several other causes of hypoglycaemia, particularly alcohol excess in free-dwelling elderly people, and terminal decline in the hospital inpatient (Gale 1985; Shilo et al 1998).

An important message for both health professionals and patients (and carers) with hypoglycaemia is to avoid it in the first place by careful prescription and review of hypoglycaemic medication, and by ensuring a regular adequate diet.

LACTIC ACIDOSIS

Lactic acidosis can be due to either biguanide therapy and other primarily metabolic disorders (Type B), or shock and tissue hypoxia (Type A) due to severe organ failure (Krentz and Nattrass 1997). This chapter concentrates on that due to biguanide therapy.

Lactic acidosis is much less common with metformin which enhances the mitochondrial oxidation of lactate (Stumvoll et al 1995), compared with older biguanides with which patients would unexpectedly tip into fatal lactic acidosis despite the absence of contraindications (Gale and Tattersall 1976; Luft, Schmulling, and Eggstein 1978).

In a review of 274 cases, it was clear that the majority of patients (approximately 67%) with biguanide-associated lactic acidosis were aged 60 or more (Luft, Schmulling and Eggstein 1978). Presenting symptoms were decreased consciousness level, abdominal discomfort and/or nausea/vomiting. Signs include

Kussmaul's respiration, hypotension and circulatory collapse. (Luft et al 1978; Krentz and Nattrass 1997).

Diagnosis is confirmed by demonstrating acidosis (arterial pH <7.2), and raised lactate level (either plasma lactate >5 mM; or anion gap greater than 18 mM) (Krentz and Nattrass 1997). Lactate levels are measured on a fluoride oxalate specimen (sugar tube) and must be rushed to the laboratory. The anion gap $(Na^+ + K^+ - Cl^- - HCO_3^-)$ may also be raised by ketones, salicylates, urea, methanol and ethylene glycol.

Survival is associated with higher pH, higher bicarbonate concentration, higher blood pressure, lower urea and lower lactate levels. Survival correlates more with plasma lactate levels than degree of acidosis (Stacpoole 1986). Survival in the elderly is at most 45% but is generally much lower (Luft et al 1978).

Treatment is unsatisfactory, and consists of fluid replacement and correction of the acidosis with intravenous bicarbonate. It is also possible to use haemodialysis to correct the acidosis and remove the offending biguanide (Krentz and Nattrass 1997). However, the mortality is still high (60–70% unless shocked, when mortality approaches 100%) (Stacpoole 1986). Dichloroacetate, which increases lactate metabolism, causes a significant biochemical improvement, but survival is still low with a 92% mortality in lactic acidosis from various causes (Stacpoole et al 1983, 1992).

Metformin-associated lactic acidosis is preventable by observing the contraindications in Table 5.5 (Monson 1993; Joint Formulary Committee 1993). By adhering to these contraindications, there have been no cases of lactic acidosis in Canada, and glibenclamide has been found to have a greater fatality rate (Campbell 1984). It cannot be emphasized too strongly that metformin-associated lactic acidosis is predictable and occurs in those with contraindications (Howlett and Bailey 1999; Brown et al 1998).

Intravenous radiological contrast media sometimes cause a transient deterioration in renal function, so it is

Table 5.5   Contraindications to metformin

Renal impairment (creatinine >120μM
Hepatic impairment, including alcohol abuse, as indicated by abnormal liver function tests
Cardiac failure, even if treated
Critical limb ischaemia
Any acute illness (e.g. warranting hospital admission)
Use of intravenous radiological contrast media

advisable to omit the metformin for 48 hours prior to the test, recheck the renal function 24 hours after the test and, if satisfactory, restart the metformin. Over the intervening period, acarbose or p.r.n. insulin may be considered. Some suggest that this is unnecessarily cautious since most subjects with metformin-associated lactic acidosis had pre-existing renal impairment (McCartney et al 1999); however, it has occurred with normal renal function with a high mortality.

There has been some debate as to whether metformin in the presence of heart failure leads to lactic acidosis or whether it is the heart failure per se which leads to lactic acidosis (Hart and Walker 1996). If a patient has evidence of biventricular failure on chest X-ray or echocardiography, the wise course of action is to avoid the use of metformin.

DIABETES AND INTERCURRENT ILLNESSES

An elderly patient with diabetes is at great risk from several other acute conditions.

Myocardial Infarction or Stroke

The DIGAMI study (Malmberg K et al 1995, 1997) showed that after myocardial infarction an insulin/glucose infusion with subsequent basal/bolus regimen improved survival in the diabetic person with Type 2 diabetes. This study is slightly complicated by several factors (Fisher 1998). Many of the control group went on to insulin, many of the intervention group came off insulin, some of the subjects may have had stress hyperglycaemia rather than diabetes. Nonetheless, many would now recommend an insulin–glucose infusion for acute myocardial infarction in diabetic subjects with appropriate blood glucose control afterwards, not necessarily with insulin. The DIGAMI protocol is given in Table 5.6, but many units use their own, less complicated glucose–insulin–potassium infusion schemes.

There is also a strong suggestion that an insulin–glucose infusion should be used after a cerebrovascular accident (Scott et al 1998, 1999). Although this is still very much at the research stage, it appears safe and may well become clinical practice.

Table 5.6 The DIGAMI regimen

Glucose–insulin infusion of 80 units soluble insulin in 500 mL of 5% dextrose–initially infused at 30 mL/h with hourly fingerprick plasma glucose and dose titration aiming for glucose level 7–10.9 mM

Plasma glucose (mM)	Adjustment to infusion rate
>15.0	Give 8 units soluble insulin IV bolus; increase rate by 6 mL/h
11.0–14.9	Increase rate 3 mL/h
7.0–10.9	Same rate
4.0–6.9	Decrease rate by 6 mL/h
<4.0	Stop, treat symptomatic hypoglycaemia; restart at 6 mL/h less when plasma glucose >7.0 mM

Source: modified from Malmberg et al (1995) by permission of the American College of Cardiology.

Difficult Oral Intake

If a subject is unable to eat, then an insulin–glucose infusion is the best way to maintain good control (having tackled any hyperglycaemic coma as above); 10% dextrose (with 10 mmol KCl per 500 mL) is infused at 100 mL/h along with an insulin infusion. The insulin infusion rate is either derived from the individual's insulin requirements, or a trial of 3 units per hour is given (Husband, Thai and Alberti 1986). The morbidly obese patient will need a higher insulin rate (e.g. 4 units per hour), and the frail thin person will need less (e.g. 2 units per hour). Monitor the fingerprick plasma glucose hourly initially, aiming for 5–10 mM, and adjust the insulin infusion appropriately (Table 5.7). Once the patient stabilizes, the frequency of testing may be partly relaxed. The initial descriptions mixed the insulin in the bag of dextrose, but it is more convenient and gives more frequent acceptable blood glucose levels to use a bag of dextrose and a separate insulin pump. Simmons et al (1994) give different regimens for different classes of patient based on a bedside estimate of their insulin requirements; this

Table 5.7 Adjusting the insulin–glucose infusion

Fingerprick glucose level	Action
Above target range	Increase insulin infusion by 25%
Within target range	Leave insulin infusion at same rate
Below target range	Decrease insulin infusion by 25%
Below 3.0 mM	Stop insulin infusion, run in 200 mL 10% dextrose over 5 min; restart insulin infusion at 50% previous rate

is eminently sensible. These infusions are known by many names depending on location.

If the patient has to be nil-by-mouth for an operation or procedure there are several scenarios (Gill and Alberti 1989). If the patient has a serious problem needing major surgery, then he or she needs resuscitation and an insulin–glucose infusion. If the patient is well controlled (FPG <10 mM) on diet, metformin, acarbose or short-acting sulphonylurea, and the procedure is short, the patient can undergo the procedure, omitting breakfast and the morning antidiabetic medication (i.e. needs to be first on the operating list), and can then have normal breakfast and usual treatment later in the morning. This does mean that these patients have to be on the main hospital site, or have good transport and support if this is being done from home. If the patient is not insulin-requiring, but is going for a prolonged operation, then it would be wise to institute an insulin–glucose infusion and set it up preoperatively. Often these matters are ignored, and the anaesthetist is left to sort it out shortly before the operation—which they do extremely well, but it is not best clinical practice.

In insulin-treated patients, an insulin–glucose infusion may be used, except in Type 2 diabetic subjects on short- or intermediate-acting insulins who can tolerate a short delay in insulin and breakfast if monitored.

Poor Glycaemic Control

If a subject has unstable blood glucose levels after any illness but is generally eating well, then a basal/bolus regimen is extremely flexible; e.g. 6 units Lyspro or Novorapid at the start of each meal, and 6 units of Insulatard at bedtime in insulin-naïve patients, or one-third of the of usual daily insulin requirement at bedtime and the remainder distributed evenly during the three main meals.

The advantage of either Lyspro or Novorapid is that they may be given at the start of the meal, rather than having to estimate a period of 20 minutes before the meal to give a standard soluble insulin. Lyspro or Novorapid can also be given at the end of the meal (Schernthaner et al 1998) when it is certain that the meal has been consumed and there is no history of gastrointestinal upset. If a meal is omitted then the Lyspro or Novorapid is omitted. The only minor problem is that the background insulin from the Insulatard does not provide a full 24-hour background insulin level, but can decline after lunch; this does not nor-

mally cause difficulties. An ultralente insulin is possibly better as a background insulin than isophane insulin given before bedtime (Zinman et al 1997), but is not as flexible and is not available as a pen device. Isophane as a BD regime to provide basal levels can be alternatively used. One of the advantages of modern pens and fine needles is easy relatively painfree injections.

It is common to hear of patients who are unwell with unstable plasma glucose levels, but who are not in coma, being subjected to either an intravenous or 4-hourly subcutaneous insulin sliding scale. The sliding scale is not to be used in this situation for several reasons. Firstly, the sliding scale corrects the plasma glucose after it has become abnormal when the objective should be to anticipate insulin requirements in advance to stabilize plasma glucose levels. Second, unless the insulin prescription for the target blood glucose matches these requirements (which is unlikely), then the regimen will always be set to avoid the target blood glucose. Third, Queale, Seidler and Brancati (1997) showed that the results of sliding-scale use were not acceptable, and others feel that their use is very limited (Gill and MacFarlane 1997).

THE EFFECT OF INTERCURRENT ILLNESS ON THE DIABETES

Intercurrent illness may affect patients with diabetes in several ways. First, associated liver or renal disease may contraindicate the use of oral agents, when insulin in a basal/bolus regimen may be used. Second, the treatment itself, (e.g. steroids) may cause hyperglycaemia, and again insulin treatment may be needed. Third, the illness may make dietary intake unreliable, and in this situation a basal/bolus regimen (omitting the bolus if the meal is omitted) is very useful. At the end of the illness, it is necessary to reassess glycaemic control and review treatment possibilities.

Oral glucocorticosteroids are a major problem, since the plasma glucose rises particularly in the afternoon. Their co-prescription is best avoided if possible; for example, use other disease-modifying agents in rheumatological diseases or use inhaled steroids for airflow limitation. With low doses, there may not be much alteration to glycaemic control, but it is frequently a problem. The plasma glucose levels rise over the afternoon (Dunning 1996), and hence hypoglycaemic medication may well be needed before lunch. A twice-daily insulin regimen does not seem to give acceptable

Table 5.8 Sick day rules for insulin-treated patients

1. Never stop your insulin
2. Drink plenty of fluids
3. Test your blood more frequently, at least before each insulin dose
4. Alter your insulin dose as follows:
   Blood test <11 mM take normal insulin
   Blood test 11.1–16.9 mM take normal insulin plus 4 units
      (of clear if choice exists)
   Blood test >17 mM take normal insulin plus 6 units (of clear if
      choice exists)
5. If blood tests persistently >17.0, or if cannot keep food down,
   or if drowsy, call your doctor
6. Do not omit food; if unable to eat meal, replace with small
   sugary drinks, such as milk, Lucozade etc., approximately
   one mugful (large cup) sipped over 4 hours

control even if the steroid dose is divided into a four times daily dose schedule. As a consequence, many of the cases managed by the author take a basal/bolus regimen in this circumstance. Deflazacort is a steroid which appears not to cause such marked hyperglycaemia (Bruno et al 1987); 6 mg is equivalent in potency to 5 mg of prednisolone, but its use so far has been limited and more clinical experience with the drug is required.

The patient and/or carers should be familiar with the 'sick day rules' (this is an unfortunate name since the rules apply to any illness, not just nausea and vomiting). If the subject is not performing home blood glucose monitoring, then he or she cannot adjust medication, but must be instructed to get professional help if drowsy, confused, have nausea or vomiting or complaining of osmotic symptoms. There are various rules published (Table 5.8), but they all aim to continue medication, continue carbohydrate intake, maintain fluid intake and increase a patient's individual insulin dosage by 10–20% of the total daily dose if hyperglycaemia occurs.

CONCLUSION

Major metabolic disturbances occur frequently enough in older subjects with diabetes to warrant greater care and attention to their management. Measurement of plasma glucose level in all older subjects admitted into hospital with acute illness is paramount. Management of both metabolic excursions and diabetes during intercurrent illness requires the input of a physician with diabetic expertise.

REFERENCES

Adrogué HJ, Barrero J, Eknoyan G (1989) Salutary effects of modest fluid replacement in the treatment of adults with diabetic ketoacidosis *JAMA* **262**, 2108–2113.

Alberti KGGM (1989) Diabetic emergencies. *British Medical Bulletin*, **45**, 242–263.

Asplund K, Wilholm B–E, Lithner F (1983) Glibenclamide-associated hypoglycaemia; a report on 57 cases *Diabetologia*, **24**, 412–417.

Asplund K, Wiholm BE, Lundman B (1991) Severe hypoglycaemia during treatment with glipizide. *Diabetic Medicine*, **8**, 726–731.

Atkin SH, Dasmahapatra A, Jaker MA, Chorost MI, Reddy S (1991) Fingerstick glucose determination in shock. *Annals of Internal Medicine*, **114**, 1020–1024.

Barnett DM, Wilcox DS, Marble A (1962) Diabetic coma in persons over 60. *Geriatrics*, **17**, 327–336.

Basu A, Close CF, Jenkins D, Krentz AJ, Nattrass M, Wright AD (1993) Persisting mortality in diabetic ketoacidosis. *Diabetic Medicine*, **10**, 282–284.

Berger W, Keller U (1992) Treatment of diabetic ketoacidosis and non-ketotic hyper-osmolar diabetic coma. *Bailliére's Clinical Endocrinology and Metabolism*, **6** (1), 1–22.

Brierley EJ, Broughton DL, James OF, Alberti KG (1995) Reduced awareness of hypoglycaemia in the elderly despite an intact counter-regulatory response. *Quarterly Journal of Medicine*, **88**, 439–445.

Brown JB, Pedula K, Barzilay J, Herson MK, Latare P (1998) Lactic acidosis rates in Type 2 diabetes. *Diabetes Care*, **21**, 1659–1663

Bruno A, Cavallo-Perrin P, Cassader M, Pagano G (1987) Deflazacort vs prednisolone: effect on blood glucose in insulin treated diabetics. *Archives of Internal Medicine*, **147**, 679–680.

Campbell IW (1984) Metformin and glibenclamide: comparative risks. *British Medical Journal*, **289**, 289.

Clarke BF, Campbell IW (1975) Long term comparative trial of glibenclamide and chlorpropamide in diet failed maturity onset diabetics *Lancet*, **i**, 246–247.

Collier A, Steedman DJ, Patrick AW, Nimmo GR, Matthews DM, MacIntyre CCA, Little K, Clarke BF (1987) Comparison of intravenous glucagon and dextrose in treatment of severe hypoglycaemia in an accident and emergency department. *Diabetes Care*, **10**, 712–715.

Croxson SCM, Burden AC (1998) Polyuria and polydipsia in an elderly population: its relationship to previously undiagnosed diabetes. *Practical Diabetes International*, **15**, 170–172.

Croxson SCM, Sinclair AJ (1995) Acute diabetic and endocrine problems. In: Sinclair A, Woodhouse K (eds) *Acute Medical Illness in Elderly People*. London Chapman & Hall, 127–150

Diabetes Control and Complications Trial Research Group (1993) The effect of intensive treatment of diabetes on the development and progression of long-term complications in insulin-dependent diabetes mellitus. *New England Journal Medicine*, **329**, 977–986.

Dunning T (1996) Corticosteroid medications and diabetes mellitus. *Practical Diabetes International*, **13**, 186–188.

Fisher M (1998) Diabetes and myocardial infarction: critical evaluation of the DIGAMI study. *Practical Diabetes International*, **15**, 101–102.

Fonseca V, Phear DN (1982) Hyper-osmolar non-ketotic diabetic syndrome precipitated by treatment with diuretics. *British Medical Journal*, **284**, 36–37.

Gale E (1985) Causes of hypoglycaemia. *British Journal of Hospital Medicine*, **33**, 159–162.

Gale E, Tattersall RB (1976) Can phenformin-induced lactic acidosis be prevented? *British Medical Journal*, **2**, 972–975.

Gale E, Tattersall R (1990a) The new patient: assessment and management. In: Tattersall RB, Gale EAM (eds) Edinburgh; Churchill Livingstone, 3–16.

Gale E, Tattersall R (1990b). Hypoglycaemia. In: Tattersall RB, Gale EAM (eds). *Diabetes: Clinical Management*. Edinburgh; Churchill Livingstone, 228–239

Gale EM, Dornan TL, Tattersall RB (1981) Severely uncontrolled diabetes in the over-fifties. *Diabetologia*, **21**, 25–28.

Garg SK, Carmain JA, Braddy KC, Anderson JH, Vignati L, Jennings MK, Chase HP (1996) Pre-meal insulin analogue insulin Lispro vs Humulin R insulin treatment in young subjects with Type 1 diabetes. *Diabetic Medicine*, **13** 47–52.

Gerich JE, Martin MM, Recant L (1971) Clinical and metabolic characteristics of hyper-osmolar nonketotic coma. *Diabetes*, **20**, 228–238.

Gill GV, Alberti KGGM (1989) Surgery and diabetes. *Hospital Update*, **15**, 327–336.

Gill G, MacFarlane I (1997) Are sliding-scale insulin regimens a recipe for diabetic instability? *Lancet*, **349**, 1555 (letter).

Hale PJ, Crase J, Nattrass M (1984) Metabolic effects of bicarbonate in the treatment of diabetic ketoacidosis. *British Medical Journal*, **289**, 1035–1038.

Hall R, Anderson J, Smart GA, Besser M (1980) *Fundamentals of Clinical Endocrinology*, 3rd edn. London: Pitman, 583–599.

Hamblin PS, Topliss DJ, Chosich N, Lording DW, Stockigt JR (1989) Deaths associated with diabetic ketoacidosis and hyperosmolar coma. *Medical Journal of Australia*, **151**, 439–444.

Hammond P, Wallis S (1992) Cerebral oedema in diabetic ketoacidosis *British Medical Journal*, **305**, 203–204.

Harrower ADB. (1994) Comparison of efficacy, secondary failure rate, and complications of sulphonylureas. *Journal of Diabetes and its Complications*, **8**, 201–203.

Hart SP, Frier BM (1998) Causes, management and morbidity of acute hypoglycaemia in adults requiring hospital admission. *Quarterly Journal of Medicine*, **91**, 505–510.

Hart SP, Walker JD (1996) Is metformin contraindicated in diabetic patients with chronic stable heart failure? *Practical Diabetes*, **13**, 18–20.

Herings RM, de Boer A, Stricker BH, Leufkens HG, Porsius A (1995) Hypoglycaemia associated with use of inhibitors of angiotensin converting enzyme. *Lancet*, **345**, 1195–1198.

Home PD, Lindholm A, Hylleberg B, Round P (UK Insulin Aspart Study Group) (1998) Improved glycemic control with insulin aspart: a multicenter randomized double-blind crossover trial in Type 1 diabetic patients. *Diabetes Care*, **21**, 1904–1909.

Howlett HCS, Bailey CJ (1999) A risk–benefit assessment of metformin in Type 2 diabetes mellitus. *Drug Safety*, **20**, 489–503.

Husband DJ, Thai AC, Alberti KGMM (1986) Management of diabetes during surgery with glucose–insulin–potassium infusion. *Diabetic Medicine*, **3**, 69–74.

Ilkova H, Glaser B, Tunckale A, Bagriacik N, Cerasi E (1997) Induction of long term glycaemic control in newly diagnosed Type 2 diabetic patients by transient intensive insulin treatment. *Diabetes Care*, **20**, 1353–1356.

Jaap AJ, Jones GC, McCrimmon RJ, Deary IJ, Frier BM (1998) Perceived symptoms of hypoglycaemia in elderly Type 2 diabetic patients treated with insulin. *Diabetic Medicine*, **15**, 398–401.

Jennings AM, Wilson RM, Ward JD (1989) Symptomatic hypoglycaemia in NIDDM patients treated with oral hypoglycaemic agents. *Diabetes Care*, **12**, 203–208.

Joint Formulary Committee (George CF, chairman) (1993) British National Formulary, no 26. London: British Medical Association and Royal Pharmaceutical Society of Great Britain, 249–284.

Khardori R, Soler NG (1984) Hyper-osmolar hyperglycaemic nonketotic syndrome. *American Journal of Medicine* **77**, 899–904.

Kitabchi AE, Murphy MB, (1988) Diabetic ketoacidosis and hyperosmolar hyperglycaemic nonketotic coma. *Medical Clinics of North America*, **72**, 1545–1563.

Krentz AJ, Ferner RE, Bailey CJ (1994) Comparative tolerability profiles of oral antidiabetic agents. *Drug Safety*, **11**, 223–241.

Krentz AJ, Nattrass M (1997) Acute metabolic complications of diabetes mellitus: diabetic ketoacidosis, hyper-osmolar nonketotic syndrome and lactic acidosis. In: Pickup JC, Williams G (eds) *Textbook of Diabetes*, 2nd edn. Oxford; Blackwell Science, 39.1–39.23.

Leutscher PDC, Svendsen KN (1991) Svær ketoacidose hos en ikke-insulinkrævende diabetes mellitus patient. *Ugeskr Læger* **153**, 2634–2635.

Lever E, Jaspan JB (1983) Sodium bicarbonate therapy in severe diabetic ketoacidosis. *American Journal of Medicine*, **75**, 263–268.

Lorber S (1995) Nonketotic hypertonicity in diabetes mellitus. *Medical Clinics of North America*, **79**, 39–52.

Luft D, Schmulling RM, Eggstein M (1978) Lactic acidosis in biguanide-treated diabetics. *Diabetologia*, **14**, 75–87.

Malmberg K and the DIGAMI (Diabetes Mellitus, Insulin Glucose Infusion in Acute Myocardial Infarction) Study Group (1997) Prospective randomised study of intensive insulin treatment on long term survival after acute myocardial infarction in patients with diabetes mellitus. *British Medical Journal*, **314**, 1512–1515.

Malmberg K, Ryden L, Efendic S, Herlitz J, Nicol P, Waldenstrom A, Wedel H, Welin L (1995) Randomized trial of insulin–glucose infusion followed by subcutaneous insulin treatment in diabetic patients with acute myocardial infarction (DIGAMI study):effects on mortality at 1 year. *Journal of American College of Cardiology*, **26**, 57–65.

Malone ML, Gennis V, Goodwin JS (1992) Characteristics of diabetic ketoacidosis in older versus younger adults. *Journal of the American Geniatics Society* **40**, 1100–1104.

Marker JC, Cryer PE, Clutter WE (1992) Attenuated glucose recovery from hypoglycemia in the elderly. *Diabetes*, **41**, 671–678.

Marri G, Cozzolino G, Palumbo R (1968) Glucagon in sulphonylurea hypoglycaemia? *Lancet*, **1**, 303–304.

Matyka K, Evans M, Lomas J, Cranston I, Macdonald I, Amiel SA (1997) Altered hierarchy of protective responses against severe hypoglycemia in normal aging in healthy men. *Diabetes Care*, **20**, 135–141.

McCartney MM, Gilbert FJ, Murchison LE, Pearson D, McHardy K, Murray AD (1999) Metformin and contrast media: a dangerous combination? *Clinical Radiology*, **54**, 29–33.

Meneilly GS, Cheung E, Tuokko H (1994a) Altered responses to hypoglycemia of healthy elderly people. *Journal of Clinical Endocrinology & Metabolism*, **78**, 1341–1348.

Meneilly GS, Cheung E, Tuokko H (1994b) Counter-regulatory hormone responses to hypoglycemia in the elderly patient with diabetes. *Diabetes*, **43**, 403–410.

Meneilly GS, Milberg WP, Tuokko H (1995) Differential effects of human and animal insulin on the responses to hypoglycemia in elderly patients with NIDDM. *Diabetes*, **44**, 272–277.

Mølbak AG, Christau B, Marner B, Borch-Johnson K, Nerup J (1994). Incidence of insulin-dependent diabetes mellitus in age groups over 30 years in Denmark. *Diabetic Medicine*, **11**, 650–655.

Monson JP (1993) Selected side effects: II. Metformin and lactic acidosis. *Prescribers' Journal*, **33**, 170–173.

Morris AD, Boyle DI, McMahon AD, Pearce H, Evans JM, Newton RW, Jung RT, MacDonald TM (1997) ACE inhibitor use is associated with hospitalization for severe hypoglycemia in patients with diabetes. DARTS/MEMO Collaboration. Diabetes Audit and Research in Tayside, Scotland. Medicines Monitoring Unit. *Diabetes Care*, **20**, 1363–1367.

Morris LR, Murphy MB, Kitabchi AE (1986) Bicarbonate therapy in severe diabetic ketoacidosis. *Annals Internal Medicine*, **105**, 836–840.

Ortiz-Alonso FJ, Galecki A, Herman WH, Smith MJ, Jacquez JA, Halter JB (1994) Hypoglycemia counter-regulation in elderly humans: relationship to glucose levels. *American Journal of Physiology*, **267**(4 Pt 1), E497–506.

Page SR, Hall M (1999) *Diabetes: Emergency and Hospital Management*. London: BMJ Books.

Popli S, Leehey DJ, Daugirdas JT, Bansal VK, Ho DS, Hano JE, Ing TS (1990) Asymptomatic, nonketotic, severe hypoglycaemia with hyponatremia. *Archives of Internal Medicine*, **150**, 1962–1964.

Potter J, Clarke P, Gale EAM, Dave SH, Tattersall RB (1982) Insulin induced hypoglycaemia in an accident and emergency department: the tip of an iceberg. *British Medical Journal*, **285**, 1180–1182.

Queale WS, Seidler AJ, Brancati FL (1997) Glycemic control and sliding scale insulin use in medical inpatients with diabetes mellitus. *Archives of Internal Medicine*, **157**, 545–552.

Ryder REJ, Hayes TM (1983) Normo-osmolar, nonketotic, hyponatremic diabetic syndrome associated with impaired renal function. *Diabetes Care*, **6**, 402–404.

Schernthaner G, Equiluz-Bruck S, Wein W, Bates PC, Sandholzer K, Birkett MA (1998) Postprandial insulin Lispro. *Diabetes Care*, **21**, 570–573.

Schiel R, Ulbrich S, Muller UA (1998) Quality of diabetes care, diabetes knowledge and risk of severe hypoglycaemia one and four years after participation in a 5-day structured treatment and teaching programme for intensified insulin therapy. *Diabetes & Metabolism*, **24**, 509–514.

Scott JF, Gray CS, O'Connell JE, Alberti KGGM (1998) Glucose and insulin therapy in acute stroke: why delay further? *Quarterly Journal of Medicine*, **91**, 511–515.

Scott JF, Robinson GM, French JM, O'Connell JE, Alberti KG, Gray CS (1999) Glucose potassium insulin infusions in the treatment of acute stroke patients with mild to moderate hypoglycaemia: the Glucose Insulin in Stroke Trial (GIST). *Stroke*, **30**, 793–799.

Shilo S, Berezovsky S, Friedlander Y, Sonnenblick M (1998) Hypoglycemia in hospitalized nondiabetic older patients. *Journal of the American Geriatrics Society*, **46**, 978–982.

Shorr RI, Ray WA, Daugherty JR, Griffin MR (1996) Individual sulfonylureas and serious hypoglycemia in older people. *Journal of the American Geriatrics Society*, **44**, 751–755.

Shorr RI, Ray WA, Daugherty JR, Griffin MR (1997a) Antihypertensives and the risk of serious hypoglycemia in older persons using insulin or sulfonylureas. *JAMA*, **278**, 40–43.

Shorr RI, Ray WA, Daugherty JR, Griffin MR (1997b) Incidence and risk factors for serious hypoglycemia in older persons using insulin or sulfonylureas. *Archives Internal Medicine*, **157**, 1681–1686.

Simmons D, Morton K, Laughton SJ, Scott DJ (1994) A comparison of two intravenous insulin regimens among surgical patients with insulin-dependent diabetes mellitus. *Diabetes Educator*, **20**, 422–427.

Small M, Alzaid A, MacCuish AC. (1988) Diabetic hyper-osmolar non–ketotic decompensation. *Quarterly Journal of Medicine*, (NS) **66**, 251–257.

Stacpoole PW (1986) Lactic acidosis: the case against bicarbonate therapy. *Annals of Internal Medicine*, **105**, 276–279.

Stacpoole PW, Harman EM, Curry SH, Baumgartner TG, Misbin RI (1983) Treatment of lactic acidosis with dichloroacetate. *New England Journal of Medicine*, **309**, 390–396.

Stacpoole PW, Wright EC, Baumgartner TG, Bersin RM, Buchalter S, Curry SH, Duncan CA, Harman EM, Henderson GN, Jenkinson S et al (The Dichloroacetate-Lactic Acidosis Study Group) (1992) A controlled clinical trial of dichloroacetate for treatment of lactic acidosis in adults. *New England Journal of Medicine*, **327**, 1564–1569.

Stahl M, Berger W (1999) Higher incidence of severe hypoglycaemia leading to hospital admission in Type 2 diabetic patients treated with long-acting versus short-acting sulphonylureas. *Diabetic Medicine*, **16**, 586–590.

Stumvoll M, Nurjhan N, Perriello G, Dailey G, Gerich JE (1995) Metabolic effects of metformin in non-insulin-dependent diabetes mellitus. *New England Journal of Medicine*, **333**, 550–554.

Sturrock ND, Page SR, Clarke P, Tattersall RB (1995) Insulin dependent diabetes in nonagenarians. *British Medical Journal*, **310**, 1117–118.

Taylor R, Foster B, Kyne-Grzebalski D, Vanderpump M (1994) Insulin regimes for the non-insulin dependent: impact on diurnal metabolic state and quality of life. *Diabetic Medicine*, **11**, 551–557.

Taylor R, Davies R, Fox C, Sampson M, Weaver J, Wood L (1999) Optimal insulin treatment for Type 2 diabetes: a multicentre randomised crossover trial. *Diabetic Medicine*, **16** (Suppl. 1), 9 (abstract A26).

Tessier D, Dawson K, Tetrault JP, Bravo G, Meneilly GS, (1994) Glibenclamide vs gliclazide in Type 2 diabetes of the elderly. *Diabetic Medicine*, **11**, 974–980.

Thomson FJ, Masson EA, Leeming JT, Boulton AJ (1991) Lack of knowledge of symptoms of hypoglycaemia by elderly diabetic patients. *Age and Aging*, **20**, 404–406.

Tronier B, Marbury TC, Damsbo B, Windfield K (1995) A new oral hypoglycaemic agent, repaglinide, minimises risk of hypoglycaemia in well controlled NIDDM patients. *Diabetologia*, **38**, A752.

UK Prospective Diabetes Study (UKPDS) Group (1998) Effect of intensive blood–glucose control with metformin on complications in overweight patients with Type 2 diabetes. *Lancet*, **352**, 854–865.

Wachtel TJ, (1990) The diabetic hyper-osmolar state. *Clinics Geriatric Medicine*, **6**, 797–806.

Wachtel TJ, Tetu-Mouradjian LM, Goldman DL, Ellis SE, O'Sullivan PS (1991) Hyper-osmolarity and acidosis in diabetes mellitus: a three-year experience in Rhode Island. *Journal of General Internal Medicine*, **6**, 495–502.

Zinman B, Ross S, Campos R, Strack T (1997) A double blind randomized controlled trial comparing NPH and ultralente as basal insulin replacement with Lispro insulin. *Diabetes*, **46** (Suppl. 1), 43 (abstract).

6

The Diabetic Foot

Matthew J. Young, Andrew J. M. Boulton
Royal Infirmary of Edinburgh and Manchester Royal Infirmary

INTRODUCTION

The St Vincent timescale (WHO/IDF 1990) to reduce the number of amputations for diabetes in Europe by 50% within three years seems a dim and distant memory to those who work with the diabetic foot. The publication of BDA/RCP guidelines in England and Wales and SIGN guidelines in Scotland have demonstrated that there is still a lack of good evidence-based randomized controlled trials on which to base diabetic footcare (specialist UK Workgroup Reports 1996; SIGN 1997). However, the fact remains that structured diabetic footcare, performed in a multidisciplinary team, has repeatedly delivered the reductions in amputation rates that were required by the St Vincent declaration. At present this is the ideal standard to which those who wish to improve the outcome for patients with diabetic foot problems should work.

Foot problems in diabetes can develop from a number of component causes. The main contributing factors include sensorimotor and autonomic neuropathy, peripheral vascular disease, limited joint mobility and high foot pressures. The existence of other long-term complications of diabetes also influences the development of foot ulceration. General practitioners, geriatricians and diabetologists need to pay particular attention to the feet of older patients to prevent significant avoidable morbidity and mortality in this vulnerable group.

Lower limb amputation is more common in older, usually Type 2, diabetic patients (Thomson et al 1991). The average age of diabetic foot clinic attenders is over 60 years, clearly demonstrating that the elderly are at particular risk of foot ulceration. Reduced mobility, particularly at the hip, in patients over 60 impairs their ability to inspect the feet and leads to the continued progression of foot lesions, often beyond a point of repair, before they are discovered (Thomson and Masson 1992). In addition, patients with severely impaired vision depend on other people for foot inspection, and when they are not easily available this may make footcare very difficult to perform adequately.

Diabetes alone probably does not add to the prevalence of bunions, clawed toes and medial arterial calcification that is seen in the elderly (Cavanagh et al 1994; Young et al 1993a). Neuropathy, however, is more prevalent in the elderly, increasing with both age and duration of diabetes. Once this is superimposed on the normal aging process, skeletal abnormalities including spontaneous fractures are significantly more common (Young et al 1993). Add the increased prevalence of peripheral vascular disease in the older Type 2 diabetic patient to the increase in neuropathy, together with difficulties in personal footcare, and it fully explains the particular predilection for foot problems that exists in older diabetic patients. The demographic changes, increasing numbers of elderly people, an increase in those who live alone and increasing levels of obesity, which are occurring within the United Kingdom, will only serve to add to the already substantial numbers of Type 2 diabetic patients who develop foot ulceration and peripheral ischaemia. Therefore, it is our challenge to reduce this excess burden of risk to a minimum by accurate detection and amelerioation of risk.

PERIPHERAL SENSORIMOTOR NEUROPATHY

Peripheral sensorimotor neuropathy is a major contributory cause in 90% of diabetic foot ulceration (Thomson et al 1991). The incidence of diabetic peripheral sensorimotor neuropathy increases with the duration of diabetes. However, as the prevalence depends on the diagnostic criteria that are used, the prevalence rates reported from different epidemiological studies vary considerably (Melton and Dyck 1987). In a prospective study of a large cohort of diabetic patients followed over 25 years, 50% exhibited objective signs of neuropathy (Pirart 1978), whilst a multicentre study which screened a large hospital-treated diabetic population found that the overall prevalence of neuropathy was 28.5% (Young et al 1993b). More than half of all the patients with Type 2 diabetes, aged over 60, were found to have neuropathy. Therefore the majority of the elderly population who have diabetes are at an increased risk of foot ulceration.

The most common symptoms of sensory neuropathy are numbness, lancinating pain, 'pins and needles', burning pain and hyperaesthesiae typically with nocturnal exacerbation. The clinical signs are usually sensory loss in a glove-and-stocking distribution (See Figure 6.1). Whilst loss of pain, fine touch and temperature sensation are related to small (often unmyelinated) fibre involvement, loss of vibration

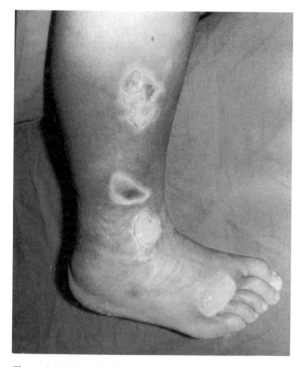

Figure 6.1   Extensive burns on the leg of a neuropathic diabetic patient who had fallen asleep in front of the gas fire to be woken by the smell of burning

perception and proprioception is believed to be related to large (usually myelinated) fibre damage. Painful symptoms are found in around 11% of all diabetic patients and can be particularly distressing.

The therapies for painful diabetic neuropathy vary from non-pharmacological interventions such as transcutaneous nerve stimulation or complimentary therapies to drugs with potentially major side-effects. In each case there is often a clear placebo effect and it is often better to start with low doses and build up to an effective dose of any drug therapy. None of the non-analgesic pharmacological agents, tricyclics, antiepileptics and antiarrhythmics, are currently licensed for this use, and the use of such agents should therefore bc cxplaincd to thc patient, in detail, including their often significant side-effect profiles, prior to their use as coanalgesics. The most commonly used drugs are tricyclic antiodepressants and antiepileptics such as carbamezepine. Gabapentin (Parke–Davis Medical, UK) has now been licensed for the treatment of painful neuropathy on the basis of promising clinical trials. Such a therapy is useful but, like all adjuvant analgesics, requires careful titration to minimize the side-effects. Capsaicin 0.075% cream (Bioglan Laboratories, UK) has been licensed for the treatment of post-herpetic neuralgia for many years and recently was licensed for the treatment of painful peripheral neuropathy. In addition to monotherapy, it can also be safely added to any existing, partially effective oral agent. Its usefulness is often limited by a poor understanding of the need to use it little and often and to persevere beyond the initial first week or two when it may even make the symptoms a little worse (Young 1998).

It must be remembered that in some patients the presenting feature of peripheral neuropathy, and indeed of diabetes itself, may be foot ulceration, as the progression to an insensitive foot may occur without any positive symptoms. It is not uncommon for neuropathic diabetic patients to present because of the smell caused by purulent discharge. Thus, the absence of symptoms must never be equated with absence of risk of ulceration. Patients may also have a curious indifference to the condition of their feet, which can be likened to sensory inattention, and this can make the importance of education about footcare difficult to impress upon them (Walsh et al 1975).

The diagnosis of diabetic peripheral neuropathy for clinical purposes is a complex issue (Young and Matthews 1998). For routine screening purposes, clinical examination using a 128 Hz tuning fork will suffice. The vibration perception threshold (VPT) can be measured quantitatively using a Neurothesiometer (Arnold Horwell, UK). Such measurements have shown to be increased in association with other measurements of diabetic peripheral neuropathy, but also increase with normal aging; therefore the use of age-related normal values have been recommended. Other authors have claimed that the increased coefficient of variation in older patients makes the measurement of vibration perception threshold unreliable and that it should be supplemented by other tests of neuropathy (Thomson, Masson and Boulton 1994). For screening purposes, however, this may not be necessary. A VPT of greater than 25 volts has been shown in cross-sectional and prospective studies to be strongly predictive of subsequent foot ulceration (Young et al 1994). In the latter study patients with a VPT > 25 V were seven times more likely to develop a foot ulcer than a patient with a VPT < 25 V over a 4-year period. This increased to 11 times when recurrent ulceration was considered, as no patient with a VPT < 25 V developed a second ulcer. This study also revealed a relationship between foot ulceration and increasing age but, even after correcting for this, vibration perception threshold remained a strong predictor of foot ulceration risk.

Monofilaments (see Figure 4.1) are a quick method for assessing the at-risk foot in leprosy and are now used extensivly in the United Kingdom. There is some doubt as to the reliability of manufacture of monofilaments and there are widely varying rates of ulcer incidence in those studies that have used monofilaments as a screening tool (Booth and Young 2000). In general a 10 g monofilament should be used in a variety of sites on the foot with a clearly defined pass/fail criteria. They remain relatively cheap to buy and easy to use and therefore are very popular with many foot clinics.

Diabetologists still tend to diagnose peripheral neuropathy on clinical grounds. This can be improved by use of a neuropathy disability score (NDS) (Young et al 1993b). The score is derived from examination of the ankle reflex, vibration sensation using a 128 Hz tuning fork, pin-prick sensation, and temperature (cold tuning fork) sensation at the great toe. Each sensory modality is scored as either normal $= 0$ or reduced/absent $= 1$ for each side and the ankle reflexes as normal $= 0$, present with reinforcement $= 1$ or absent $= 2$ per side. Thus the total maximum abnormal score is 10. A score of 6 or over can be regarded as indicative of significant peripheral neuropathy. Such a score correlates well with vibration perception

threshold measurements, which, as described above, predict foot ulceration in diabetic patients. If a Neurothesiometer is available then a vibration perception threshold of greater than 25 V in both feet will predict up to 84% of those patients who will develop foot ulceration over the next four years.

Motor fibre loss is another significant result of peripheral neuropathy leading to small muscle atrophy in the foot. As a consequence, there is an imbalance between flexor and extensor muscle function resulting in clawing of the toes, prominent metatarsal heads and anterior displacement of the metatarsal footpads (Figure 6.2). Abnormally high foot pressures usually develop under these areas and, as discussed below, can lead to foot ulceration in the susceptible foot.

In addition the gait pattern is significantly altered in patients with diabetic neuropathy (Cavanagh et al 1992) and this may alter the foot pressure distribution making the foot more prone to the effects of high pressure. Gait problems, with increasing falls, and the risks of injury to the feet, are increased in neuropathic diabetic patients. Such problems are more pronounced in elderly neuropathic patients, and worse in those with visual handicap, increasing the risk of foot ulceration.

AUTONOMIC NEUROPATHY

Autonomic neuropathy results in a wide spectrum of problems in the cardiovascular, gastrointestinal and genitourinary systems and is known to be associated with the development of foot ulceration in diabetic patients (Gillmore, Allen and Hayes 1993). In the foot, denervation of the sweat glands leads to dry, atrophic skin and callus formation. Severe cracking of the skin often occurs under these circumstances and facilitates microbial infections. Regular use of emollient creams or ointments, often twice a day, is required to keep the skin supple and reduce the risk of such fissures.

Loss of sympathetic tone in small vessels also leads to reduced resistance and increased arteriovenous shunting. Venous PO_2 and pressure is raised in the neuropathic limb to a level approaching that of arterial blood, and has been measured at higher levels than in the endoneurium (Purewal et al 1995). Thus in a diabetic patient with autonomic neuropathy, but without coexisting vascular disease, the blood flow is increased at rest and distended dorsal foot veins can be seen. Initially, the overall increase in blood flow increases capillary pressure. However, over time this leads to microvascular sclerosis; and when taken in conjunc-

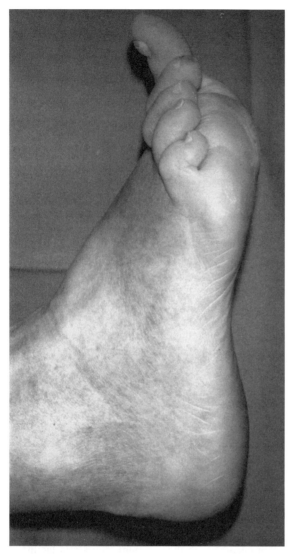

Figure 6.2 At-risk foot showing prominent metatarsal heads and clawed toes

tion with the increased shunting in the diabetic neuropathic foot, it may lead to inadequate nutritional flow and subsequent tissue ischaemia, greatly increasing the risk of ulceration (Flynn and Tooke 1992). The coexistence of autonomic neuropathy and macrovascular disease may cause a further deterioration in the level of tissue oxygenation.

PERIPHERAL VASCULAR DISEASE

Both the micro- and macrocirculation in the lower extremities are affected by diabetes. In the micro-

circulation the skin capillary pressure is increased in patients with Type 1 diabetes, either of recent onset or of long duration, and this abnormality reverses when the diabetes control improves (Saudeman, Shore and Tooke 1992). This increase in the capillary pressure is probably responsible for the loss of the blood flow autoregulation, increased arteriovenous shunting, impaired hyperaemic response, changes in capillary blood flow and basement membrane thickening seen in diabetic patients. This microvascular sclerosis may contribute to nephropathy, retinopathy and probably neuropathy, but the direct role in the development of foot ulceration remains unclear.

Macrovascular disease is more common in diabetic patients. Peripheral vascular disease is estimated to occur 20 times more often in diabetic patients than in non-diabetic patients (Ganda 1984). Lipid disorders (Uusitupa 1990), platelet dysfunction (Colwell and Halushka 1980), increased coagulation (Juhan-Vague, Alessi and Vague) and endothelial cell dysfunction (Bossaler 1987) have been implicated in the pathogenesis of the atherosclerosis (Colwell, Lopes-Virella and Halnshka 1981). Peripheral vascular disease usually has the same clinical presentation as that seen in non-diabetic patients, with intermittent claudication, rest pain, ulceration and gangrene being the main clinical features (Levin 1988); but the symptoms may be masked by coexisting peripheral neuropathy and significant ischaemia may develop in the absence of pain.

Although the femoropopliteal segments are most often affected, as in non-diabetic patients, smaller vessels below the knee, such as the tibial and peroneal arteries, are more severely affected in diabetic than in non-diabetic patients (LoGerfo and Coffman 1984). This means that overall vascular diasease in diabetic patients is more likely to lead to amputation even though, level for level, the outcome of revascularization is similar to the non-diabetic population. In addition, the presence of simultaneous cardiac and cerebrovascular disease means that long-time survival after such procedures is often shorter. Medial arterial calcification is another common finding in diabetic patients and can be recognised on X-ray films by its 'pipe-stem' appearance. Medial arterial calcification is reported to be associated with diabetic peripheral somatosensory and autonomic neuropathy, but few previous studies have examined the distribution of medial arterial calcification quantitatively within the diabetic foot. Medial arterial calcification is significantly associated with an increased prevalence of cardiovascular mortality (Lachman et al 1977; Nillson et al 1967; Janka, Stadl and Mehnert 1980), although this may also be related to the increase in medial arterial calcification associated with diabetic nephropathy, an independent marker of increased mortality in diabetes (Jensen et al 1987). Diabetes alone does not increase the prevalence of medial arterial calcification in matched groups of controls and non-neuropathic subjects, but there is significantly heavier arterial calcification in the feet of neuropathic diabetic patients (Young et al 1993a). Vibration perception threshold, duration of diabetes and serum creatinine are all independent predictors of the degree of medial arterial calcification. Medial arterial calcification, when present, is known to alter the pulse waveform and falsely elevate ankle pressures in diabetic patients (Gibbons and Freeman 1987). Therefore it has been suggested that toe systolic pressure measurements might replace ankle pressure measurements as an index of arterial inflow to the diabetic foot, as the ankle pressure index, measured by Doppler ultrasound, may be misleadingly high despite the presence of occlusive peripheral vascular disease. If the ankle systolic is more than 75 mmHg above the brachial systolic, then this is highly indicative of medial arterial calcification and the poor reliability of the ankle pressure to indicate lower extremity arterial disease (Orchard and Strandness 1993). However, it is also possible that medial arterial calcification is falsely elevating the ankle pressure into the normal range in some neuropathic patients. Therefore a normal ankle pressure should be interpreted with caution, and perhaps with a plain radiograph of the foot, particularly in elderly and in neuropathic diabetic patients. A low ankle pressure, and an ankle pressure index of <0.9, suggests arterial occlusive disease and the need for further investigation (Orchard and Strandness 1993). However, with all of the problems associated with ankle pressure measurements, foot pulses are still the best clinical guide to the presence of peripheral vascular disease in diabetes. Diabetic patients with neuropathy may have significant ischaemia with no pain because of the loss of pain sensation. The absence of foot pulses indicates vascular disease even if the popliteal pulse is present and there is no complaint of claudication or rest pain. Any areas of cyanosis or peripheral necrosis also indicate arterial insufficiency.

Diabetic patients with evidence of peripheral vascular disease should be referred for vascular assessment with arterial reconstruction or angioplasty where appropriate (Gibbons and Freeman 1987). The best advice for any stable claudicant with no evidence of tissue loss is to 'stop smoking and keep walking'. There is considerable evidence that in order to be effective the patient should walk to the point of claudicating and even some distance with claudication. It is believed that this might encourage the proliferation of collateral circulation (Hiatt et al 1990).

Although the long-term benefit is a disputed area amongst vascular surgeons, reconstructive surgery for diabetic patients with claudication should be considered if walking distance reduces, even before the onset of tissue loss. Reducing claudication distance is a sign of impending critical ischaemia in diabetic patients who have a greater tendency to early and more aggressive progression of arterial disease. Most vascular teams will not consider patients with stable claudication and will generally wait for the development of critical limb ischaemia prior to intervention. However, diabetic patients also have a higher amputation rate than non-diabetic patients for similar initial grades of arterial disease (McAllister 1976). With such clear evidence that tissue loss has a significantly adverse effect on limb prognosis, surgery before the onset of critical ischaemia has its advocates in many centres and should be encouraged.

As an additional consideration, peripheral autonomic neuropathy is usually present in patients with foot ulceration. Patients can therefore be said to have performed auto-sympathectomy. Surgical sympathectomy is still attempted in a number of diabetic patients but, because of the pre-existing peripheral autonomic changes, and associated medial arterial calcification, it is unlikely to produce substantial benefit.

LIMITED JOINT MOBILITY

Diffuse collagen abnormalities are common in diabetic patients (Larkin and Frier 1986). The main pathogenic mechanism for these abnormalities is glycation of collagen which results in thickening and increased cross-linking of collagen bundles (Goodfield and Millard 1988). One of the clinical manifestations of this change is thick, tight and waxy skin, leading to restriction of joint movements. Patients with limited joint mobility are unable to oppose the palms of their hands (the prayer sign; see Figure 6.3) (Lundbaek 1957). The term 'cheiroarthropathy' was used to describe this condition; but as other joints, including those in the shoulder, hip and foot, can also be affected,

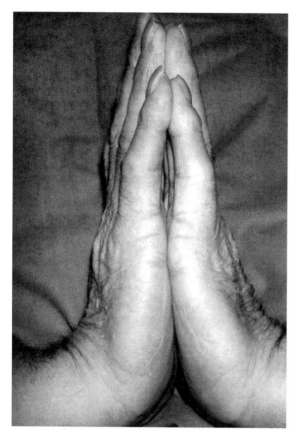

Figure 6.3   The prayer sign

a more appropriate term is 'limited joint mobility', and this is now in general use (Rosenbloom et al 1981; Campbell et al 1985). Limited joint mobility in the foot mainly involves the subtalar joint, which provides the foot with shock-absorbing capacity during walking (Delbridge et al 1988). This results in increased plantar foot pressures and, in the neuropathic foot, maybe a contributory factor to the development of foot ulceration (Fernando et al 1991). Limited extension of the great toe, 'hallux rigidus', can also predispose to ulceration by limiting the adaptive extension of the toe during the final 'toe-off' phase of walking, thus increasing the vertical and shear forces on the toe.

FOOT PRESSURE ABNORMALITIES

The two main factors responsible for the development of high foot pressures, motor neuropathy and limited joint mobility, have already been discussed. Callus formation, which itself is a result of high foot pressures and dry skin, may also act as a foreign body and results

in further increases of these pressures (Young et al 1992). In contrast, the patient's age and bodyweight do not significantly influence the foot pressure probably because foot contact surface area also increases with weight (Veves et al 1991; Cavanagh, Sims and Sanders 1991).

Intermittent moderate stress on healthy tissue for an excessive time, as in the case of abnormal pressures applied on the plantar surface of the foot during excessive walking, can lead to tissue inflammation and, finally, to ulceration. At the microscopic level, it is believed that pressure overcomes the nutritive capillary blood flow of the skin and this leads to localized tissue necrosis and breakdown (Boulton 1990). The demonstration of increased arteriovenous shunting in the diabetic foot (Gilmore et al 1993), and the reports of an impaired hyperaemic injury response in neuropathic patients (Rayman et al 1986; Walmsley, Wales and Wiles 1989) may also contribute to the increased risk of ulceration. Studies in dogs have shown that repetitive moderate trauma leads to the eventual breakdown of the skin and ulceration (Koziak 1959). Thermography of the feet of patients with diabetic neuropathy has shown hot spots of inflammation in areas of high foot pressures and repetitive trauma (MacFarlane et al 1993). Sensory dysfunction is crucial for the development of neuropathic ulceration. In a non-neuropathic subject, the pain which accompanies the inflammation will usually force the individual to rest the foot before it progresses to ulceration, whereas a patient with loss of pain awareness will continue to walk long after an ulcer has developed. Therefore, high foot pressures alone, in the absence of sensory neuropathy, do not result in foot ulceration. This can be illustrated in patients with rheumatoid arthritis, in whom joint involvement in the feet results in high foot pressures comparable to those found in diabetic patients, but not ulceration (Masson et al 1989).

The measurement of foot pressures is not routine in most clinics. Careful visual inspection and palpation of the foot can detect most high pressure areas, and accomodative insoles can therefore be made to redistribute pressure away from vulnerable areas without the need for expensive foot pressure measuring systems.

OTHER RISK FACTORS

History of Previous Foot Problems

A history of previous foot problems in diabetic patients strongly suggests that the patient is at high risk for future problems, especially lower limb amputation. Studies of patients with traumatic or diabetic amputations have shown that amputation alone does not cause an increase in the loads under the remaining foot. However in a neuropathic diabetic patient amputation is associated with high pressure under the remaining foot, probably related to neuropathy and limited joint mobility in that foot (Veves, Van Ross and Boulton 1992).

In a prospective study of the prediction of foot ulceration using vibration perception thresholds, recurrent ulceration was common, affecting over 50% of the patients. In addition, in an audit of dressing policy at the Manchester Foot Hospital the median number of ulcers per patient was 2 (range 1–12) (Knowles et al 1993), again suggesting that over half the patients reulcerated despite preventative care and advice. The likely causes for this are unknown, but it appears that those patients who do not wear their recommended shoes (which are usually supplied), or do not follow the appropriate advice, are those who subsequently reulcerate. Strategies to increase footwear acceptibility and compliance can reduce reulceration rates.

Reduced Resistance to Infection

There are many reasons for impaired resistance to infection in a diabetic ulcer. Diabetes is associated with impaired neutrophil function, particularly in the presence of a high blood glucose, and macro- and microcirculatory abnormalities lead to relative hypoxia in the wound (Pecoraro et al 1991). Multiple microbes, often a mixture of aerobic and anaerobic bacteria, are usually found in cultures from foot ulcers. The commonest pathogenic organisms in diabetic foot ulcers are *Staphylococcus* and *Streptococcus*. The streptococci are often faecal in origin. The clinical relevance of organisms grown from superficial swabs is variable as other organisms may colonize the wound surface and the quality of the sample and the method of transport and culture markedly influence the reliability of the result (Louie, Gartlett and Tally 1976). The treatment of infections associated with foot ulceration is detailed further in the management of foot ulceration.

Smoking and Alcohol

Smoking is known to be associated with foot ulceration, probably by increasing the prevalence of vascular disease (Delbridge, Appleberg and Reeves 1983).

Recurrent neuropathic foot ulceration has been reported as being more common in patients with a high alcohol consumption (Young et al 1986).

Other Complications of Diabetes

Foot pressures in patients with nephropathy are higher than in diabetic patients without renal impairment. In combination with neuropathy, which is also more common in such patients, this imposes a serious risk for foot ulceration (Fernando et al 1991a).

THE CLASSIFICATION OF ULCERATION

The most widely used and validated foot ulcer classification system is the Meggitt–Wagner system (Young 2000). It calls patients with risk factors but no ulcer 'grade 0', the 'at-risk' foot. The classification divides foot ulcers into five categories. Grade 1 are superficial ulcers limited to the dermis. Grade 2 are transdermal with exposed tendon or bone without osteomyelitis or abscess. Grade 3 are deep ulcers with osteomyelitis or abscess formation. Grade 4 is given to feet with localized gangrene confined to the toes or forefoot. Grade 5 applies to feet with extensive gangrene.

A significant problem with the Meggitt–Wagner classification is that it does not differentiate between those grade 1–3 ulcers which are associated with arterial insufficiency. Such ulcers might be expected to heal less well. Neither does it differentiate those grade 1 and 4 ulcers which are significantly infected and which might also be expected to have a poorer prognosis. Despite this, the Meggitt–Wagner classification has been shown to give an accurate guide to risk of amputation in a number of studies and remains the standard by which other classifications have to be judged.

The most successful recent system is that of the Texas group which uses depth and ischaemia as its main classification criteria and therefore is able to predict the progression from ulceration to amputation with some accuracy (Lavery, Armstrong and Harkless 1996). Despite this, there are over a dozen classification systems in use in different centres. With such a variety of classification systems available it is clear that no one system offers an ideal compromise between comprehensive applicability and simplicity. The reviewers of classification systems usually want each system to include their own particular facet. For example, the Texas system was reviewed by Levin

(1998), who noted that site of ulceration was missing despite the fact that this has been shown to be an uncertain predictor of outcome. A good classification system would seem to require some allowance for patient factors and inclusion of a deformity index, particularly in relation to ulceration in association with Charcot feet (see later). At present, most of the current classifications force the user to become totally foot-centred at the expense of the patient as a whole. Whilst this is not likely to create problems in multidisciplinary practice, it is a possible cause of fragmented care where the foot clinic is separate from diabetology and other support. Addressing the social and diabetes factors of patients is likely to improve foot ulcer outcomes (LoGerfo and Coffman 1984), and this is particularly true of the elderly living alone.

THE AT-RISK FOOT

(Tables 6.1 and 6.2)

The mainstay of risk reduction must lie with footcare education and the amelioration of other risk factors if present. Footcare education should be concise and repeated regularly in order to have the maximum effect on patient behaviour (Barth et al 1991). Video presentations have been shown to be effective at imparting knowledge about footcare (Knowles et al 1992), but they should not supplant one-to-one or small-group education. The main aspects of footcare education include the need for regular, at least once daily, inspection of the feet for new lesions and the need to have shoes measured each time they are acquired. These are two aspects which appear, from experience, to be regularly overlooked in the majority of patients with ulcers. Although education is the potential saviour

Table 6.1 At-risk groups for diabetic foot ulceration

Patients with:
   a history of previous ulceration
   peripheral neuropathy
   peripheral vascular disease
   limited joint mobility
   bony deformities
   diabetic nephropathy
   visual impairment
   a history of alcohol excess
Patients who live alone
Elderly patients

Table 6.2 General principles of foot care education

1. Target the level of information to the needs of the patient. Those not at risk may require only general advice about foot hygiene and shoes
2. Assess the ability of the patient to understand and perform the necessary components of footcare. If this is limited then the spouse or carer should be involved at the beginning of the process.
3. Suggest a positive approach to footcare with 'dos' rather than 'don'ts' as the principle of active rather than passive footcare is more likely to be successful and acceptable to the patient:
   Inspect the feet daily
   Report any problems immediately
   Have your feet measured every time new shoes are brought
   Buy shoes with a square toe box and laces
   Inspect the inside of shoes for foreign objects every day before putting them on
   Attend a fully trained podiatrist regularly
   Cut your nails straight across and not rounded
   Keep your feet away from heat (fires, radiators and hotwater bottles) and check the bathwater before stepping into it
   Always wear something on your feet to protect them and never walk barefoot
4. Repeat the advice at regular intervals and check that it is being followed
5. Disseminate advice to other family members and other healthcare professionals involved in the care of the patient

of the diabetic foot, there is a considerable body of evidence to suggest that whilst knowledge about diabetic foot problems may increase, attitudes to, and compliance with, the necessary care may remain unchanged.

The limitations of current education and preventative methods are highlighted by the number of patients who have recurrent ulceration, even in specialist clinics. The lack of perceived vulnerability in neuropathic patients has been highlighted as one reason for this (Stuart and Wiles 1992, 1993). Until this is addressed effectively, education programs may be limited in their success.

Hospital shoes are the second line of risk reduction for those patients with deformity which increases foot ulcer risk. The attendance of a dedicated orthotist as part of the diabetic footcare team can significantly improve shoe acceptibility and compliance amongst patients and reduce recurrence rates in those with healed ulcers.

As mentioned repeatedly in this text, the elderly pose particular problems when trying to impart effective footcare advice and strategies. Many are unable to perform routine footcare because of poor eyesight and reduced mobility which make it difficult to inspect the foot, and so a spouse or carer should be taught how to provide footcare. There is a particular problem when the patient lives alone, especially if they are partially sighted, and this may be insoluble despite home support services.

SUPERFICIAL ULCERS: GRADE 1

Superficial plantar ulcers are predominantly neuropathic in origin, and form at sites of pressure such as metatarsal heads or plantar prominences including the rocker bottom of advanced midfoot Charcot neuro-

arthropathy (see later). Ulceration of the dorsum of clawed toes in shoes that are too shallow at the toe-box or the lateral and medial aspects of toes are more commonly seen in neuroischaemic patients, but any pressure point can ulcerate in any patient, particularly callused plantar areas (Murray et al 1996). Superficial ulcers are believed to form when pressure leads to a reduction in skin blood flow, to autolysis and to a breakdown in the dermal layer which results in the formation of an ulcer. (Figures 6.4 and 6.5).

Neuropathy allows diabetic patients to continue to stress the skin, by walking or continuing to wear the same tight shoes even after the ulcer has formed. Continued walking inevitably leads to a deterioration in the foot. The causative factor, which may be unknown to the patient, may be deduced from the site or nature of the ulcer. In particular, any assessment of the patient with a foot ulcer should pay careful attention to their shoes. Bedrest causing heel ulcers, and trauma, including the heat of hotwater bottles or inappropriate self-'chiropody', are easily recognized causes of ulceration (Boulton 1990).

The relief of pressure is the principal mode of management of superficial ulcers regardless of origin. Metatarsal head ulceration can be unloaded in a variety of ways. Bedrest, with adequate heel protection, is perhaps the most effective, but is difficult to enforce, carries its own risks and, especially if in hospital, is expensive. For this reason a number of ambulatory methods of off-loading ulcer sites have been devised. It must be stressed to the patient that such devices are supplied only for minimal walking such as to the toilet

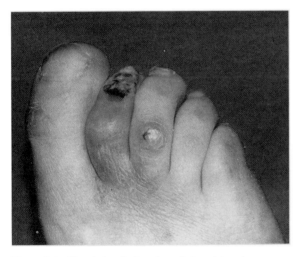

Figure 6.4 Shoe-induced ulceration of clawed toes in a neuropathic diabetic patient

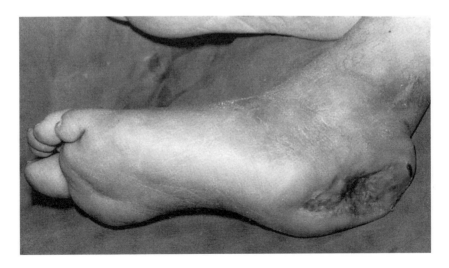

Figure 6.5 Heel ulcer due to pressure from resting on unprotected heels in a neuropathic patient

indoors and not for trips to the shops etc. There is often a problem in the patient group of elderly men or women who live alone, especially if they abuse alcohol or have no carers. In such patients the advice to stop excess walking may not always be followed.

The majority of ambulatory ulcer care systems comprise some form of pressure-redistributing insole in either a temporary shoe or cast (Pollard and Le Quesne 1983). Removable casts, such as the 'Scotch-cast' boot (Burden et al 1983), may be abused by patients not wearing them, but this is sometimes preferable to the problems of iatrogenic injury from a non-removable (by the patient) total contact cast (Mueller et al 1989). Shoe-induced dorsal and digital ulcers can be easily unloaded by the provision of, or by recommencing the wearing of, appropriately fitting wide and extra-depth shoes with or without insoles and toe spacers or props as required. (Figure 6.6).

Callus should be debrided at every clinic visit. This not only unloads the plantar ulcer but encourages healing. The formation of excessive callus is a sign that the patient is still walking. Low levels of callus formation are also seen in neuroischaemic patients; this too may be debrided with care. Whilst bleeding is a sign that viable tissue has been reached during the debridement of neuropathic ulcers, the neuroischaemic ulcer should not be traumatized if possible.

The presence or absence of infection is difficult to determine in a diabetic foot ulcer. Necrosis, slough and erythema are not universal and systemic features are rare. Culture from the ulcer surface is likely to produce a mixed growth of dubious significance. Culture from ulcer scrapings during debridement, or better, deep surgical debridement, may provide a more reliable guide to the principal organism responsible for the infection; however, this too may be misleading and the broad-spectrum antibiotics are the first choice in the treatment of infected ulcers. The provision of 'prophylactic' antibiotics has its advocates, but the case for their use is not clear from the currently available published evidence. Whilst it is common practice, their use is debatable in purely neuropathic ulcers with clean wounds in a patient who is able to rest, to report any changes during regular visits to the foot clinic, and who can obtain same-day clinic access in emergencies. Neuropathic ulcers which are not overtly infected might be managed expectantly with antibiotics as an optional component of therapy. In neuroischaemic ulceration, the additional ischaemic risk and potential for foot-threatening infections should encourage the use of long-term antibiotics (Foster, McColgan and Edmonds 1998).

If prophylactic antibiotics are not instituted then they should be started with the minimum of clinical suspicion. The choice of antibiotics is also difficult, but in general most opinion seems to support the use of broad-spectrum monotherapy; co-amoxiclav is regularly used in the authors' and many other units, as is clindamycin, which is also a useful antibiotic for foot infections.

X-rays of the foot are recommended to detect osteomyelitis in the majority of patients with ulcers which are either deeper than grade 1 on inspection, have a history of penetrative trauma, are associated with swelling and redness, or are not healing after a month.

It is important to measure the size of the ulcer in order to gauge the progress of healing. The minimum measurement should be the diameter of the ulcer in two planes at right-angles. Tracing the perimeter and/or photographs are also useful to measure progress. Failure of the ulcer to heal should prompt an investigation as to the effectiveness of any pressure-reduction system, including whether it is being used and whether the patient is able to rest sufficiently at home (Cavanagh, Ulbrecht and Caputo 1998).

If all of these aspects are satisfactory then the question of vascular insufficiency should be addressed. Even in apparently purely neuropathic ulcers there may be an underlying element of vascular impairment which, without correction, might significantly impede

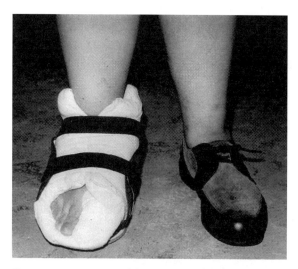

Figure 6.6 'Scotch-cast' boot (right foot) and extra-depth shoe (left foot) used in the prevention and treatment of diabetic foot ulceration

the healing of recalcitrant ulceration. The successful treatment of vascular insufficiency can dramatically improve healing rates.

Dressings alone will not heal an ulcer without adequate pressure relief. Newer 'active' dressings have been advocated in the treatment of chronic venous ulcers but have not been widely adopted in diabetes. The dry dressing is still in common use, but a moist wound environment encourages granulation tissue (Porter 1992).

The use of wound healing factors and biosynthetic skin replacements are in their infancy but may hold great promise for the future. Autologous, blood-derived, wound healing factor has been used for many years, particularly in the United States, but adequate controlled studies in diabetic patients are uncommon (Krupski et al 1991). Becaplermin (Regranex, Jann-sen-CIlag, UK) has been shown to increase the healing rate and total percentage of healed ulcers compared with placebo (Young 1999). The biosynthetic dermal replacement Dermagraft (Smith and Nephew, UK) has had some promise in clinical trials of patients with neuropathic diabetic foot ulcers (Gentzkow et al 1996). The market for these products must, however, remain the difficult-to-heal ulcer, and in most cases appropriate care and pressure relief will achieve healing of superficial ulcers of neuropathic and neuroischaemic origins.

The Myth of the Non-healing Ulcer?

Many reports have tried to categorize ulcers as healing and non-healing. It is important to be able to identify those patients in whom treatment is failing and for whom a new approach should be used. If no objective measure of ulcer healing is used then there is no possibility that such patients will be detected, and once again the need for measurement and standardized descriptions of ulcers cannot be stressed too highly.

It is clear that the primary reasons for failure of the neuropathic plantar diabetic foot ulcer to heal are inadequate or inappropriate pressure relief, inadequate debridement and infection control, failure to recognize or treat vascular insufficiency, or patient non-compliance. It is only when all of these factors have been addressed, including angiography and reconstruction where necessary, or by the implementation of non-weight-bearing regimes using in-patient bedrest or a non-removable cast, that an ulcer can truly be described as non-healing. Such ulcers will be rare (Cavanagh et al 1998).

Once an ulcer is healed that patient is left in the highest category of all for predicting future ulcer risk. Education, footcare, chiropody, footwear and careful follow-up are all necessary to try to prevent the recurrence of foot ulceration.

DEEP ULCERS: GRADES 2 AND 3

Deep ulcers are usually superficial ulcers that have continued to be traumatized by an insensate patient. Continued walking on plantar ulcers or wearing of inappropriate shoes advances the cycle of tissue destruction and enlarges the ulcer cavity. If this process continues it may lead to the involvement of underlying tendons (Meggitt–Wagner grade 2) and eventually to bone, causing osteomyelitis (grade 3). Occasionally, penetrating injuries will cause the primary formation of a deep abscess.

X-rays of the feet should be routine in all patients with deep ulcers. If osteomyelitis is suspected but is not apparent on initial plain radiographs, then further investigations with Tc99m radioisotopes and labelled white cell scanning should be performed. CT and MRI scanning are also used in centres with ready access to such facilities. Levin (1992) has suggested that if the ulcer can be probed to bone then this is likely to be complicated by osteomyelitis in all cases, and therefore empirical treatment has been advocated.

As with superficial ulcers, pressure relief is still the mainstay of treatment of deep ulceration, but the treatment of sepsis and aggressive surgical debridement is increasingly important. If the patient is systemically well and there is no evidence of spreading infection, then the patient can often be managed as an outpatient. The use of total contact casts is, however, contraindicated in patients with oedema secondary to deep infection owing to the risk of swelling within the cast, leading to cast trauma. Regular debridement down to the ulcer base is required. Bleeding points demonstrate adequate debridement in the neuropathic foot. In the foot with coexisting ischaemia debridement should be less aggressive. The patient may need admission for investigation and treatment of osteomyelitis, surgical debridement or intravenous antibiotics.

Diabetes control should be optimized if possible, as there is evidence to suggest that healing is impaired with poor blood glucose control; although this does not necessarily mean a need for insulin in a non-insulin dependent patient.

Podiatric debridement and conservative care will heal over 60% of such ulcers (Pittet et al 1999). If surgical debridement is required then it should aim to remove all the infected tissue in one operation. This may necessitate partial amputation, commonly of a metatarsal and associated toe (the 'ray amputation'— see Figure 6.7) which should then heal well if the blood supply is adequate (McKeown 1994). The removal of all the infected and/or necrotic tissue should produce an improvement in the patients' metabolic state and, in neuropathic patients with adequate blood supply, even extensive tissue loss will heal. Local operations in neuroischaemic patients can lead to larger non-healing wounds, so it is important to ensure the vascular status of the patient prior to forefoot and other surgery. If vascular disease is suspected from the absence of pulses, the site of the ulcer, failure to heal despite adequate therapy or the presence of local gangrene, a vascular opinion should be obtained before any decision to operate. Where indicated, restoration of impaired blood flow may remove the need for amputation or at least markedly reduce its scope.

Previous concerns about the long-term patency of arterial grafts in diabetic patients should be discounted. There is evidence to show that a successful arterial bypass operation has the same graft survival rate in diabetic patients as in patients without diabetes (Stipa and Wheelcock 1971). Once healing has been achieved, subsequent graft failure may not lead to loss of the limb as the vascular requirements of healed tissue seem to be lower than that of healing ulcers.

Slough is commonly seen in neuroischaemic ulcers and impedes healing by blocking the formation of granulation tissue. Chemical debridement with desloughing agents such as hydrogels or hydrofoams seems to help in the early stages of healing if there is adherent slough. Necrotic eschar is probably best removed mechanically. An alternative is larval debridement which has been effective in removing slough and necrotic debris from wounds in a number of case reports. This method is usually used in neuroischaemic ulcers to debride recalcitrant slough. If larvae are used it may take more than one application to clear the ulcer of slough.

Antibiotics should be universal in all deep ulcers and again should, at least initially, be broad-spectrum

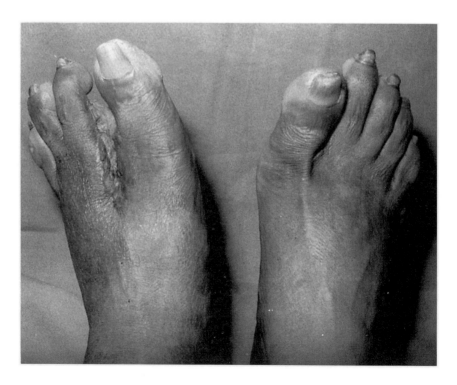

Figure 6.7   Ray amputation of second toe and associated metatarsal

until a definitive pathogen is isolated. The average number of potential pathogens isolated from a wound swab is over two organisms (Hunt 1992). The deeper the tissue which is cultured, or the growth of an organism from the blood stream, increases the reliability of the pathogenicity of the isolate. Combination therapy for initial blind treatment has traditionally been ampicillin, flucloxacillin and metronidazole intravenously, or ciprofloxacin and metronidazole. Clinical trial evidence for the use of ciprofloxacin and clindamycin as combination therapy in oral or intravenous dosing also seems to be effective. Outpatient treatment might be with these antibiotics or clindamycin alone, which is a useful oral antibiotic for the treatment of mild to moderate infections, and in the long-term treatment of osteomyelitis.

Dressings should conform to the cavity left by a deep ulcer. Deep ulcers often have tendons at their bases and they should not be allowed to get too dry. Once again, the choice of dressing is rarely based upon any clinical trial. Theoretical concepts would point to the use of a moist wound-healing environment with enough absorbency to deal with wound exudation. Foam dressings are the authors' current choice as a primary or secondary dressing for such ulcers.

If the patient has been admitted, once the initial infection is controlled then outpatient care, using off-loading casts or similar, can be restarted. The clinical progress of these ulcers is slow but eventually complete healing can be achieved. Regular measurement of the ulcer is important to gauge progress above the usual 'It looks better/the same/worse' notes which are commonplace in most clinical records. Failure to improve should again prompt a search for the reasons behind the lack of appropriate healing.

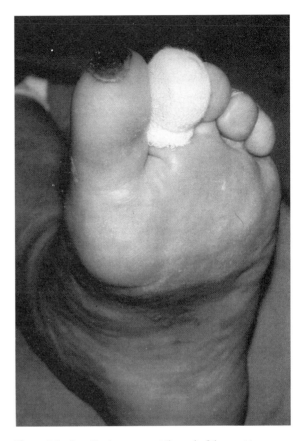

Figure 6.8 Localized gangrene at the end of the great toe

LOCALIZED GANGRENE: GRADE 4

Localized gangrene is commonly seen at the ends of toes (Figure 6.8) and at the apex of the heel. These are regions where there are endarteries with little collateral circulation if a feeder branch artery fails. As well as being a sign of global arterial insufficiency in the foot and therefore of neuroischaemia, digital necrosis can occur as a result of infection in a purely neuropathic foot, leading to an infective vasculitis and digital artery closure (Edmonds et al 1992).

Vascular assessment is mandatory for all patients with localized gangrene. No clinical arterial insufficiency may be found in patients with toe gangrene alone; but if treatable arterial insufficiency is found then correction will significantly reduce the amount of tissue loss. Angioplasty and proximal reconstructive surgery is as effective in diabetic patients as non-diabetic patients. However, the vascular disease of diabetic patients is often below the trifurcation of the popliteal artery.

Interventional radiology with angioplasty can now tackle tibial and peroneal disease. The technique of percutaneous transluminal angioplasty using an inflatable balloon was first described by Gruntzig (1976). Positioned at the site of an atheromatous narrowing within an artery, the balloon stretches the vessel, thus splitting the plaque and restoring luminal area. Re-endothelialization then has to occur over the fissured plaque, and it is usual to use intravenous heparin to prevent thrombotic occlusion in the first 24 hours after angioplasty. In general, the success rate for recanalization of an arterial occlusion by angioplasty is proportionate to the length of stenosis or thrombosis.

Recanalization can usually be achieved in over 90% of short stenoses in appropriately skilled hands (Mansell, Gregson and Allison 1992). Even a good technical result with total recanalization of an occluded vessel does not always lead to clinical improvement in the limb if the distal run-off is poor, and this may require further treatment to the distal vessels. Angioplasty has been performed at the level of the tibial and peroneal arteries since 1982 and may be the therapy of first line in elderly diabetic patients with other medical conditions or in whom a vein is not available for distal bypass (Dean 1984). Arterial tears and early thrombotic occlusion are the main adverse events associated with angioplasty. Fortunately the incidence of these problems is low.

There remains a problem with long-term reocclusion. Even in technically successful angioplasties with good run-off, intimal hyperplasia or recurrence of native disease lead to reocclusion rates which approach 50% overall depending on the duration of follow-up. However, these rates are similar in diabetic and non-diabetic patients. Re-angioplasty may be possible, and, even if a vessel does re-stenose or occlude, there may have been sufficient duration of improved circulation to facilitate healing or to allow a plane of tissue viability to establish or even the closure of the lesion (Figure 6.9). Once a lesion is closed the blood supply requirements may be lower than those for an ulcerated limb, and limb salvage rates are usually higher than patency rates in most series.

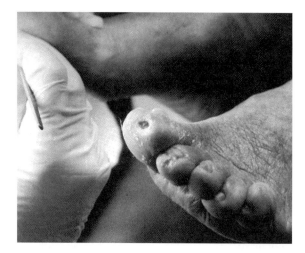

Figure 6.9 Gangrene has separated to leave a clean ulcer, which subsequently healed well

There is evidence that in iliac vessels, or situations where re-stenosis is likely, stenting the artery wall can prevent re-occlusion (Palmaz, Laborde and Rivera 1992). Iliac angioplasty with or without stenting can also be employed to increase arterial inflow to the limb and improve the chances of a lower bypass remaining patent. Reconstructive surgery, particularly with *in situ* or reversed saphenous vein as a conduit, can now be performed at the level of the dorsalis pedis artery to restore pulsitile flow below the tibial arteries (Estes and Pomposelli 1996). The availability of such techniques is often limited to regional centres, and indeed this may be appropriate in order to achieve the best limb salvage rates from what are highly specialized surgery and angioplasty.

Indications for Revascularization

Many surgeons talk of an aggressive limb salvage approach in the management of the ischaemic diabetic limb (Gibbons 1994). Such an approach is often, and probably should always be, based on appropriate patient selection. The patient should be expected to have a reasonable life expectancy. It should be remembered that concomitant cardiac and cerebrovascular disease is likely to result in death in over 50% of vascular disease patients within 5 years regardless of whether they have diabetes. (Sigurdsson et al 1999). It is the practice of many American surgeons to attend to these vascular beds at the same time as, or prior to, revascularization of the lower limbs. Such a policy requires greater resources than are likely to be available in most state-funded healthcare systems. In general, the patient must be able to undergo what is usually a lengthy operation, particularly for distal bypass, and pre-existing lung or cardiac pathology may limit the ability of the patient to withstand the operation or limit its effectiveness. If the patient has a low functional capacity with poor potential for rehabilitation beyond a wheelchair, then such an approach is not tenable. Similarly, if the patient is not able or motivated to walk, or will not stop smoking, then the graft patency will be jeopardized.

If surgery to vessels below the knee is required then this has to be performed with a vein as the conduit. Synthetic grafts, even with vein cuffs, have such low patency rates as to render attempts at below-knee reconstructive surgery using such materials pointless (Cheshire et al 1992). If the leg veins are varicosed or have been harvested for coronary grafting, then arm vein can be used but this adds to the technical aspects and duration of the operation. If a short length of vein can be found, popliteal artery to foot bypass may be almost as successful as femoral artery to distal bypass (Pomposelli et al 1991). Similarly, the patient must have suitable anatomy with adequate inflow and a patent foot vessel to graft on to. If the nature and extent of infection and necrosis is such that it encroaches upon the potential graft site, then again the likelihood is that the graft will fail. This once again highlights the need for control of infection.

Any centre which wishes to perform reconstructive surgery, and particularly distal surgery, needs to operate a graft surveillance program in order to assess the clinical progress of patients and to audit results. In the follow-up period, the other vascular trees, coronaries, carotids and the other limb may need attention to reduce the coexisting morbidity and mortality and to improve patient outcome.

The nature of diabetes as a systemic disorder usually implies that in those patients requiring reconstructive surgery there are other associated complications. This is particularly true of the elderly patient with diabetes. Intensive care time is often longer in diabetic patients, and the perioperative management of diabetes control, cardiac and renal impairment, and radiological investigation require a team approach to the management of surgery in such patients (Hirsch and White 1988).

Proximal Arterial Reconstruction

These operations are divided into inflow procedures, usually aorto-iliac surgery, where synthetic graft materials are usually used, and where, because of high flow rates, the graft patency is excellent. For aorto-bifemoral grafts the 5-year patency rate is commonly over 85%. The patency of aorto-bifemoral grafts is the same in the diabetic and non-diabetic patient, but, because of associated cardiovascular disease, overall patient survival rates are lower in diabetic patients, but this is not usually significantly so (Sigurdsson et al 1999).

Reconstructive surgery below the inguinal ligament is usually referred to as an outflow procedure. The usual operation is the femoro-popliteal bypass graft around a superficial femoral occlusion. Synthetic graft materials can be used for these operations but vein grafts have better secondary patency rates. Regardless of the conduit used, the long-term patency depends on the flow rate through the graft, which in turn is influ-

enced by the run-off vessels. In most series the 5-year patency averages 70%, although reoperation and redo angioplasty rates are higher in diabetic patients in some series (Bartlett, Gibbons and Wheelcock 1986). Despite the predilection for vascular disease to be multi-level and to affect the infra-popliteal vessels in diabetes, there appears to be no significant difference in patency rates between diabetic and non-diabetic patients. This may be due to patient selection, but there also is some evidence that femoral disease and distal disease do not always coexist in diabetic patients. In addition, owing to high coexisting mortality, graft patency may exceed the life expectancy of the patient (Bartlett et al 1986).

Distal Reconstructive Operations

These operations are all outflow procedures performed to vessels below the popliteal artery. As outlined above, autologous vein is the only suitable conduit for these procedures, which can limit the suitability of many patients for surgery. In general these are operations performed for limb salvage. The flow rate may mean that in many cases the graft may have failed by one year. However, the limb be saved if the lesion has closed. In selected centres, 5-year limb salvage rates approach 85% despite a graft patency of only 68%, and are at least 50% in unselected British centres (Sigurdsson et al 1999). Infection should be treated promptly to prevent rapidly spreading gangrene and systemic infection leading to a severely ill and toxic patient. The antibiotic regimens outlined above under deep ulcers should also be appropriate for these patients. Well-circumscribed, localized, usually digital, necrosis with viable tissue borders can often be left to separate undisturbed. This is usually termed 'auto-amputation'. The wound left behind should then be treated as a neuroischaemic ulcer in the usual way and usually heals well.

More extensive or spreading necrosis in a toxic patient, particularly if there is no reversible arterial lesion, may require primary amputation. This decision should be taken only after review by a vascular surgeon, as arterial reconstruction or angioplasty can markedly improve the level at which the amputation stump is viable.

The remaining foot of an amputee is at an exceedingly high risk of ulceration and further surgery. General aftercare should be as for other ulcers but with particular attention to the intact foot. A partial amputation of a toe or ray leads to biomechanical changes within the foot which are often very different from normal and frequently produces new pressure points at risk of ulceration. Transmetatarsal or Lisfranc amputations are often very poorly functioning amputations in diabetic patients.

Amputation, at whatever level, results in special orthotic needs which must be addressed by the footcare team. Insoles and orthoses all require careful and regular review to ensure that they are functioning correctly in order to reduce the significant reulceration and amputation rate of diabetic amputees.

EXTENSIVE GANGRENE: GRADE 5

Extensive necrosis of the foot is due to arterial occlusion and failure of arterial inflow. It usually presents with multiple areas of necrosis. It is usually seen in the context of the neuroischaemic foot. Primary amputation is the usual treatment for extensive gangrene. However, the extent of amputation can sometimes be reduced by pre-amputation arterial reconstructive surgery. For this reason, the counsel of perfection is that a vascular assessment should be performed in all patients prior to amputation. Femoro-popliteal or similar bypass operations might improve the viability of a distal stump or convert an above-knee to a below-knee amputation. Again this may not always be possible in diabetic patients, because the arterial disease is often below the popliteal trifurcation, and if the necrosis extends beyond the dorsalis pedis artery it will preclude distal bypass.

Metabolic and infection control should be attended to as a priority, as these patients are often very ill owing to the toxic effects of the necrotic tissue burden. In addition, coexistent coronary and cerebral vascular disease often makes the anaesthetic choice difficult and regional anaesthesia is commonly used for amputation surgery in diabetic patients. Close cooperation between the medical, surgical and anaesthetic teams is likely to produce the best survival outcomes for these patients.

If the patient survives the immediate perioperative period then the mortality rate in patients following major amputation is over 50% at one year. Care of the remaining foot is particularly important to prevent further amputation which usually results in confinement to a wheelchair. Significant improvements in preservation of the remaining limb can be achieved if the patient returns to the diabetic foot clinic for follow-up after amputation (Abbott, Carrington and Boulton 1996). The patient is likely to die from other major vessel problems, particularly coronary artery and cerebrovascular disease, and treatment for these conditions—including aspirin, lipid modification and blood pressure control—should also be addressed in the follow-up period.

THE DIABETIC CHARCOT FOOT

The devastating effects of Charcot neuroarthropathy in the diabetic foot have been well described in the literature (Sinha, Munichoodappa and Kozak 1972; Cofield, Morrison and Beabout 1983; Sammarco 1991). Diabetes is now believed to be the leading cause of Charcot neuroarthropathy in the developed world (Fryckberg 1987). Eighty percent of the patients who develop Charcot neuroarthropathy have a known duration of diabetes of over 10 years. The long duration of diabetes prior to the initiation of the Charcot process probably reflects the degree of neuropathy that is usually present in these patients. Autonomic neuropathy appears to be a universal finding in diabetic Charcot patients (Marshall Young and Boulton 1993). The duration of diabetes appears to be more important than age alone, but this is compounded in Type 2 diabetic patients who frequently have a long prodromal disease duration prior to diagnosis.

The initiating event of the Charcot process is often a seemingly trivial injury, which may result in a minor periarticular fracture (McEnery et al 1993) or in a major fracture (Johnson 1967; Connolly and Jacobsen 1985), despite the inability of the patient to recall the injury in many cases. Following this there is a rapid onset of swelling, an increase in temperature in the foot and often an ache or discomfort. The patient may have noticed a change in the shape of the foot, and others describe the sensation, or the sound, of the bones crunching as they walk. The blood supply to the Charcot foot is always good; indeed there are case reports of the Charcot process starting in patients following arterial bypass surgery (Edelman et al 1987). It is assumed that autonomic neuropathy plays a part in the increased vascularity of bone, possibly by increased arteriovenous shunting (Edmonds et al 1985), and this increases osteoclastic activity, resulting in the destruction, fragmentation and remodelling of bone. It is these processes which, if left untreated, lead to the characteristic patterns of deformity in the Charcot foot, including the collapse of the longitudinal and trans-

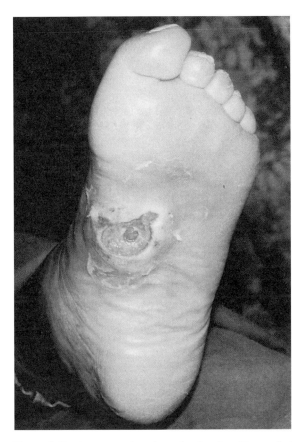

Figure 6.10 Anteroposterior view of sole of a Charcot foot showing a plantar prominence which has ulcerated

verse arches leading to a rocker bottom foot (see Figures 6.10 and 6.11).

Charcot neuroarthropathy passes from this acute phase of development through a stage of coalescence, in which the bone fragments are reabsorbed, the oedema lessens and the foot cools. It then enters the stage of reconstruction, in which the final repair and regenerative modelling of bone takes place to leave a stable, chronic Charcot foot (Eichenholtz 1966). The time course of these events is variable but is often up to a year. Intervention must be made in the earliest phase to prevent subsequent deformity and to reduce the risk of amputation (Gazis, Macfarlane and Jeffcoate 2000).

Radiographs of the foot should be performed to make the initial diagnosis (Figure 6.12). The characteristic appearances of bone destruction, fragmentation, loss of joint architecture and new bone formation should be determined. Confirmation of Charcot neuroarthropathy can be made through bone scans, CT scans or MRI scans, but this is usually not required in the majority of clinical settings.

The management of the Charcot foot has always been difficult and varies from the expectant to the markedly interventional (Lesko and Maurer 1989). The first principles of management are rest and freedom from weight-bearing. Non-weight-bearing is useful to reduce the activity but this frequently restarts when walking is recommenced. In the United States, in particular, the practice of prolonged, (one year or more) immobilization in a plaster of Paris cast is the

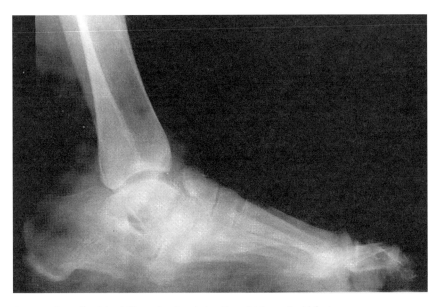

Figure 6.11 Charcot neuroarthropathy: lateral X-ray showing destruction of talus and mid-foot

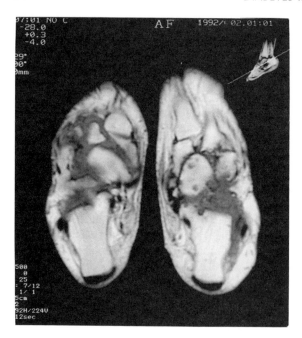

Figure 6.12   Magnetic resonance image of the talus and mid-foot of the patient in Figure 6.11. Note the bilateral Charcot changes. Such changes are often difficult to interpret, even by experienced radiologists

usual treatment. The total-contact cast is usually the method employed, but this requires frequent changes as the oedema reduces. Plaster casting will stabilize the foot; but again, whilst casting reduces activity initially, when the plaster is finally removed after 6–12 months the acute destructive process may restart. Surgical fusion of the joints of the foot in their anatomical positions has usually met with little success during the active phase.

Surgery may still be used, for example to remove a plantar prominence once the process has finally settled (Tom and Pupp 1992; Young 1999a,b). The end of the active phase can be assessed by following skin temperature and radiographic change (Sanders and Frykberg 1991). In the United Kingdom, total-contact casting or bedrest are still the mainstays of treatment. The Scotch-cast boot (Figure 6.6) can also be used to rest the active Charcot foot, and is particularly useful to provide pressure redistribution of a rocker bottom foot with an ulcer at its apex.

As yet there is no definitive treatment aimed at the underlying overactivity of osteoclasts in the active destructive phase of Charcot neuroarthropathy. Two clinical studies, including a randomized placebo-controlled trial, of the use of intravenous pamidronate

(Aredia, Ciba–Geigy) have now been performed in acute Charcot neuroarthropathy. In patients with acute destructive phase Charcot neuroarthropathy, treatment with intravenous bisphosphonate caused a rapid resolution of symptoms and signs, including foot temperature, and a marked improvement in the biochemical markers of bone turnover, particularly alkaline phosphatase concentrations (Selby, Young and Boulton 1994; Jude et al 2000). Such therapy should therefore be considered in addition to the use of rest and casting outlined above.

CONCLUSION

The diabetic foot syndrome is a significant cause of morbidity and mortality in elderly diabetic patients. However, by recognizing the known risk associations, and taking measures to reduce their effect, the incidence of foot ulceration can be significantly reduced. If, in turn, foot ulceration is managed in a systematic and appropriate manner the incidence of amputations because of ulceration can be significantly reduced. This is the ultimate goal in treating diabetic foot problems. Clear evidence of the success of a multidisciplinary approach should lead to its adoption more widely than is currently the case.

REFERENCES

Abbott CA, Carrington AL, Boulton AJM (1996) Reduced bilateral amputation rate in diabetic patients: effect of a foot care clinic. *Diabetic Medicine*, **13** (Suppl. 7), S45.

Barth R, Campbell LV, Allen S, Jupp JJ, Chisholm DJ (1991) Intensive education improves knowledge, compliance, and foot problems in Type 2 diabetes. *Diabetic Medicine*, **8**, 111–117.

Bartlett FF, Gibbons GW, Wheelcock FC (1986) Aortic reconstruction for occlusive disease: comparable results in diabetics. *Archives of Surgery*, **121**, 1150–1153.

Booth J, Young MJ (2000) Differences in performance of commercially available 10 g monofilaments. *Diabetes Care*, **22** in press.

Bossaler C (1987) Impaired muscarinic endothelium dependent relaxation and cyclic guanosine 5'-monophosphate formation in atherosclerotic human coronary artery and rabbit aorta. *Journal of Clinical Investigations*, **79**, 170.

Boulton AJM (1990) Diabetic foot. Neuropathic in origin? *Diabetic Medicine* **7**, 852–858.

Burden AC, Jones GR, Jones R, Blandford RL (1983) Use of the 'Scotchcast boot' in treating diabetic foot ulcers. *British Medicine Journal*, **286**, 1555–1557.

Campbell RR, Hawkins SJ, Maddison PJ, Reckless JPD (1988) Limited joint mobility in the diabetes mellitus. *Annals of the Rheumatic Disease*, **44**, 93–97.

Cavanagh PR, Derr JA, Ulbrecht JS, Maser RE, Orchard TJ (1992) Problems with gait and posture in neuropathic patients with insulin dependent diabetes mellitus. *Diabetic Medicine*, **9**, 469–474.

Cavanagh PR, Sims DS Jr, Sanders LJ (1991) Body mass is a poor predictor of peak plantar pressure in diabetic men. *Diabetes Care*, **14**, 750–755.

Cavanagh PR, Ulbrecht JS, Caputo GM (1998) The non-healing diabetic foot wound: fact or fiction? *Ostomy Wound Management* **44** (3A Suppl.), 6S–12S.

Cavanagh PR, Young MJ, Adams JE, Vickers KL, Boulton AJM (1994) Radiographic abnormalities in the feet of neuropathic diabetic patients. *Diabetes Care*, **17**, 201–209.

Cheshire NJW, Wolfe JHN, Noone MA, Davies BA, Drummond M (1992) The economics of femorocrural reconstruction for critical leg ischaemia with and without autologous vein. *Journal of Vascular Surgery*, **15**, 167–175.

Cofield RH, Morrison MJ, Beabout JW (1983) Diabetic neuroarthropathy in the foot: patient characteristics and patterns of radiographic change. *Foot and Ankle*, **4**, 15–22.

Colwell JA, Halushka PV (1980) Platelet function in diabetes mellitus. *British Journal of Haematology*, **44**, 521–526.

Colwell JA, Lopes-Virella M, Halnshka PV (1981) Pathogenesis of atherosclerosis in Diabetus Mellitus. *Diabetes Care*, **4**, 121–133.

Connolly JF, Jacobsen FS (1985) Rapid bone destruction after a stress fracture in a diabetic (Charcot) foot. *Nebraska Medical Journal*, **70**, 438–440.

Dean MRE (1984) Percutaneous transluminal angioplasty of the popliteal and posterior tibial arteries. In: Vecht RJ (ed) *Angioplasty*. London: Pitman, 34–47.

Delbridge L, Appleberg M, Reeves TS (1983) Factors associated with the development of foot lesions in the diabetic. *Surgery*, **93**, 78–82.

Delbridge L, Perry P, Marr S, Arnold N, Yue DK, Turtle JR, Reeve TS (1988) Limited Joint Mobility in the Diabetic Foot: Relationship to neuropathic ulceration. *Diabetic Medicine*, **5**, 333–337.

Edelman SV, Kosofsky EM, Paul RA, Kozak GP (1987) Neuroosteoarthropathy (Charcot's joints) in diabetes mellitus following revascularisation surgery: three case reports and a review of the literature. *Archives of Internal Medicine*, **147**, 1504–1508.

Edmonds M, Foster A, Greenhill M, Sinha J, Philpott-Howard J, Salisbury J (1992) Acute septic vasculitis not diabetic microangiopathy leads to digital necrosis in the neuropathic foot. *Diabetic Medicine*, **9** (Suppl. 1), 85.

Edmonds ME, Clarke MB, Newton S, Barrett J, Watkins PJ (1985) Increased uptake of bone radiopharmaceutical in diabetic neuropathy. *Quarterly Journal of Medicine*, **57**, 843–855.

Eichenholtz SN (1966) *Charcot Joints*. Springfield, IL: Charles C Thomas.

Estes JM, Pomposelli FB (1996) Lower extremity arterial reconstruction in patients with diabetes mellitus. *Diabetic Medicine*, **13** (Suppl. 1), S43–S57.

Fernando DJS, Hutchison A, Veves A, Gokal R, Boulton AJM (1991) Risk factors for non-ischaemic foot ulceration in diabetic nephropathy. *Diabetic Medicine*, **8**, 223–225.

Fernando DJS, Masson EA, Veves A, Boulton AJM (1991b) Relattionship of limited joint mobility to abnormal foot pressures and diabetic foot ulceration. *Diabetes Care*, **14**, 8–11.

Flynn MD, Tooke JE (1992) Aetiology of diabetic foot ulceration: a role for the microcirculation? *Diabetic Medicine*, **9**, 320–329.

Foster A, McColgan M, Edmonds M (1989). Should oral antibiotics be given to 'clean' foot ulcers with no cellulites? *Diabetic Medicine*, **15** (Suppl. 2), A27 (abstract).

Fryckberg RG (1987) Osteoarthropathy. *Clin Podiatr Med Surg* **4**, 351–376.

Ganda OP (1984) Pathogenesis of accelerated atherosclerosis in diabetes. In: Kozak GP, Hoar CS et al (eds) *Management of Diabetic Foot Problems*. Philadelphia: WB Saunders, pp 17–26.

Gazis A, Macfarlane RM, Jeffcoate WJ (2000) Delay in diagnosis of the Charcot foot. *Diabetic Medicine*, **17** (Suppl. 1), 80.

Gentzkow GD et al (1996) Use of Dermagraft, a cultured human dermis, to treat diabetic foot ulcers. *Diabetes Care*, **19**, 350–352.

Gibbons GW (1994) Vascular surgery: its role in foot salvage. In: Boulton AJM, Connor H, Cavanagh PR (eds). *The Foot in Diabetes*. Chichester: John Wiley, 177–190.

Gibbons GW, Freeman D (1987) Vascular evaluation and treatment of the diabetic. *Clinics in Podiatric Medicine and Surgery*, **4**, 377–381.

Gilmore JE, Allen JA, Hayes JR (1993) Autonomic function in neuropathic diabetic patients with foot ulceration. *Diabetes Care*, **16**, 61–67

Goodfield MJB, Millard LG (1988) The skin in diabetes mellitus. *Diabetologia* **31**, 567–575.

Gruntzig A (1976) Die perkutane Rekanalization chronischer Arterieller Veschlusse (Dotter Princip) mit einem neuen Dilationskatheter. *ROFO*, **124**, 80.

Hiatt WR, Regensteiner JG, Hargaten ME et al (1990) Benefit of exercise conditioning for patients with peripheral arterial disease. *Circulation*, **81**, 602–609.

Hirsch IB, White PF (1988) Medical management of surgical patients with diabetes. In: Levin ME, O'Neal LW (eds) *The Diabetic Foot*. St Louis: CV Mosby, 423–432.

Hunt JA (1992) Foot infections are rarely due to a single microorganism. *Diabetic Medicine*, **9**, 749–752.

Janka HU, Stadl E, Mehnert H (1980) Peripheral vascular disease in diabetes mellitus and its relation to cardiovascular risk factors: screening with Doppler ultrasonic technique. *Diabetes Care*, **3**, 207–213.

Jensen T, Borch-Johnsen K, Kofoed-Enevoldsen A, Deckert T (1987) Coronary heart disease in young Type 1 (insulin-dependent) diabetic patients with and without diabetic nephropathy: incidence and risk factors. *Diabetologia* **30**, 144–148.

Johnson JTH (1967) Neuropathic fractures and joint injuries: pathogenesis and rationale of prevention and treatment. *Journal of Bone and Joint Surgery* **49A**, 1–30.

Jude EB, Selby PL, Donohue M, Foster A, Mawer B, Adams JE, Edmonds ME, Page S, Boulton AJM (2000) Pamidronate in diabetic Charcot neuroarthropathy: a randomised placebo controlled trial. *Diabetic Medicine*, **17** (Suppl. 1), 81.

Juhan-Vague I, Alessi MC, Vague P (1991) Increased plasma plasminogen activator inhibitor 1 levels: a possible link between insulin resistance and and atherosclerosis. *Diabetologia*, **34**, 457–462.

Knowles A, Westwood B, Young MJ, Boulton AJM (1993) A retrospective study to assess the outcome of diabetic ulcers that have been dressed with Granuflex and other dressings. In: *Proceedings of the Joint Meeting of the Wound Healing Society and the European Tissue Repair Society*, Amsterdam, August 1993, P68.

Knowles EA, Kumar S, Veves A, Young MJ, Fernando DJS, Boulton AJM (1992) Essential elements of footcare education are retained for at least a year. *Diabetic Medicine*, **9** (Suppl. 2), S6.

Koziak M (1959) Etiology and pathology of ischaemic ulcers. *Archives of Physical Medicine and Rehabilitation*, **40**, 62–69.

Krupski WC, Reilly LM, Perez S, Moss KM, Crombleholme PA, Rapp JH (1991) A prospective randomized trial of autologous platelet-derived wound healing factors for the treatment of chronic nonhealing wounds: A preliminary report. *Journal of Vascular Surgery*, **14**, 526–536.

Lachman AS, Spray TL, Kerwin DM, Shugoll GI, Roberts WC (1977) Medial calcinosis of Mönckeberg: a review of the problem and a description of a patient with involvement of peripheral, visceral and coronary arteries. *American Journal of Medicine*, **63**, 615–622.

Larkin JG, Frier BM (1986) Limited Joint Mobility and Dupuytrens contracture in diabetic, hypertensive and normal populations. *British Medical Journal*, **292**, 1494.

Lavery LA, Armstrong DG, Harkless LB (1996) Classification of diabetic foot wounds. *Journal of Foot and Ankle Surgery*, **35**, 528–531.

Lesko P, Maurer RC (1989) Talonavicular dislocations and midfoot arthropathy in neuropathic diabetic feet: natural course and principles of treatment. *Clinical Orthopaedics*, **240**, 226.

Levin ME (1988). The diabetic foot: pathophysiology, evaluation and treatment. In: Levin ME and O'Neal LW (eds) *The Diabetic Foot*. St Louis: CV Mosby, 1–50.

Levin S (1992) Digest of current literature. *Infectious Disease in Clinical Practice*, **1**, 49–50.

Levin ME (1998) Classification of diabetic foot wounds. *Diabetes Care*, **21**, 681.

LoGerfo FW, Coffman JD (1984) Vascular and microvascular disease of the foot in diabetes. *New England Journal of Medicine*, **311**, 1615–1619.

Louie TJ, Gartlett JG, Tally FP (1976) Aerobic and anaerobic bacteria in diabetic foot ulcers. *Annals of Internal Medicine*, **85**, 461–463.

Lundbaek K (1957) Stiff hands in long term diabetes. *Acta Medica Scandinavica* **158**, 447–451.

MacFarlane IA, Benbow SJ, Chan AW, Bowsher D, Williams G (1993) Diabetic peripheral neuropathy: the significance of plantar foot temperatures as demonstrated by liquid crystal contact thermography. *Diabetic Medicine*, **10** (Suppl. 1), P104.

Mansell PI, Gregson R, Allison SP (1992) An audit of lower limb angioplasty in diabetic patients. *Diabetic Medicine* **9**, 84–90.

Marshall A, Young MJ, Boulton AJM (1993) The neuropathy of patients with Charcot feet: is there a specific deficit? *Diabetic Medicine*, **10** (Suppl. 1), 101.

Masson EA, Hay EM, Stockley I, Veves A, Betts RP, Boulton AJM (1989) Abnormal foot pressures alone may not cause ulceration. *Diabetic Medicine*, **6**, 426–428.

McAllister FF (1976) The fate of patients with intermittent claudication managed conservatively. *American Journal of Surgery* **132**, 593–595.

McEnery KW, Gilula LA, Hardy DC, Staple TW (1993) Imaging of the diabetic foot. In: Levin ME, O'Neal LW, Bowker JH (eds) *The Diabetic Foot*, 5th edn. St Louis: Mosby Year Books, 341–364.

McKeown KC (1994) The history of the diabetic foot. In: Boulton AJM, Connor H, Cavanagh PR (eds) *The Foot in Diabetes*, 2nd edn. Chichester: John Wiley, 5–14.

Melton LJ, Dyck PJ (1987) Clinical features of the diabetic neuropathies: Epidemiology. In: Dyck PJ, Thomas PK et al (eds) *Diabetic Neuropathy*. Philadelphia: WB Saunders, 27–35.

MJ Young (1999b) The management of neurogenic arthropathy: a tale of two Charcots. *Diabetes and Metabolism Research Review*, **15**, 59–64.

Mueller MJ, Diamond JE, Sinacore DR et al (1989) Total contact casting in treatment of diabetic plantar ulcers. *Diabetes Care*, **12**, 384–388.

Murray HJ, Young MJ, Hollis S, Boulton AJM (1996) The association between callus formation, high pressures and neuropathy in diabetic foot ulceration. *Diabetic Medicine*, **13**, 979–82.

Nillson SE, Lindholm H, Bülow S, Frostberg N, Emilsson T, Stenkula G (1967) The Kristianstad survey 63–64 (Calcifications in arteries of lower limbs). *Acta Medica Scandinavica*, **428** (Suppl.), 1–46.

Orchard TJ, Strandness DE (1993) Assessment of peripheral vascular disease in diabetes. *Diabetes Care*, **16**, 1199–1209.

Palmaz JC, Laborde JC, Rivera FJ (1992) Stenting of the iliac arteries with the Palmaz stent: experience from a multicentre trial. *Cardiovascular Interventional Radiology*, **15**, 291–297.

Pecoraro RE, Ahroni JH, Boyko EJ, Stensel VL (1991) Chronology and determinants of tissue repair in diabetic lower-extremity ulcers. *Diabetes*, **40**, 1305–1313.

Pirart J (1978) Diabetes mellitus and its degenerative complications: a prospective study of 4400 patients observed between 1947 and 1973. *Diabetes Care*, **1**, 168–188.

Pittet D, Wyssa B, Clavel C, Kursteiner K, Vaucher J, Lew PD (1999) Outcome of diabetic foot infections treated conservatively; a retrospective cohort study with long term follow up. *Archives of Internal Medicine*, **159**, 851–856.

Pollard JP, Le Quesne LP (1983) Method of healing diabetic forefoot ulcers. *British Medicine Journal*, **286**, 436–437.

Pomposelli JB, Jepson SJ, Gibbons GW, Campbell DR, Freeman DV, Miller A, LoGerfo FW (1991) A flexible approach to infrapopliteal vein grafts in patients with diabetes mellitus. *Archives of Surgery*, **126**, 724–729.

Porter M. Making sense of dressings. *Wound Management*, **2**, 10–12.

Purewal TS, Goss DE, Watkins PJ, Edmonds ME (1995) Lower limb venous pressure in diabetic neuropathy. *Diabetes Care*, **18**, 377–381.

Rayman G, Willams SA, Spencer PD, Smaje LH, Wise PH, Tooke JE (1986) Impaired microvascular response to minor skin trauma in Type 1 diabetes. *British Medical Journal*, **292**, 1295–1298.

Reiber GE, Pecoraro RE, Koepsell TD (1992) Risk factors for amputation in patients with diabetes mellitus. *Annals of Internal Medicine*, **117**, 97–105.

Rosenbloom AL, Silverstain JM, Lezotte DC, Richardon K, McCallum M (1981) Limited joint mobility in childhood diabetes indicates increased risk for microvascular disease. *New England Journal of Medicine* **305**, 191–194.

Sammarco GJ (1991) Diabetic arthropathy. In: Sammarco GJ (ed) *The Foot In Diabetes*. Philadelphia: Lea and Fabiger.

Sandeman DD, Shore AC, Tooke JE (1992) Relation of skin capillary pressure in patients with insulin-dependent diabetes mellitus to complications and metabolic control. *New England Journal of Medicine*, **327**, 760–764.

Sanders LJ, Frykberg RG (1991) Diabetic neuropathic osteoarthropathy: the Charcot foot. In: Frykberg RG (ed) *The High Risk Foot in Diabetes*. New York: Churchill Livingstone, 297–338.

Selby PL, Young MJ, Boulton AJM (1994) Pamidronate in the treatment of diabetic Charcot neuroarthropathy. *Diabetic Medicine*, **11**, 28–31.

SIGN (1997) *Management of Diabetic Foot Disease*. Edinburgh: SIGN.

Sigurdsson HH, Macaulay EM, McHardy KC, GG Cooper (1999) Long-term outcome of infra-inguinal bypass for limb salvage: are we giving diabetic patients a fair deal? *Practical Diabetes International*, **16**, 204–206.

Sinha S, Munichoodappa CS, Kozak GP. Neuroarthropathy (Charcot joints) in diabetes mellitus. *Medicine (Baltimore)*, **51**, 191–210.

Specialist UK Workgroup Reports (1996) St Vincent and improving diabetes care: report of the Diabetic Foot and Amputation Subgroup. *Diabetic Medicine*, **13** (Suppl 4): S27–S42.

Stipa S, Wheelcock FC (1971) A comparison of femoral artery grafts in diabetic and non-diabetic patients. *American Journal of Surgery*, **121**, 223–228.

Stuart L, Wiles PJ (1993) Knowledge and beliefs towards footcare among diabetic patients: a comparison of qualitative and quantitative methodologies. *Diabetic Medicine*, **9** (Suppl. 2), S3.

Stuart L, Wiles PJ (1993) The influence of a learning contract on levels of footcare. *Diabetic Medicine*, **10** (Suppl 3), S3.

Thomson FJ, Masson EA (1992) Can elderly diabetic patients co-operate with routine foot care? *Age and aging*, **21**, 333–337.

Thomson FJ, Veves A, Ashe H, Knowles EA, Gem J, Walker MG, Hirst P, Boulton AJM (1991) A team approach to diabetic foot care: the Manchester experience. *The Foot*, **1**, 75–82.

Thomson FJ, Masson EA, Boulton AJM (1992) Quantitative vibration perception testing in elderly people: an assessment of variability. *Age and aging*, **21**, 171–174.

Tom RK, Pupp GR (1992) Talectomy for diabetic Charcot foot: an alternative to amputation. *J Am Podiatr Med Assoc* **82**, 447–453.

Uusitupa MIJ (1990) Five year incidence of atherosclerotic vascular disease in relation of general risk factors, insulin level, and abnormalities of lipoprotein composition in non-insulin-dependent and non-diabetic subjects. *Circulation*, **82**, 27–36.

Veves A, Fernando DJS, Walewski P, Boulton AJM (1991) A study of plantar pressures in a diabetic clinic population. *The Foot*, **1**, 89–92.

Veves A, Van Ross ERE, Boulton AJM (1992) Foot pressure measurements in diabetic and non-diabetic amputees. *Diabetes Care*, **15**, 905–907.

Walmsley D, Wales JK, Wiles PG (1989) Reduced hyperaemia following skin trauma: evidence for an impaired microvascular response to injury in the diabetic foot. *Diabetologia*, **32**, 736–739.

Walsh CH, Soler NG, Fitzgerald MG, Malins JM (1975) Association of foot lesions with retinopathy in patients with newly diagnosed diabetes. *Lancet*, **i**, 878–880.

WHO/IDF (1990) Diabetes care and research in Europe: the St Vincent Declaration. *Diabetic Medicine*, **7**, 360.

Young MJ (1998) Capsaicin as topical therapy for painful diabetic neuropathy. *The Diabetic Foot*, **1**, 147–150.

Young MJ (1999a) Becaplermin and its role in healing neuropathic diabetic foot ulcers. *The Diabetic Foot*, **2**, 105–107.

Young MJ (1999b) The management of neurogenic arthropathy–A tale of two Charcots. *Diabetes Metabolism Research and Reviews*, **15**, 59–64.

Young MJ (2000) Classification of ulcers and its relevance to management. In Boulton AJM, Cavanagh PR, Connor H (eds) *The Foot in Diabetes*, 3rd edn. Chichester: John Wiley, in press.

Young MJ, Matthews CF (1998) Screening for neuropathy - can we achieve our ideals. *The Diabetic Foot*, **1**, 22–25.

Young MJ, Cavanagh PR, Thomas G, Johnson MM, Murray H, Boulton AJM (1992) The effect of callus removal on dynamic plantar foot pressures in diabetic patients. *Diabetic Medicine*, **9**, 55–57.

Young MJ, Adams JE, Anderson GF, Boulton AJM, Cavanagh PR (1993a) Medial arterial calcification in the feet of diabetic patients and matched non-diabetic control subjects. *Diabetologia*, **36**, 615–621.

Young MJ, Boulton AJM, Macleod AF, Williams DRR, Sonksen PH (1993b) A multicentre study of the prevalence of diabetic peripheral neuropathy in the United Kingdom hospital clinic population. *Diabetologia*, **36**, 150–154

Young MJ, Breddy JL, Veves A, Boulton AJM (1994) The use of vibration perception to predict diabetic neuropathic foot ulceration: a prospective study. *Diabetes Care*, **17**, 557–560.

Young RJ, Zhou YQ, Rodriguez E, Prescott RJ, Ewing DJ, Clark BF (1986) Variable relationship between peripheral somatic and autonomic neuropathy in patients with different syndromes of diabetic polyneuropathy. *Diabetes*, **35**, 192–197.

7

Erectile Dysfunction

Aaron Vinik, Donald Richardson
Eastern Virginia Medical School

INTRODUCTION

Erectile dysfunction (ED) is defined as the consistent inability to attain and maintain an erection adequate for sexual intercourse, usually qualified by being present for several months and occurring at least half the time. The former term, impotence, while descriptive of the denigrated state many afflicted men feel, has been abandoned in an attempt to lessen the psychologic burden and foster discussion. ED in diabetes is a common and troublesome complication associated with a decreased quality of life and depression, and is a marker of cardiovascular disease and early demise. The prevalence of erectile dysfunction increases with advancing age in both diabetics and non-diabetics; as diabetes is a model of advanced aging, the incidence is increased at any age.

The pathophysiology of ED in diabetes is complex, with major contributions from neuropathy, vasculopathy, and endothelial dysfunction, both vasodilatory and vasoconstrictive. Some lost functions—including hormonal, neural and vasodilatory deficits—can now be replaced, although successful intercourse is not assured. In addition, because of the high incidence of cardiovascular disease, precautions concerning exercise-induced ischemic events may be indicated.

An estimated 10–15 million men in the United States (or over 10%) have ED, while the economic impact on the British economy is estimated in billions of pounds. One in every three men will experience the problem. The prevalence of ED in diabetic men has been estimated to be 35–75%. After the age of 60, 55–95% of diabetic men are affected, compared with approximately 50% in an unselected population in the Massachusetts Aging Male Survey (Vernet et al 1995; Guay, Bansal and Heatly 1995; Figure 7.1). Indeed, diabetes mellitus is frequently the most common single

diagnosis associated with ED during sequential case finding; conversely ED may be the presenting symptom of diabetes and precede and herald the other complications, especially the development of generalized vascular disease and premature demise from coronary artery disease.

PATHOPHYSIOLOGY OF ED IN DIABETES

Physiology of Tumescence and Detumescence

The flaccid penis is restrained by the tonic contraction of the vascular smooth muscle in the cavernosal arterioles and sinusoids under the influence of noradrenergic sympathetic neurons, allowing only a small amount of blood (1–4 mL/100 g tissue) to enter the penis. Penile erection is produced by the relaxation of these vessels combined with restriction of venous return, both of which result in engorgement of the sinusoids. It requires intact arterial blood flow via the iliac, femoral, pudendal, cavernosal and helicene arteries. The cavernosal smooth muscle surrounds a complex vascular network consisting of endothelial cell lined sinuses, or lacunae, and the helicene arteries. The corpora are enclosed by a dense non-distensible fibrous sheath, the tunica albuginea, and communicate with each other via a medial septum. Subtunical vessels pierce this sheath, coalescing to form the emissary veins, which provide the venous drainage of the corpora into the dorsal vein (Figure 7.2).

The autonomic innervation of the penis is (Figure 7.3) mainly from the thoracolumbar sympathetic (T12–L2) and parasympathetic sacral spinal cord segments (S2–S4), while sensory innervation is via the pudendal nerve (S2–S4). In the proper androgenic

Diabetes in Old Age. Second Edition. Edited by A. J. Sinclair and P. Finucane. © 2001 John Wiley & Sons Ltd.

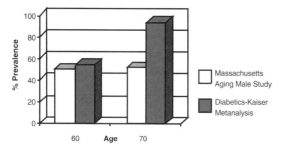

Figure 7.1   Prevalence of ED

milieu, with either psychic or physical stimulation of the brain or genitals, these autonomic nerves are activated releasing cholinergic and non-cholinergic neurotransmitters; simultaneous reduction in adrenergic tone is responsible for the orchestrated vasodilatation of the helicene arteries and relaxation of the cavernosal smooth muscle. Recently it has become apparent that the endothelium plays an important role since cholinergic activation is dependent upon endothelial release of the potent vasodilators nitric oxide (NO) and pros-

taglandin E1 (PGE1). NO relaxes smooth muscle by activating guanyl cyclase. The resulting increased cyclic GMP concentrations reduce calcium influx into the smooth muscle; this is the proximate cause of relaxation. Neuropeptides such as VIP and oxytocin may be released from the nerves per se (Table 7.1). Penile blood flow increases markedly, and sinusoidal filling results in compression of the subtunical vessels, occluding outflow and producing the remaining (critical) engorgement of the corpora. Contraction of the ischiocavernosis muscles increases intracavernosal pressure and adds to the rigidity.

Both penile NO containing neurons and the spinal motor neurons innervating the striated erectile muscles (bulbocavernosus and ischiocavernosus) are androgen-dependent, and in diabetes NO is depressed in direct correlation with testosterone. Thus there appears to be two mechanisms outside the brain, which would support an extralibidinous role for androgens in penile tumescence.

Detumescence is initiated by the sympathetic discharge associated with orgasm and ejaculation. Phos-

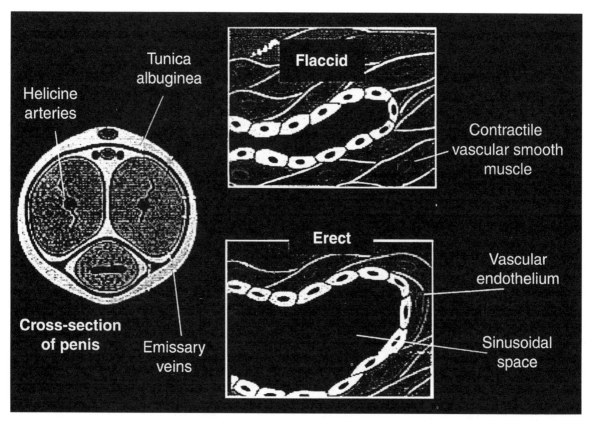

Figure 7.2   Schematic of the anatomic structure of the penis

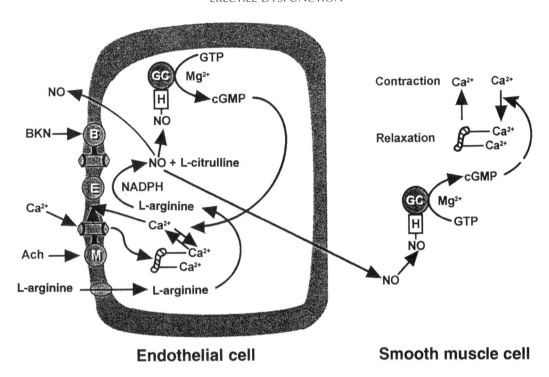

Figure 7.3 Schematic of the interaction between endothelial cells and smooth muscle. GC, guanyl cyclase; cGMP, cyclic guanosine monophosphate; NO, nitric oxide; GTP, guanyl triphosphate; Ach, acetylcholine; BKN, bradykinin

Table 7.1 Autonomic and nonadrenergic/noncholinergic modulators of erectile function

Modulator	Detumescence	Tumescence
Acetylcholine		Yes
Norepinephrine (alpha$_1$-adrenergic)	Yes	
Peptide histidine methionine		Yes
Neuropeptide Y	Yes/No	Yes/No
Somatostatin	Yes/No	Yes/no
Calcitonin gene-related peptide		
Substance P	Yes	
Histamine	Yes	Yes
Vasoactive intestinal peptide		Yes
Prostanoids:		
Prostaglandin E1		Yes
Prostaglandin F2 alpha	Yes	
Thromboxane A2	Yes	
Calcium	Yes	
Endothelin 1	Yes	
Endothelial-derived relaxing factor (NO)		Yes
Prostanoids	Yes	Yes

phodiesterase (isoenzyme 5) reduces cGMP levels and allows the return of calcium. Detumescence is heralded by the return of tone to the cavernosal smooth muscle with reduction of size of the vascular sinuses and release of the compression of the subtunical vessels. This allows the corpora to drain and the penis to return to flaccidity. The major regulator of detumescence is norepinephrine acting via postsynaptic alpha$_1$-adrenergic nerves modulated by presynaptic alpha$_2$-receptor activity. It is for this reason that detumescence can be achieved with infusion of an alpha-adrenergic agonist such as phenylephrine and that erection can be achieved with an alpha-adrenergic blocking drug such as phentolamine. Exceptions to this rule abound and people with severe autonomic adrenergic insufficiency do not have priapism, suggesting once again that there are alternate modulators of corporeal detumescence. A recent candidate is endothelin, a potent smooth muscle contractor, which is elevated in patients with diabetes or vascular disease, and may of itself contribute to ED.

Etiology of ED

The etiology of ED in diabetes is multifactorial and appears to involve any or all of the mechanisms required to produce tumescence, plus iatrogenic and psychogenic factors in some individuals. Neuropathy, especially parasympathetic autonomic, and vascular disease at all levels including endothelial elaboration and sensitivity to the vasodilators, seem to be present in most affected men. Damage to elastic sinusoidal tissue, increased reactive oxidizing substances, and reduced NO production by advanced glycation end-products (AGEs) due to poor glycemic control, have also been shown. Reduced androgen levels due to obesity or illness may contribute but are not limiting in most patients. Complications and concomitant risk factors, including hypertension, hyperlipidemia and depression, and their treatment, all play a role.

The partnership between the sympathetic and para-sympathetic nervous system, the endothelium and smooth muscle function may be disrupted by neuro-pathy and vascular disease, as are common in diabetes. In diabetes the development of autonomic neuropathy is in part responsible for the loss of cholinergic acti-vation via NO and PGs. The association of diabetes with atherosclerosis and microvascular disease further compounds the problem, and recent data indicate that circulating levels of the potent vasoconstrictor, en-dothelin may be increased in diabetes. Thus, ED in diabetes derives from a host of abnormalities, with diabetes and vascular disease together causing 70% of all ED. Other causes—such as multiple sclerosis and kidney disease, surgery and injuries to the penis, prostate, bladder, pelvis and spinal cord, and drugs such as alcohol, medicines, antihypertensing anti-histamines, antidepressants, tranquilizers, appetite suppressants and cimetidine used for peptic ulcer disease—are less frequent offenders. A partial list of particular drug culprits is offered in Table 7.2.

Symptoms and Diagnosis

The symptoms of organic ED are gradual in onset and progress with time. The earliest complaints are de-creased rigidity with incomplete tumescence before total failure. It occurs with all partners and there is no loss of libido. Morning erections are lost. Sudden loss of erections with a particular partner, while maintain-ing morning erections and nocturnal penile tumes-cence, suggest a psychogenic cause. Psychogenic factors may, however, be superimposed on organic dysfunction in diabetes. The neurologic manifestations are those of dysfunction of the autonomic nervous system (ANS) and include constipation, diarrhea, or-thostasis, gustatory sweating, and post-prandial full-ness. ANS dysfunction can be diagnosed simply on the basis of loss of beat-to-beat variation in heart rate with

Table 7.2 Drugs commonly used in diabetic patients and known to cause ED

Antihypertensive agents
Beta-blockers
Thiazide diuretics
Spironolactone
Methyldopa, clonidine, reserpine
Lesser: ACE inhibitors, calcium-channel blockers

Agents acting on the CNS
Phenothiazines
Haloperidol
Tricyclic antidepressants
Selective serotonin reuptake inhibitors (usually ejaculatory delay, but anorgasmia may lead to ED)

Drugs acting on the endocrine system
Estrogens
Antiandrogens
Gonadotropin antagonists
Spironolactone
Cimetidine
Metoclopramide
Fibric acid derivatives
Alcohol, marijuana

deep slow (6 breaths/minute) respiration. Vascular disease is usually manifested by buttock claudication but may be due to stenosis of the internal pudendal artery. A penile/brachial index of < 0.7 indicates diminished blood supply. A venous leak manifests as unresponsiveness to vasodilators and needs to be evaluated by penile Doppler sonography.

Diagnosis of the causes of ED is made by a logical stepwise progression. In all instances a careful history for the rapidity of onset of ED, morning erections, uniformity of sexual dysfunction with all partners, evidence of autonomic nerve dysfunction, vascular insufficiency, hormonal inadequacy, and drugs used in the treatment of satellite disorders must be appraised. Physical examination must include an evaluation of the ANS, vascular supply and the hypothalamic/pituitary gonadal axis. All patients should receive penile injec-tion of a vasodilator intracavernously for diagnostic purposes and choice of therapeutic options. Proble-matic cases should be tested for nocturnal penile tumescence (NPT). Normal NPT defines psychogenic ED and a negative response to vasodilators implies vascular insufficiency.

Relationship of Hypogonadism and Diabetes

Normal gonadal function is required for phenotypi-cally male development of the genital tract, and for maintenance of some elements of male sexual behavior. The most clearly androgen-dependent aspects include libido (sexual interest, appetite or drive), sexual activity, and spontaneous nocturnal or daytime erections. Recent studies also indicate that low normal, (not supernormal or even average) levels of testosterone are required for sexual function. In normal young males rendered hypogonadal with a GnRH antagonist (Nal-Glu), sexual acts, fantasies and desire were significantly diminished, both clinically and statistically (Guay et al 1995). Spontaneous erections also decreased by approximately 40% within 6 weeks of treatment. In this experiment, replacement with testosterone prevented these changes, suggesting that an intact male gonadal system is required to maintain sexual function in men. However, visual, and possibly tactile, stimulus-bound erections are not impaired in men rendered hypogonadal after infancy, implying that androgen action is not required to maintain the capacity for erection. Nonetheless, any deficiency of androgens related to diabetes is of concern for those who provide for patients with erectile dysfunction. Insulin-dependent diabetes has occasionally been associated with hypogonadism. Most cases seem to be due to the hypogonadism of malnutrition and respond to improved control. Likewise, some specific conditions associated with diabetes mellitus—such as hemachromatosis, the Laurence–Moon–Biedl, Alstrom, and Cushing's syndromes—also typically produce hypogonadism, either primary or secondary; but decisions relating to replacement therapy in any of the above are usually easy and unrelated to erectile dysfunction. These will not be considered further here.

The vastly more common Type 2 diabetes seems to be frequently associated with a hypogonadotropic hypogonadism not related to poor control (Barrett-Connor, Khaw and Yen 1990; Andersson et al 1994). This secondary hypogonadism can best be ascribed to the truncal obesity so closely tied to Type 2 diabetes, rather than to the abnormalities of glucose metabolism (e.g. Seidell et al 1990; Khaw, Chir and Barrett-Connor 1992; Tchernof et al 1995). This seems to be due to a lower output of pulsatile GnRH, both in amplitude and frequency of pulses, and consequently of LH (Giagulli, Kaufman and Vermeulen 1994). This decrease in central gonadotropin output has been shown to be mediated by elevated levels of estrogens (estrone and estradiol) produced by the aromatase enzyme found in fat of both sexes, and is derived from adrenal (androstenedione) and testicular (testosterone) androgen. How much this contributes to ED in diabetes is still

uncertain; but it must be recognized and if of sufficient magnitude should be treated.

Physiology of Normal Hypothalamic–Hypophyseal–Testicular Axis

Gonadotropin-releasing hormone (GnRH) pulses, occurring every few hours, stimulate release of pituitary luteinizing (LH) and follicle stimulating (FSH) hormones. LH induces the secretion of testosterone from the Leydig cell (see Figure 7.4) compartment of the testes, while FSH induces spermatogenesis. Feedback is at both pituitary and hypothalamic levels by both androgens and estrogens. The latter result from conversion of androgens by the aromatase enzyme in both testicular and fatty tissue (estradiol (E2) from testosterone). Adrenal androgens, resulting from a separate pituitary axis (ACTH), also contribute androstenedione, a potent androgen, which is also converted to estrone (E1). Inhibin, a peptide hormone, is produced by the Sertoli cells and inhibits FSH.

Pathophysiology of Hypogonadotropic Hypogonadism of Obesity in NIDDM

Increased fat aromatase in adipose tissue converts more androgen (testosterone and androstenedione) to estrogens (E2 and E1, respectively), resulting in greater negative feedback at both central sites. The overall result is diminished gonadotropins with consequent moderate reductions in testosterone secretion.

EVALUATION OF ED

Initial assessment of the patient with ED should be carried out in the presence of the significant other or the sexual partner if possible. An attempt should be made to interview the partner and obtain an impression of the overall relationship and the impact that return of erections will have on the relationship. Extreme care must be exercised in these situations, since in many instances the wish of the male is to be able to have erections and feel more a complete man than the actual desire to have sexual relations. A satisfactory evaluation for ED will include: medical and sexual history; physical and psychological evaluations; blood tests to assess diabetes control, lipid, testosterone, and thyroid hormones (prolactin only if reduced libido or testosterone). More extensive testing for unclear cases would

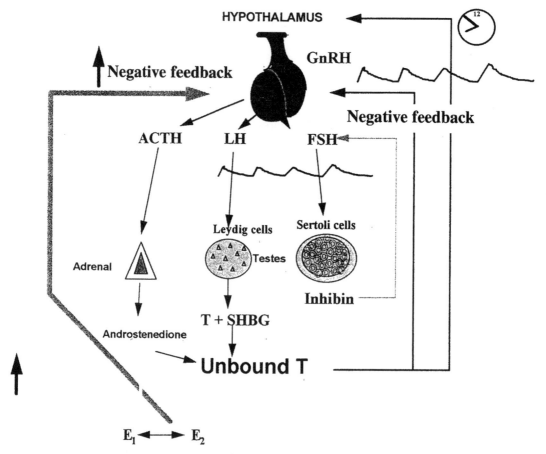

Figure 7.4 Physiology of normal hypothalamic–hypophyseal–testicular axis

include NPT for nocturnal erections (absence of erections during sleep suggests a physical cause of impotence); tests to assess penile, pelvic, and spinal nerve function; and tests to assess penile blood supply and blood pressure.

History

The major problem in history taking for males with ED is that neither the practitioners nor the patients are comfortable with sexually explicit questions. This is all the more regrettable since a careful history will usually lead to the right diagnosis. The use of a questionnaire such as the International Index of Erectile Function provides some objectivity and has been statistically tested as an instrument (Rosen, Riley and Wagen 1995).

It is important to establish the type of problem. For example, is there partial or complete loss of rigidity? Is the problem really one of premature or retrograde ejaculation? The natural sequence in diabetes is for a slow progression from poor quality of the erection culminating often many years later in total failure. There is no loss of libido, which should alert one to the possibility of the presence of an endocrine or psychogenic component. Unlike psychogenic ED (in which the onset is often sudden and maximal ab initio, occurs with a particular partner, and is associated with persistence of morning, nocturnal and reflex erections due to a distended bladder), ED in diabetes affects all partners, with loss of morning, nocturnal or reflex erections, and is progressive. It is therefore important to evaluate past and present relationships. Many patients with psychogenic ED suffer from performance anxiety with a new partner and have often done perfectly well with a long-established partner with whom they have a comfortable relationship.

It must not be forgotten that the health of the partner must be considered when entering into a discussion of sexual function. Deteriorating physical and psychological health of the female companion can wreak havoc with the sexual performance of the male, as can deterioration of the relationship. Performance anxiety and marital disharmony are major causes of ED, which may be neglected if the patient is diabetic. They can perpetuate an organic problem and sabotage treatment if they are not addressed. Depression is rife amongst patients with diabetes, as it is in ED (Shabsigh, Klien and Seidell 1998) especially that complicated by neuropathy, retinopathy and nephropathy; it can place an additional burden on the sexual performance of the male. Illness on the part of the partner can likewise compromise the normal participation in a sexual relationship.

It is important to ascertain whether there has been surgery, trauma or radiation to the pelvis, and especially to inquire after symptoms of prostatism and the ramifications of treatment with surgery, radiation, orchidectomy, long-acting GnRH agonists, and anti-androgens.

A history of sexual development, stages of androgenization (e.g. deepening of the voice, growth of a beard and pubic hair, changes in penile and scrotal development) need to be pursued in younger people with IDDM. Other endocrine conditions associated with ED include hyper- and hypothyroidism, and it is well to ask about heat and cold intolerance.

The association of vascular disease of the penis and generalized vascular disease requires an inquiry into angina, myocardial infarction, strokes, claudication and amputations for vascular insufficiency.

Since a major cause of ED in diabetes is autonomic insufficiency, it behooves one to ask about the major symptom complexes of autonomic neuropathy, such as nausea, vomiting, bloating with meals, constipation, diarrhea, urinary incontinence, dizziness on standing, gustatory sweating and night blindness (or the inability to drive a car at night because of the failure of pupillary adaptation to oncoming headlights).

Physical Examination

The physical examination should establish the level of sexual development, with emphasis on the size of the penis, the maturity of the scrotal sac and the size of the testes. Evidence of virilization should be sought (e.g. the presence of pubic hair, a beard, a thyroid cartilage and deepening of the voice). If hypogonadism is apparent, then absence of sense of smell, in Kallman's syndrome, optic fundus examination, breast exam, measurement of arm span to height ratio as an indicator of hypogonadism, and inspection of the hands for klinedactylly may identify the rarer genetic forms of sexual infantilism such as Laurence–Moon–Biedl syndrome.

Vascular status must be evaluated with measurement of blood pressure, cardiac exam, presence of pulses or bruits over vessels, and if suspicious a penile brachial index measured using Doppler ultrasound. An index < 0.7 suggests significant compromise of penile blood flow.

Lastly and probably most important is a thorough examination of the somatic and autonomic nervous systems (Vinik et al 1996). Autonomic neuropathy causing ED is almost always accompanied by loss of ankle jerks and absence or reduction of vibration sense over the large toes. More direct evidence of impairment of penile autonomic function can be obtained by demonstrating normal perianal sensation, assessing the tone of the anal sphincter during a rectal exam, and ascertaining the presence of an anal wink when the area of the skin adjacent to the anus is stroked, or contraction of the anus when the glans penis is squeezed (the bulbocavernosus reflex). These measurements are easily and quickly done at the bedside and reflect upon the integrity of sacral outflow segments S2, S3 and S4 which represent the sacral parasympathetic divisions. More sophisticated testing of the autonomic nervous system can be done by measuring the change in postural blood pressure and the change in heart rate with deep breathing.

At this point the cause of ED is usually obvious and there is no need for further testing. When there are subtleties in the presentation, hormonal measurement of free testosterone and prolactin as well as gonadotropins and TSH should be made. In most institutions further expensive testing is avoided and the decision is simply to administer oral sildenafil or intracavernous prostaglandin, or suggest a vacuum tumescence device. A normal response to a small dose of intracavernous alprostadil indicates the presence of neuropathy with competent vasculature and at least reasonable vasodilatory capacity. Resistance to the low dose or absence of an erection is compatible with vascular insufficiency and indicates a need to consider higher doses of the intrapenile drugs, vacuum devices or prostheses. Older men are not usually so interested in aggressive treatment, especially those lacking a healthy or interested partner. If aggressive therapy is felt appropriate, and the easier and less invasive measures fail, distinguishing a precise diagnosis using nocturnal penile tumescence (NPT) can be done, either in a sleep lab or with the NPT portable device.

Pharmaco-diagnostic Testing

A breakthrough in the diagnosis of ED was accomplished with the discovery of pharmacologically inducible erection by intracavernosal injection (ICI) of one of the vasoactive compounds: papaverine, papaverine/phentolamine and PGE1 (Junemann and Alken 1989). In patients with psychogenic impotence, erections can be obtained virtually 100% of the time. Similarly in neurogenic impotence, the response to ICI is about 95%. Failure of response implies vascular insufficiency, which can be arterial or venous incompetence. It is not surprising then that patients with diabetes respond about 65–70% of the time, in keeping with a predominantly neurogenic cause of their ED and compatible with a significant arterial component; i.e. a normal erectile response implies normal veno-occlusive function but not necessarily arterial function. A negative response may, however, reflect anxiety in the office setting. To overcome this problem it is advisable on initial ICI testing to administer the drug in the office and allow the patient to go home and report on the degree of ED. Re-dosing is in order with increasing doses to eliminate the refractoriness of people with diabetes because of the arterial element. Simultaneous evaluation of penile blood flow with synchronized pharmaco-penile-duplex ultrasonography (PPDU), cavernosometry and enhancement of the erectile response by genital self-stimulation, vibratory stimulation, visual erotic stimulation or application of a penoscrotal tourniquet, may overcome the element of anxiety and embarrassment. In general, however, this does not apply to people with diabetes who have come to recognize that theirs is principally an organic problem. Prolonged erection tends to occur in young patients and those with psychogenic disorders and does not seem to require a reduction in dose of vasodilators.

Since Gaskell and others introduced Doppler for evaluating penile blood flow it has been combined with pharmacodynamic testing to assess anatomic and functional parameters of ED (Gaskell 1971); but PPDU (Lue et al 1985) has replaced duplex ultrasound as a means of evaluating veno-occlusive function, and pudendal angiography and cavernosometry are second-line tests reserved for patients in whom surgical repair is being considered—for the most part not applicable to the diabetic patient. Cavernosometry is the primary modality available for evaluating veno-occlusive function, but because it is an invasive test it is reserved for those individuals in whom surgical repair is being considered. Veno-occlusive failure usually occurs in younger patients with anatomic abnormalities such as ectopic veins, or abnormal venous communications between the corpora cavernosa and the corpus spongiosum.

TREATMENT OPTIONS

There are in essence three treatment options for the elderly diabetic male with ED: (1) no pharmacological treatment, but hygienic measures including withdrawal from offending medications, perhaps coupled with psychosexual counselling; (2) medical treatment; and (3) surgery.

'No Treatment'

Before considering any form of treatment every effort should be made to have the patient withdraw from drugs liable to promote ED, including alcohol (the Bard pointed out that alcohol enhances the desire but decreases the performance), and eliminate smoking even to the extent of using nicotine substitution therapy. Reconditioning in inactive persons can be suggested (careful, we are discussing elderly diabetics with a high risk of asymptomatic coronary artery disease!), perhaps after an exercise tolerance test. Control of glycemia and dyslipidemia is recommended, if only to avoid further insult to the already deranged tissues.

Choices of antihypertensive medication should be made on the basis of the least offensive agent (Table 7.3) and antidepressant medications can be selected for those with minimal tendency to compromise sexual function (Table 7.4). This decision will usually be made in patients with long-standing disorder who, with the understanding and compassion of the significant other, have given up the thought of sexual relations and have transferred their energies to other avenues of reward. There are also those patients who have serious underlying vascular or other disease, which limits their physical activity, who should not be pursuing the level

Table 7.3 Sexual dysfunction with selected antihypertensive agents

Drug	Percentage of patients with ED	Comments
Thiazide	4–30%	
Spironolactone	3–20%	Dose-dependent; gynecomastia common
Sympatholytics (methyldopa, clonidine, reserpine, guanethidine)	8–80%	Decreased libido
Beta-adrenergic blockers	0–43%	Dose-dependent; lowest with beta$_1$-specific (pindolol, nadolol, atenolol); may occur with eye drops
Alpha-blockers	Minimal	May induce priapism
Labetolol	Minimal	Ejaculatory changes common
ACE inhibitors and antagonists	Minimal	—
Vasodilators (hydralazine, minoxidil)	Minimal	Some patients report aphrodisiac effects of hydralazine
Calcium-channel antagonists	Minimal	—

Table 7.4 Sexual dysfunction with selected antidepressants

Tricyclics	Significant	Also decreased libido; anorgasmia; may be less with desipramine
Selective serotonin reuptake inhbitors	8–16%	Also decreased libido; ejaculatory changes reported
Benzodiazepines	Reported	—

of exertion that is required to generate sexual satisfaction. ED may protect the older male with ischemic heart disease from foolhardy pursuits.

Whatever the decision, it is important to establish the alternative techniques to intercourse the couple have established, and if not to educate them to the possible means of jointly achieving satisfaction despite the ED. In many instances loss of this area of interpersonal reward is simply due to ignorance of the possibilities. Psychosexual counselling is mandatory in these situations. Sexual therapy is vital for people with diabetes since the chronic condition is fraught with situational stresses, performance anxiety and problems in relationships, especially new ones in which the sexual partners have not yet found a happy common ground. Depression is rife in people with diabetes and its chronic complications, and attention must be given to counselling and if necessary pharmacological management of the depression which may enhance sexual performance in its own right.

The development of ED may severely affect compliance with a drug regimen, and all men placed on antihypertensive medications should be counselled in this regard. The prevalence of ED may range from 9% in patients on diuretics to 30% in patients on combination drugs. Thus, in hypertensive patients a rise in blood pressure should lead to the suspicion that he has stopped taking his medication because of the loss of potency!

Medical Treatment

A number of drugs have been shown to have some measure of success in men with diabetes and ED. First and foremost the patient should be removed if possible from drugs that are known to cause ED (Table 7.2).

Erectogenic Drugs

Yohimbine and trazodone, alpha$_2$-antagonist and 5HT agonists respectively, have a long history of use for ED but have been shown to be ineffective.

Sildenafil, the phosphodiesterase Type 5 inhibitor, has been available for some years. It has been a huge financial and therapeutic success, having been given to upwards of 4 million men in the US alone. It has demonstrated reasonable efficacy and safety in men with diabetes. Sildenafil prevents breakdown of cGMP and so prolongs/improves smooth muscle relaxation. It does require that NO be released first to stimulate cGMP production; as noted above this can be a particular problem in diabetes owing to endothelial dysfunction. Sildenafil has been evaluated in men over 65 years of age. While not as effective as in those less than 65 (67% versus 75% improved erections), it is vastly superior to placebo (17%). Side-effects are generally infrequent and well tolerated; these include headache (16%), flushing (10%), dyspepsia, and nasal congestion. It is metabolized by, and is a weak inhibitor of, cytochrome P450 3A4, so that some drug interactions have been identified (potentiation of calcium-channel blockers, 'statins' etc.).

Because nitric oxide donors such as nitrates, either short- or long-acting, can produce severe hypotension when administered to patients taking sildenafil, patients on nitrates or who will probably require them for treatment of CAD should not be treated with the drug. In part because of this concern, and also because of media reporting, some concern about safety of use in men with ED and the attendant CVD risk factors (age and diabetes in this case) has been raised. Post-marketing data in nearly 5000 patients showed no increased death rate compared with placebo (0.53 deaths/10 patient-years versus 0.57/10 patient-years on placebo). Nonetheless, warnings are appropriate for patients on nitrates which are clearly contraindicated, and for other patients in whom sildenafil is potentially hazardous. These include men with active coronary ischemia not on nitrates (e.g. positive exercise test), men with congestive heart failure and lowish blood pressure, patients on complicated medical regimens which may result in drug interactions, and patients on drugs which are potent inhibitors of P450 3A4 such as erythromycin and cimetidine (Cheitlan, Hutter and Brindis 1999). We must remember that these patients are highly likely to have undiagnosed CAD due to multiple risk factors. Even in the general population there is an increased risk for MI during the 2 hours after sexual activity. This is a relative risk 2.5 times that during other periods but still an absolutely low risk (one chance in a million) of triggering myocardial infarction by sexual activity. (Muller, Mittleman and Maclure et al 1996).

Apomorphine is a short-acting dopamine receptor agonist that has been used in a sublingual form as a central dopamine agonist to enhance erectile capability. Acting proximally to the penis it may enhance neurotransmitter and NO release, and may therefore synergize with sildenafil. Apomorphine successfully induced erection in one-half of the patients tested in a very small series (Lal et al 1989), but more research is needed to establish a place for the agent. Side-effects relate to its emetic properties. Although tentatively approved in the US, problems with nausea and nausea-induced vasovagal syncope (with one case of skull fracture) are worrisome.

Phentolamine, while apparently available for oral therapy in Mexico, and with some evidence of efficacy (Goldstein et al 1998), does not appear to be coming to

market for oral use in the near future. This alpha-blocker is discussed below in its established role of intracavernous therapy.

Androgens. While there are many reasons to replace androgens in hypogonadal men other than as correction of erectile dysfunction (Bondil 1992), most patients seeking assistance in this regard are not worried about bone density, hand-grip strength, or hematocrit. Unfortunately, the track record for testosterone replacement therapy in diabetic patients, who if hypogonadal most frequently fall into the category of obesity-related secondary hypogonadism as discussed above, is not stellar. Direct replacement with fortnightly testosterone enanthate (200 mg IM) improved long-term sexual function in only 17% of 78 obese NIDDM patients. Correction of the underlying excess estrogenic feedback of the obesity using clomiphene citrate, allowing total and free testosterone to rise to normal, did not produce any meaningful improvement in subjective and objective measures of sexual activity. Finally, in the experiment alluded to earlier, in which normals underwent suppression of the HPT axis using GnRH antagonists, replacement with testosterone in doses producing subnormal concentrations (8.9 pM) allowed normal sexual function, suggesting that normal levels are well above that required to maintain sexual function in men (Barrett-Connor et al 1990). Similar levels are typical of those seen in obese males, which predicts that their testosterone concentrations are adequate to support libido and erections; thus no major improvement would be expected with hormone augmentation.

While the exact degree of erectile function, which is androgen-dependent, remains uncertain, androgen replacement therapy does provide a return to normal sexual function for many hypogonadal men with or without diabetes mellitus. In hypo- or hyper-gonadotropic hypogonadal men, testosterone given by any of several routes results in a two- to three-fold increase in measures of nocturnal penile tumescence and sexual activity (Bondil 1992). Clearly, therefore, any deficiency of androgens related to diabetes is of concern for those who provide for patients with erectile dysfunction.

The use of androgens in men with normal testosterone levels is not recommended, but replacement therapy for those with a documented low level of testosterone may be worth a trial, especially if in addition to the ED the patient has loss of libido. Administration of androgens to people with ED and normal gonadal function is usually not beneficial (Hubert 1990; Guay et al 1995; Bondil 1992). In normal young men or older men with prostate cancer, suppression of testosterone by GnRH agonists to the range associated with castration reduces spontaneous erections by up to 90%. ED is not a universal feature, as it has been known since the time of Caesar that some male castrates remain potent.

Care must be exercised in any patient, but especially the elderly diabetic, before testosterone is given. Absence of prostatic hypertrophy and cancer with levels of PSA < 2 unit/ML is required. Other precautions that need to be taken are the ability of testosterone to increase RBC mass, occasionally precipitating congestive heart failure in those at risk, or stroke. Another possible caveat for the use of androgens is with an established lipid disorder; for example the high triglycerides and low HDL-C levels in NIDDM may be accentuated by the androgen and require modification of drug therapy for the dyslipidemia to avoid increasing the risk of a macrovascular event. There are, however, several studies that suggest that androgens may actually improve lipoprotein profiles or, at least not cause worsening (Bondil 1992). It probably is wise, nonetheless, to at least determine the lipoprotein profile before and 6 months after starting treatment with an androgen.

Androgens that can be used are long- or short-acting and can be given by the transcutaneous route as Testoderm or Androderm. The older version of the former (scrotal patch) should be avoided, as it requires shaving the scrotum to allow adherence to the skin and produces higher levels of DHT (dihydrotestosterone; responsible for lowering HDL cholesterol and stimulating the prostate). Favored IM androgens are those without a methyl group and include testosterone cypionate and enanthate. Doses do vary with the individual and the degree of insufficiency fortnightly and 100–200 mg fortnightly initially can be tailored to the patients' needs. Patients can usually sense whenever the drug is wearing off in anything from 2 weeks to a month, and the frequency of dosing be adjusted according to libido and general well-being and strength. Oral testosterone undecanoate is popular in Europe but not available in the USA. Topical testosterone cream (Androgel) should be available in the immediate future, and should, like the patches, provide more stable levels of testosterone. Elderly men or those with some enlargement of the prostate should be treated initially with a lower dose (e.g. 50 mg every 14 days). Serum levels of testosterone do decline with age and may

contribute to the loss of libido, muscle strength and mass, and preliminary studies suggest that androgen therapy may restore lean body mass, muscle strength, libido and decrease bone turnover. There cannot, however, be justification for treating older people with androgens simply on the basis of these possible benefits without clear documentation of hypogonadism.

Patients with low or inappropriately normal gonadotropins in the face of low testosterone levels—i.e. those with secondary hypogonadism due to obesity (no pituitary tumor)—may undergo a trial of therapy, as long as the prostate exam, PSA, or voiding symptoms do not preclude treatment. If, as usual, minimal long-term benefit is shown, the trial can be discontinued in 6–12 weeks, unless other compelling reasons, such as osteoporosis, mandate permanent treatment.

Self-injection Therapy

Over the past decade there have been a number of reports on the use of intracavernosal treatment of ED with a wide variety of drugs. These include the smooth muscle relaxants papaverine and glyceryl trinitrate; alpha-adrenergic blockers phenoxybenzamine and phentolamine; the calcium antagonist verapamil; polypeptides; the beta-adrenergic agonists isoprenaline; antipsychotics/antidepressants trazodone and chlorpromazine; prostaglandins (Chaudhuri and Wiles 1995). Of these the vasoactive agents papaverine, phentolamine and prostaglandin E1 (PGE_1) are currently in use. These vasoactive substances stimulate the natural erectile process by inhibiting sympathetic tone and relaxing corporeal smooth muscle. Alprostadil and papaverine relax the smooth muscle of the corpora cavernosa, and phentolamine is a competitive inhibitor of alpha-adrenergic receptors. The major problem with papaverine is corporeal fibrosis, which may resemble a Peyronie's type deformity and is usually the result of repeated injections. Systemic adverse events include vasovagal reactions with bradycardia, hypotension, dizziness and flushing. These are uncommon and can be treated with atropine. Complications include local infections, hematomas and pain; occasionally systemic effects with abnormalities of liver functions are encountered, which revert with discontinuation of the drug. Because of the vascular cross-communication between the corporal bodies, injection into one causes bilateral tumescence.

Alprostadil is a prostaglandin (E_1) derived from polyunsaturated fats and is naturally occurring in the body. It has been shown to have alpha-adrenergic blocking properties, dilating blood vessels, and it relaxes smooth muscle directly via a prostacyclin receptor. A number of studies have now reported on the effects of alprostadil in diabetic patients. In one study of 577 men, 69% completed the 6-month study and 87% reported that their sexual activity was satisfactory. However, of the 31% who did not complete the study, pain or lack of efficacy were prominent complaints. Of the 683 men tested, 50% had pain of some degree. The commonly used mixture is alprostadil, papaverine and phentolamine, commonly referred to as 'trimix'. Although urologists have used these drugs for a decade or more, the FDA only approved alprostadil for this use in 1995. While pain may be more frequent with alprostadil than the mixture, the incidence of prolonged erection (5%) and priapism (1%) are rare and make it the drug of choice. A more recent $alpha_1$-antagonist for intracavernosal injection, moxisylate, is effective in improving erections 90% of the time, with 50% of these erections suitable for penetration (Costa and Motter 1995). There have been recent attempts to solve this problem with the introduction of an intra-urethral suppository system using alprostadil (MUSE) (Padma-Nathan et al 1995; (Kim and McVary 1995). As successful as intracavernous therapy had become up to 50% of men discontinue eventually because of pain, loss of effect, or lack of interest (Lakin et al 1990; Gerber and Levin 1991).

Indications for self-injection therapy. Ideal candidates for self injection therapy are lean individuals, with recent onset of ED, who seek help, in whom the cause is predominantly neuropathic, who are not on anticoagulants and in whom the relationship with the significant other is such that no extra burden is placed upon the relationship by the need to introduce the new form of foreplay. Both parties must clearly be agreeable before embarking on the pursuit. It is also useful during the course of the physical exam, to pinch the side of the penis as a forewarning of what to expect when the injection is given.

The most effective and well-studied agents are papaverine, phentolamine and prostaglandin. Priapism is most frequently seen with papaverine. Treatment of priapism with an oral adrenergic agent such as pseudorphedrine can be tried, followed by intracavernosal noradrenaline in case of failure, but can be hazardous in those receiving monoamine-oxidase inhibitors. Use of penile vasodilators can also be problematic in those patients who cannot tolerate transient hypotension;

who have severe psychiatric disease; who have poor manual dexterity; who have poor vision; or who are taking anticoagulants. Liver function should be checked in those on papaverine. Prostaglandin can be used to decrease the side-effects such as pain, corporeal fibrosis, fibrotic nodules, hypotension and priapism. The drugs are contraindicated in those people with gross obesity and those taking anticoagulants.

The skin should be cleansed properly and the index and middle fingers should occlude the venous drainage by squeezing in an inverted V at the base of the penis. The injection is then given through a 25–27-gauge insulin-type needle laterally to avoid injection into the dorsal vein or the urethra. Massage of the penis enhances action of the erection. The first injection is always given in the consulting room and allows for dose titration if necessary and for treatment of any complications such as prolonged erection or priapism. The patient can then be instructed on dose escalation and the use of enhancing procedures. Application of a constriction band to the base of the penis can enhance the quality of the erection, while some people require provocative visual images to elicit an appropriate response. The quality of the erection is almost always better in the home as opposed to the inhibiting circumstances found in most ambulatory care settings.

Men must be warned to call immediately if an erection persists for longer than 4 hours. The patient should also receive written instructions of what to do under the circumstances so that another doctor can administer the treatment if necessary. Simple measures such as immersion in a cold bath or exercising may be effective. Oral pseudoephedrine has been used to deflate priapetic penes successfully. If this fails, decompression can be achieved by injecting an alpha-adrenergic agonist such as metaraminol or phenylephrine; and if this fails, 20–300 mL of blood can be withdrawn from the corpus cavernosum.

Vacuum Devices

When medical treatment fails, vacuum tumescence devices will work irrespective of the cause of the ED. Erection is induced by negative pressure drawing blood into the corpora and retaining the blood by application of a constriction band to the base of the penis and obstructing the venous drainage. The apparatus consists of a plastic cylinder to which a vacuum pump is attached. The constriction band is made of soft transparent silicone rubber and is rolled over the cylinder and left in place at the base of the penis during intercourse. Care must be taken to place the band at the base of the penis so as to avoid a constriction band and a rigid penis pivoting around a lax base. The band should not be left in place for more than 30 minutes.

Some complain that the penis feels cold, or that they have pain with ejaculation. Most find the technique highly acceptable, especially those who have tried injection therapy without success. Partners can often be enticed into treating the application of the device as a form of sexual play before intercourse, and the successful couples invariably have learned to add this element to their sexual relations.

Surgery for ED

Penile prostheses

There are three varieties of prosthetic devices that have been used for those who fail medical therapy: semirigid, malleable and inflatable. The semirigid or malleable rods are implanted into the corpora cavernosa, but leave the penis constantly erect. This is no handicap for some but for most it constitutes an embarrassing situation when wearing shorts or a bathing suit. A possible solution to the problem is the use of an inflatable prosthesis, whereby the pump is housed in the scrotal sac and the inflatable portion is placed in the corpora. These are surgical procedures that require general anesthesia. The main problems are mechanical failure, infection and erosions. Men with diabetes (and spinal cord injuries or urinary tract infections) have an increased risk of prosthesis-associated infection, which in most instances requires removal of the device. Before the advent of injection therapy the authors were enthusiastic about the use of penile prostheses, but with vacuum therapy and penile injection now freely available we almost never insert a prosthesis.

Revascularization

While the great majority of patients with diabetes have ED secondary to autonomic neuropathy, there remains a proportion of people with severely compromised blood flow. The tests outlined above used to establish the diagnosis have been incompletely validated: therefore it is difficult to select patients with a predictable good outcome. If vascular insufficiency is documented then the inferior artery can be anastomosed to the dorsal artery of the penis or the deep cavernosal artery. When venous incompetence prevails then venous leakage can be treated by ligation of the deep dorsal vein of the penis and circumflex arteries. These procedures unfortunately are frequently unsuccessful owing to associated problems such as neuropathy, failure of endothelial vasodilator production, etc.; and the severity and extent of vascular disease in diabetics renders revascularizing procedures less successful (Wiles 1992). The only person the authors would now contemplate for revascularization is the individual who is young, with recent-onset diabetes, in whom it is likely that fairly localized insufficiency is at the root of the ED. In general, older patients with diabetes have diffuse extensive vascular disease in the pelvis with marked calcification of the pudendal vessels, making them poor candidates for an arterial anastomosis.

Possible New Treatments for ED

Combination therapy using intraurethral alprostadil combined with prazocin, an alpha$_1$-antagonist, or with the rings from vacuum retention devices, have been successful in 68% and 75% respectively. These studies are neither masked nor peer-reviewed trials and further research is clearly ongoing. Non-prescription use of the NO donor arginine, in very large quantities (16 grams/day orally) has had similar results in a similar trial. Topical alprostadil as a gel for the glans penis is under investigation.

What is the potential for reversing neuropathy, the major cause of ED in the patient with diabetes? There are exciting developments on the horizon for the use of aldose reductase inhibitors, linolenic acid and aminoguanidine. The agents may overcome the impact of metabolic abnormalities in diabetes that have not been prevented by glycemic control, and show promise for reversing established neuropathy. Aminoguanidine is expected to inhibit the production of AGEs. Various growth factors; such as nerve growth factor (NGF) and neurotropin 3 (NT3), are capable of causing nerve regeneration of autonomic nerves, thereby restoring the normal physiologic regulation of erection; their use remains unfulfilled (Vinik et al 1995).

SUMMARY

ED is nearly universal in older diabetic men and is associated with decreased life satisfaction and self-esteem. It is also associated with multiple risk factors for coronary heart disease, including insulin resistance, dyslipidemia and hypertension. Discussion of this topic should be attempted with every male patient. Treatment should be directed at the underlying cause. Hormonal abnormalities should be corrected, but that alone may not be the answer. Drugs should be changed to those with no (or a lower) potential for ED, and glycemic control should be optimized. For psychogenic dysfunction the patient should be referred to a therapist with expertise in treating sexual dysfunction. Patients responsive to sildenafil (above 70% in nonorganic cases, lower in elderly diabetics but still a good first-line choice) have this, and misaprostil urethral suppositories and intracavernous injections as therapeutic options. Those who are unresponsive usually have vascular disease and require prostheses or vascular surgery. No attempt should ever be made to treat ED without first consulting the significant other, and careful thought about the risk/benefit ratio for all the pharmacological and surgical therapies is very appropriate.

REFERENCES

Andersson B, Marin P, Lissner L, Vermeulen A, Bjorntorp P (1994) Testosterone concentrations in women and men with NIDDM. *Diabetes Care*, **17**, 405–411.

Barrett-Connor E, Khaw KT, Yen SSC (1990) Endogenous sex hormones in older adult men with diabetes mellitus. *American Journal of Epidemiology*, **132**, 895–901.

Bondil P (1992) The combination of oral trazodone-moxisylyte. Diagnostic and therapeutic value in impotence: report of 110 cases. *Progress in Urology*, **2**, 671–674.

Chaudhuri A, Wiles P (1995) Optimal treatment of erectile failure in patients with diabetes. *Drugs*, **49**, 548–554.

Cheitlan M, Hutter A, and Brindis R (1999) Use of sildenafil in patients with cardiovascular disease. *Journal of the American College of Cardiology*, **33**, 273–282.

Costa P and Motter N (1995) Efficiency and side-effects of moxisylate in impotent patients: a double-blind, placebo-controlled study. *Proceedings of the American Urological Association*, **153**, 147A.

Gaskell P (1971) The importance of penile blood pressure in cases of impotence. *Canadian Medical Association Journal*, **105**, 1047.

Gerber GS, Levin LA (1991) Pharmacological erection program using prostaglandin E-1. *Journal of Urology*, **146**, 786–789.

Giagulli VA, Kaufman JM, Vermeulen A (1994) Pathogenesis of decreased androgen levels in obese men. *Journal of Clinical Endocrinology and Metabolism*, **79**, 1310–1316.

Goldstein, I and the Vasomax Study Group (1998) Efficacy and safety of oral phentolamine (Vasomax) for the treatment of minimal erectile dysfunction. In: *Annual Meeting of the American Urological Association*, **919**, (abstract).

Guay AT, Bansal S, Heatly GJ (1995) Effect of raising endogenous testosterone levels in impotent men with secondary hypogonadism: double blind placebo-controlled trial. *Journal of Clinical Endocrinology and Metabolism*, **80**, 3546–3552.

Hubert W (1990) Psychotropic effects of testosterone. In: Nieschlag EB, Behre HM, (eds) *Testosterone: Action, Deficiency, Substitution*. Berlin: Germany, Springer-Verlag, p 51–71.

Junemann KP, Alken P (1989) Pharmacotheraphy of ED: a review. *International Journal of Impotence Research*, **1**, 71.

Khaw KT, Barrett-Connor E (1992) Lower endogenous androgens predict central adiposity in men. *American Journal of Epidemiology*, **2**(5), 675–682.

Kim ED, McVary KT (1995) Topical prostaglandin-E_1 for the treatment of erectile dysfunction. *Journal of Urology*, **153**, 1828–1830.

Lakin MM, Montague DK, VanderBrug-Medendorp S, Tesar L, Schover LR (1990) Intracavernous injection therapy: analysis of results and complications. *Journal of Urology*, **143**, 1138–1141.

Lal S, Tesfaye Y, Thavandayil JX, et al (1989) Apomorphine: clinical studies on erectile impotence and yawning. *Progess in Neuropsychopharmacological and Biological Psychiatry*, **13**, 329–339.

Lue TF, Hricak R, Marich KW, et al (1985) Vasculogenic impotence evaluated by high-resolution ultrasonography and pulsed Doppler analysis. *Radiology*, **155**, 777.

Muller J, Mittleman A, Maclure M (1996) Triggering myocardial infarction by sexual activity. *JAMA*, **275**, 1405–1409.

Padma-Nathan H, Bennett A, Gesundheit N, et al (1995) Treatment of erectile dysfunction by the medicated urethral system for erection (MUSE). *Journal of Urology*, **153**, 472A (abstract).

Rosen R, Riley A, and Wagner, G (1995) A multidimentional scale for the assessment of erectile dysfunction. *Urology*, **46**, 697–706.

Seidell JC, Bjorntorp P, Sjostrom L, Kvist H, Sannerstedt R (1990) Visceral fat accumulation is positively associated with insulin, glucose and C-peptide levels but negatively with free testosterone levels. *Metabolism*, **39**, 897–901.

Shabsigh R, Klien L, and Seidman, S (1998) Increased incidence of depressive symptoms in men with ED. *Urology*, **52**, 848–853.

Tchernof A, Despres JP, Belanger A, Dupont A, Prud'homme D, Moorjani S, Lupien PJ, Labrie F (1995) Reduced testosterone and adrenal C19 steroid levels in obese men. *Metabolism*, **44**, 513–519.

Vernet D, Cai L, Garbin H, Babbit ML, Murray FT, Fajfer J, Gonzales-Cadavid NF (1995) Reduction of penile nitrogen oxide synthase in diabetic BB/WOR (Type I) and BBZ/WOZ (Type II) rats with erectile dysfunction. *Endocrinology*, **136**, 5709–5717.

Vinik AI, Newlon PG, Lauterio TJ, Liuzzi FJ, Depto AS, Pittenger GL, Richardson DW (1995) Nerve survival and regeneration in diabetes. *Diabetes Reviews*, **3**, 139–157.

Vinik AI, Suwanwalaikorn S, Holland MT, Liuzzi FJ, Colen LB, Stansberry KB (1996) Diagnosis and management of diabetic autonomic neuropathy. In: DeFronzo RA, (ed). *Current Management of Diabetes Mellitus*. St Louis, Mosby-Year Book, Inc. (in press).

Wiles PG (1992) Erectile impotence in diabetic men: aetiology, investigation and management. *Diabetic Medicine*, **9**, 888–892.

8

Mortality and its Predictors
in Type 2 Diabetes

M. Muggeo, G. Zoppini, E. Brun, E. Bonora, G. Verlato
University of Verona

INTRODUCTION

Type 2 diabetes mellitus in elderly patients has been considered in the past a relatively benign condition with a small effect on life expectancy. More recently, it has become evident that this condition must be taken as seriously as in younger patients (Morley 1998). Type 2 diabetes mellitus is not only an established cardiovascular risk factor, but it should be considered a cardiovascular disease itself with heavy implications in cardiovascular pathophysiology (Grundy et al 1999). This emerging concept is based primarily on population studies that explored the relation between diabetes and cardiovascular diseases (Haffner et al 1990; Stamler et al 1993; Wilson 1998; Lehto et al 2000; Lowel et al 2000).

The onset of Type 2 diabetes, often asymptomatic, is easily overlooked and this causes a delay in diagnosis (Harris 1992), which may worsen the outcome especially in elderly subjects (De Fronzo 1992; Cook et al 1996). Indeed, in these patients diabetes is sometimes revealed by hyperosmolality in the context of an acute disease, such as myocardial infarction or pneumonia, and contributes to an increase in the in-hospital mortality rate. In the elderly, there is a sort of 'hyperglycaemia unawareness' owing to the general belief that hyperglycaemia in this age is almost a 'physiological abnormality', not associated with chronic complications (Muggeo 1998). Instead, this disease is a critical health problem in the elderly for two main reasons: first, its prevalence increases with age and reaches of about 12% after 65 years (Figure 8.1) (Muggeo et al 1995a); and second, in western populations the proportion of elderly subjects is progressively growing (Harris et al 1987). The large majority ($\geq$95%) of elderly diabetic patients have Type 2 diabetes mellitus (Travia et al 1991; Cacciatori et al 1991; Muggeo et al 1995a).

With the current trend, it has been estimated that in the near future the number of elderly diabetic patients will consistently increase. This will require a large proportion of the available resources (Weinberges et al 1990). The most common outcome of Type 2 diabetic patients, regardless of age, is a fatal or non-fatal vascular complication in the form of coronary artery disease, peripheral vascular disease or stroke (Laakso 1996; Lehto et al 1996).

The aim of this chapter is to summarize the present knowledge, based also on personal research (the Verona Diabetes Study, VDS), regarding the assessment of the mortality risk profile in elderly Type 2 diabetic patients, and to show how this profile changes on going from middle to old age.

MORTALITY

Diabetes mellitus increases mortality risk and reduces life expectancy. Accordingly, Figure 8.2 shows that diabetic patients from Verona experienced higher mortality rates than the general population at all ages (Muggeo et al 1995a).

When the excess mortality related to diabetes is measured by the standardised mortality ratio (SMR), the adverse effects of diabetes appears to be inversely related to both actual age and age at diagnosis (Table 8.1). In the Verona study the SMR ranged between 2 and 3.5 in middle-aged diabetic subjects, was around 1.75 in patients aged 65–74 years, and declined, although remaining above unity, in patients older than 75

Diabetes in Old Age. Second Edition. Edited by A. J. Sinclair and P. Finucane. © 2001 John Wiley & Sons Ltd.

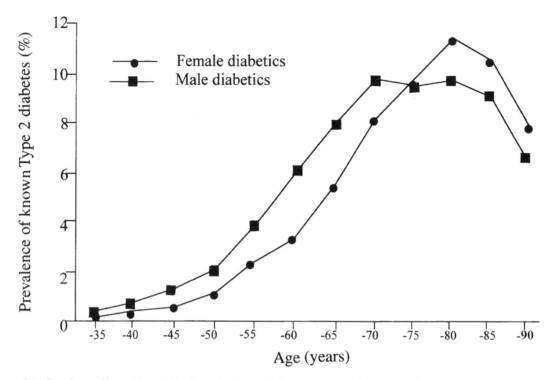

Figure 8.1 Prevalence of known Type 2 diabetes in the Verona Diabetes Study, according to sex and age

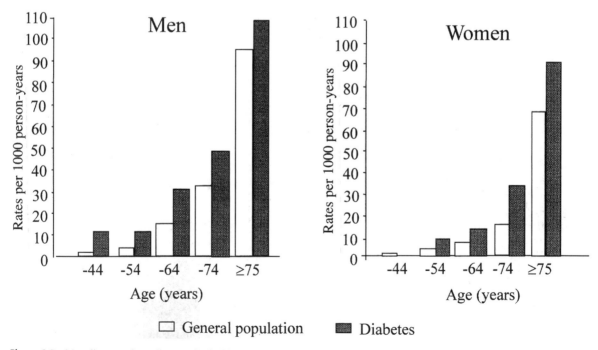

Figure 8.2 Mortality rates from all causes in the Verona Type 2 diabetic population, as compared with the general population of Verona, according to sex and age

Table 8.1 Mortality in the Verona diabetic cohort as a function of actual age and age at diagnosis

	Male	Female
Actual age (years)		
45–54	2.33 (1.38–3.69)	3.43 (1.43–6.77)
55–64	2.13 (1.76–2.56)	2.33 (1.63–3.22)
65–74	1.50 (1.30–1.72)	2.27 (1.92–2.66)
≥ 75	1.13 (1.00–1.28)	1.32 (1.20–1.44)
Age at diagnosis (years)		
35–44	1.79 (1.30–2.40)	2.65 (1.68–3.97)
45–54	1.37 (1.14–1.64)	1.79 (1.43–2.22)
55–64	1.20 (1.01–1.40)	1.27 (1.08–1.47)
65–74	1.23 (1.02–1.47)	1.34 (1.16–1.54)
≥ 75	1.10 (0.73–1.59)	1.52 (1.20–1.90)

Table 8.2 Comparison of relative risk of all-cause mortality in Type 2 diabetc patients

Authors	Country	Age (yr)	RR
Zwaag et al (1983)	US	45–54	2.07
		55–64	1.57
		65–74	1.26
		≥ 75	1.07
Waugh et al (1989)	UK	45–64	2.3
		65–74	1.7
		≥ 75	1.3
Ford and DeStefano (1991)	US	45–64	3.9
		65–74	2.4
		≥ 75	1.8
Wong et al (1991)	UK	45–64	3.0
		65–74	1.6
		≥ 75	0.9
Muggeo M (1995a)	Italy	45–54	2.6
		55–64	2.2
		65–74	1.8
		≥ 75	1.25
Gu et al (1998)	US	45–64	2.2
		65–74	1.5
Bruno et al (1999)	Italy	≤ 60	2.62
		60–69	1.86
		70–79	1.37
		≥ 80	1.12

years (Figure 8.3). This trend has been confirmed to a large extent by other investigations (Table 8.2). However, it is still controversial whether the effect of diabetes on mortality persists in patients aged over 75, as some studies found an SMR close to or below unity.

When the excess mortality is expressed as the absolute difference between mortality rates, which is more suited to estimating the burden of diseases for society, the largest impact of diabetes on mortality is often observed in the age group 65–74 years (Figure

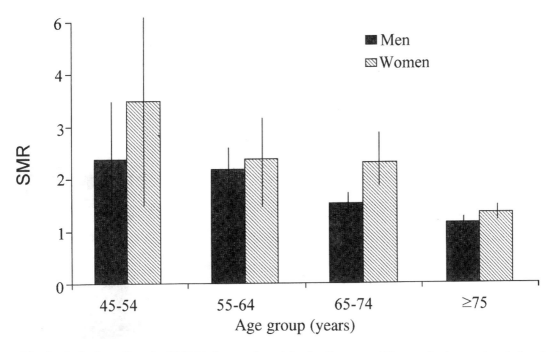

Figure 8.3 Standardized mortality ratios (SMRs) to the general population for all-cause mortality, according to sex and age in the cohort of Type 2 diabetic patients of Verona

8.2). Thus, healthcare planners should bear in mind that even a small percentage reduction in the mortality rate in this age range can eventually prolong the survival of many patients (Fullet et al 1983; Muggeo et al 1995a; Sinclair, Robert and Croxson 1997).

The age modulation of the excess mortality due to diabetes could partly explain the pattern of diabetes prevalence according to age. As shown in Figure 8.1, the prevalence of diabetes decreases after 80 years, and this trend might reflect a selection resulting from the excess mortality in younger diabetic patients. An alternative explanation could be that people aged over 80 years in 1986, having been born at the beginning of the last century, were exposed to a less diabetogenic environment.

It is difficult to compare mortality studies carried out in the past, as they present a large variation in study design, identification sources, diagnostic criteria (fasting glycemia versus OGTT), target population (known versus newly diagnosed diabetes), etc. For instance, clinical-based cohorts possibly are not representative of the overall diabetic population, since diabetic patients attending hospital clinics are generally selected for severity of disease. Similarly, patients living in particular institutions are not fully comparable with the general population (i.e. Rancho Bernardo versus USA general population) (Barrett-Connor and Wingard 1983). Ethnicity can also be responsible for the discrepancies observed in mortality risk reported for older patients.

Another problem arising in mortality studies is that death certificates are not fully reliable in assessing diabetes mortality because of under-reporting. Particularly in elderly subjects, diabetes is often listed as a contributory cause rather than an underlying cause of death, or is even not mentioned at all (Balkau and Papoz 1992; Fuller 1994). Thus, the general feeling is that the impact of diabetes on mortality is largely underestimated and this may lead to a less aggressive attitude in treating the disease.

The few European population-based studies on known diabetes have reported an excess mortality even in the older age groups (Muggeo et al 1995a; Sinclair et al 1997; Bruno et al 1999). This pattern was confirmed, at least up to the age of 75 years, also when elderly diabetic subjects were screened by OGTT, which allows identification also of the so-called 'undiagnosed' diabetic patients (Croxson et al 1994).

The onset of Type 2 diabetes mellitus often goes undetected for an interval which has been estimated at 4–7 years (Harris 1992). The prevalence of un-

diagnosed diabetes increases with age in parallel with that of diagnosed diabetes, so that the prevalence of the two remains approximately equal at all ages. In elderly Type 2 diabetic patients, undiagnosed diabetes exposes them to the risk of dying from acute complications. In fact, the risk of dying from ketoacidosis and hyperosmolar coma increases progressively with age, and often the acute complications coincide with the diagnosis of diabetes (Basu et al 1993). In this regard, it is quite striking that subjects who had died from hyperosmolar/nonketotic coma were found to have a long history of diabetic symptoms without a diagnosis of diabetes prior to admission. These findings underline the necessity to intensify the efforts to detect Type 2 diabetes mellitus in older people to reduce the in-hospital mortality from acute complications.

When specific causes of death were analysed, cardiovascular mortality maintained its high contribution to the overall mortality, especially in the 65–74 age group (Fuller et al 1983; Waugh et al 1989; Bruno et al 1999; De Marco et al 1999).

PREDICTORS OF MORTALITY

Many factors are documented to increase the risk of cardiovascular mortality in young diabetic patients (Rosengren et al 1989; Rossing et al 1996), but very few studies have addressed this topic in older patients (Ford and De Stefano 1991). Since the strength of predictors of mortality can change with age (Frost et al 1996), further studies are needed.

Recognition of the predictors of mortality is the first step in planning an intervention aimed at reducing mortality. Predictors can be divided into unmodifiable and modifiable factors. The former include age, gender and family history; the latter include cigarette smoking, high blood pressure, high blood glucose, elevated total and low-density lipoprotein cholesterol, obesity, diabetes treatment, model of diabetes care and so on. For the purpose of this review it is more useful to classify these predictors into the classic, which are shared by both the diabetic and non-diabetic population, and the diabetes-specific, which are specifically correlated with the disease, its natural history, treatment and complications (Table 8.3).

Classic Cardiovascular Risk Factors

When evaluating cardiovascular risk factors, age represents the strongest predictor of mortality: "the older

Table 8.3 Predictors of cardiovascular mortality in Type 2 diabetes

---

Classic
Age and sex
Lipid, blood pressure, BMI
Smoking, lifestyle etc.
Diabetes-specific
Duration, age of onset, severity of the disease
Treatment and level of care
Long-term glucose control (i.e. FPG, HbA_{1c}
Long-term glucose instability (FPG, post-prandial peaks, recurrent hypoglycemia)

---

the subject the higher the absolute risk of dying". Moreover, age often behaves as a confounder or as an effect modifier when assessing the importance of other risk factors.

The leading cause of death in the Verona diabetes study was cardiovascular disease, which accounted for 42% of the overall mortality. As previously observed for all-cause mortality, the overall cardiovascular mortality was higher in men than in women at all ages, both in the diabetes cohort and in the general population. However, when the SMR was considered, the impact of diabetes on mortality was higher in women than in men, especially in the 65–74 age group (De Marco et al 1999). The 16-year follow-up of the Framingham study demonstrated an equal risk among diabetic men and women in terms of cardiovascular morbidity, but mortality was more pronounced in diabetic women (Kannel and McGee 1979). The higher mortality rate in women from all causes and from ischaemic heart diseases was also found in other studies (Barrett-Connor 1997). All these data suggest that diabetes results in partial or complete loss of the 'female survival advantage' (Pyorala, Laakso and Uusitupa 1987). However, the interplay among sex, diabetes and cardiovascular mortality has not been fully explained, but many factors, such as overweight, hypertension and compliance to treatment, may account for it.

The role of smoking, high blood pressure, low HDL cholesterol, high total cholesterol and obesity have not been studied extensively in elderly subjects. Among the surveys of elderly subjects, only a small number were prospective and the results controversial. Some studies suggest that the risk factors remain the same, while others found a smaller association or even no association at all (Castelli et al 1989; Beaglehole 1991; Krumholz et al 1994; Rossing et al 1996). Surveys showing positive associations consisted largely

of subjects belonging to the 'young-old' age group (60–70 years), while negative studies recruited subjects aged 70 and over. In a Finnish study, smoking, high systolic blood pressure and low HDL cholesterol predicted cardiovascular events among elderly non-diabetic subjects, while total cholesterol did not (Kuusisto et al 1994). The risk factors for cardiovascular events remained substantially similar when non-diabetic subjects with previous myocardial infarction were excluded from the analysis. On the contrary, the same study found that in elderly Type 2 diabetic patients none of the classic cardiovascular risk factors, including smoking, hypertension, low HDL cholesterol and high total cholesterol, predicted cardiovascular mortality even when the parameters of glycaemic control were removed from the multivariate model. Although these results were obtained after a relatively short follow-up period, it is interesting to note that the levels of most cardiovascular risk factors were significantly elevated in Type 2 diabetic patients aged 75 years and over. Similar results were reached in the Verona diabetes study: neither smoking nor hypertension predicted cardiovascular mortality in Type 2 diabetic patients aged 75 years and over (Muggeo et al 1997). Similarly, in this study the stronger predictor of cardiovascular events was related to long-term metabolic control. This loss of strength of classic cardiovascular risk factors in predicting mortality in elderly subjects could be due to a selection phenomenon related to the fact that elderly people must be regarded as a cohort of 'survivors', since those patients with both diabetes and high level of cardiovascular risk factors presumably do not reach an old age. Moreover, regarding smoking, it should be acknowledged that in the Verona study the category of ex-smokers was not separately considered, and was included in the non-smoker group. This can lead to an underestimation of the real impact of smoking, because the category of ex-smokers can include patients affected by severe conditions for which smoking was stopped. Paradoxically the actual smokers can be 'healthier' than the other categories.

In the Verona study the effect of body mass index (BMI) on mortality was addressed in a cohort of 5920 Type 2 diabetic patients. BMI was categorized in quintiles and the multivariate analysis was carried out using the first quintile as the reference category. It was found that the relation between all-cause mortality and BMI tended to be U-shaped. This pattern was more pronounced and statistically significant in women. The U-shaped relationship could be observed also for cardiovascular mortality. No relationship between mortality from malignancy and BMI was found in men, while in women a J-shaped pattern was observed.

In most studies of cardiovascular risk factors, a single value of the parameters, measured at the baseline, is usually used. This approach could blunt the effect of the parameter under study, as single determinations present greater random variability than parameters derived from repeated measurements at different periods. Moreover, the analysis could be biased by the 'regression-to-the-mean' effect: owing to the interplay between inter-individual and intra-individual variability, the actual level of a risk factor is usually overestimated in those subjects with the highest values and underestimated in those with the lowest values. In this regard, more information could be obtained from studies in which serial determinations over time of each parameter were used in the analysis, instead of using a single value collected at the baseline of the study. In the Verona diabetes study, data were collected with this second approach for BMI and for glycaemic control. Survival probability was higher in those patients whose weight and metabolic control remained approximately stable.

Diabetes-specific Predictors

The excess mortality in Type 2 diabetes is only partially explained by the classic risk factors. Other fac-

tors specifically related to the natural history of diabetes strongly affect survival. Age of onset, duration of the disease, long-term glucose control, severity of the disease and presence of chronic complications, mode of therapy and the chosen model of care all contribute to patient survival.

Duration and Severity of the Disease

Duration of diabetes is computed from the time of diagnosis, which does not coincide with the biological onset of the disease. There is a latency period of 4–7 years between the biological onset of Type 2 diabetes and its clinical recognition (Harris et al 1993). During this period the mortality risk is similar or even higher than the mortality risk of known diabetic patients, as hyperglycaemia and other risk factors remain untreated (Wingard and Barrett-Connor 1995). This can explain why in the Verona diabetes study patients with duration of disease 0–4 years already showed a 23% increase of mortality risk (SMR = 1.23; 95%CI 1.19–1.27) (Brun et al 2000). In univariate analysis, mortality risk increases with the duration of diabetes, but when the changes in therapy over time are taken into account, the effect of diabetes duration loses its predictive value in relation to mortality. This suggests that the progression of diabetes and its severity are better described by the changes of therapy rather than by the time elapsed since diagnosis. Figure 8.4 clearly shows

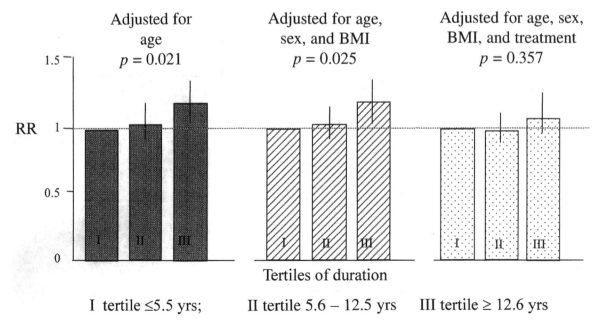

Figure 8.4 Relation between duration of diabetes and mortality in multivariate analysis with and without adjustment for treatment

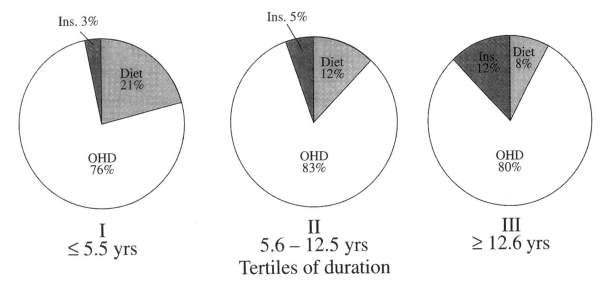

Figure 8.5   In the Verona Diabetes Study the percentage of patients treated with diet decreased with duration of diabetes; conversely the proportion of insulin-treated patients increased

that when the risk of mortality is computed accounting only for age and duration, this latter is a predictor of mortality. However, when other confounders are accounted for, the effect of duration is no longer significant. With increasing duration of diabetes the proportion of patients treated with diet progressively decreases, as observed both in the Verona study (Figure 8.5) and in the UKPDS (1998). Conversely the proportion of patients requiring insulin treatment increases four-fold from the first to the third tertile of duration. Figure 8.6 shows that mortality is significantly associated with therapy: use of oral agents and, even more strikingly, use of insulin is associated with a significant increase in mortality as compared

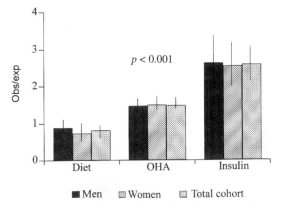

Figure 8.6   Standardized mortality ratios (SMRs) according to diabetes treatment

with diet, and this further supports the concept that mode of treatment is a potent marker of severity of the disease. Severity of the disease includes not only the degree of hyperglycaemia, but also the clustering of other risk factors (Stamler et al 1993), as well as the presence of chronic complications. Figure 8.7 shows that the prevalence of diabetic complications at baseline was significantly higher in patients who died in the following 5 years as compared with diabetic patients still alive after 5 years.

Duration of diabetes in Finnish subjects aged 65–74 years was found to be a strong predictor of cardiovascular events (Kuusisto et al 1994). This study, owing to the high (40.2%) prevalence of newly detected Type 2 diabetic patients at the baseline, allowed a better evaluation of the importance of the duration of the disease with respect to cardiovascular risk. It is reasonable to think that mechanisms associated with long-lasting hyperglycaemia underlay this relation. These findings on cardiovascular events along with the above reported evidence strongly suggest that diabetic patients should be identified and treated at the earliest stages of the disease in order to reduce the incidence of complications and, hence, mortality.

Metabolic Control

In studies on general populations including also diabetic patients (Haffner et al 1990; Stamler et al 1993;

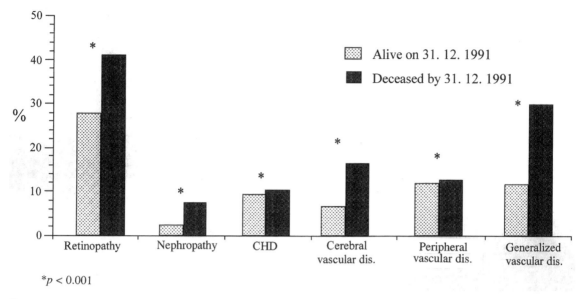

Figure 8.7 Prevalence of diabetic complications at baseline was significantly higher in diabetic patients who died in the subsequent 5 years; *p* < 0.001

Balkau et al 1998), it has been clearly shown that glycaemia and, of course, diabetes are associated with increased risk of mortality, primarily from cardiovascular diseases. There is a strong relationship between the degree of metabolic control, as measured by a single determination of fasting plasma glucose or HbA_{1c} at baseline, and the incidence of microvascular complications. A poor metabolic control also amplifies the effect of other diabetes-specific risk factors, such as duration of diabetes (Kuusisto et al 1994) and microalbuminuria (Gall et al 1995). However, intensive treatment of hyperglycemia, resulting in a reduction of HbA_{1c} from 7.9% to 7%, was associated with an impressive decrease in microvascular complications with a moderate reduction in cardiovascular events, such as fatal and non-fatal myocardial infarction (UKPDS 1998).

The weaker association between HbA_{1c} and cardiovascular mortality could be due to the fact that the assessment of long-term glucose control by FPG or HbA_{1c} does not fully reflect the complex interrelation between everyday glucose control and outcomes. For instance, a frequent recurrence of hyperglycaemic spikes and hypoglycaemic episodes could disproportionately increase the overall glycaemic risk. This additional risk, related to the 'valley and peak phenomenon', is not detected by a single determination of fasting plasma glucose or HbA_{1c}. The latter

correlates with the mean glucose level of a given patient and does not reveal the excursions of plasma glucose over time.

To detect 'glycaemic variability' we have suggested computation of the coefficient of variation $(CV = (SD/mean) \times 100)$ of a time series of fasting plasma glucose (FPG) determinations (Muggeo et al 1995b, 1997, 2000). This parameter offers additional information on the impact of long-term glucose control on mortality. In fact, in a cohort of 566 elderly Type 2 diabetic patients, grouped in tertiles of coefficient of variation of FPG over a 3 year-period (1984–86), the subsequent 5-year mortality was greater in patients of the third tertile (Muggeo et al 1995b). This association was stronger than that between the mean of fasting plasma glucose (M-FPG) and mortality (see the right panel of Figure 8.8). Interestingly, the higher mortality experienced by the patients of the third tertile of CV-FPG was explained by an excess in cardiovascular mortality. These patients showed a longer duration of diabetes, a more frequent use of insulin and tolbutamide, a higher M-FPG, and a higher number of hypoglycaemic events than did patients belonging to the first and the second tertiles (Muggeo et al 1997).

The association between CV-FPG and mortality was confirmed in a larger cohort of Type 2 diabetic patients aged 56–74 years (left panel of Figure 8.8). In these patients, CV-FPG during 1984–86 was a stronger

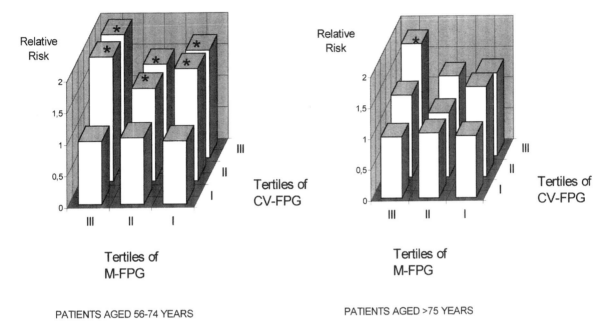

Figure 8.8 Relative risk of all-cause mortality, by tertiles of M-FPG and CV-FPG

predictor of 10-year mortality (1987–96) than M-FPG, which appeared as an independent predictor of mortality only when CV-FPG was not included in multivariate survival analysis (Muggeo et al 2000) (Figure 8.9). Of course, these results do not necessarily mean that the severity of hyperglycemia is not important in determining the outcome in Type 2 diabetes; but they do indicate that the prognostic value of M-FPG is lower than that of CV-FPG. Indeed, these data suggest that CV-FPG might be more reliable than M-FPG in assessing the relationship between long-term glucose control and survival. On the other hand, CV-FPG might be a feature of glucose control 'variability' distinct from hyperglycemia. The cardiovascular risk associated with glucose variability includes both the known poor outcome related with recurrent hypoglycaemia, and the deleterious effects associated with recurrent acute hyperglycaemia. The former predisposes to several adverse events such as trauma, myocardial infarction and arrhythmia (Frier 1993); the latter induces several changes in coagulation (Ceriello 1998), endothelial function (Giuliano et al 1997), activation of circulating adhesion molecules (Marfella et al 2000), and electrocardiographic QTc abnormalities (Marfella et al 2000), which all contribute to increase the cardiovascular risk of these patients, mainly in the post-prandial state (Ceriello 2000).

All these data underline the importance of glycaemic peaks occurring in diabetic patients especially after meals. In the Diabetes Intervention Study, carried out in 1139 Type 2 diabetic patients by Hanefeld et al (1996); the cumulative incidence of cardiovascular events during 11 years of follow-up was significantly correlated with post-prandial blood glucose rather than with fasting blood glucose at baseline, suggesting that post-prandial glucose levels could better describe the glycaemic risk for cardiovascular diseases. Recent population studies carried out in Europe (DECODE 1999) and in the USA (Sievers, Bennett and Nelson 1999) have demonstrated that both in non-diabetic and in Type 2 diabetic patients 2-hour OGTT plasma glucose, and not fasting plasma glucose, is a strong predictor of mortality. On the contrary, in a 10-year prospective study of patients with newly diagnosed Type 2 diabetes, cardiovascular mortality increased three-fold in patients included in the highest blood glucose tertile at baseline when compared with patients included in the lowest blood glucose tertile (Uusitpa et al 1993). The 8- to 10-year follow-up study of the Wisconsin cohort reported that high glycated haemoglobin (HbA$_{1c}$) was associated with increased mortality, mainly due to vascular causes, both in younger-onset and in older-onset diabetic people after controlling for other risk factors (Moss et al 1994).

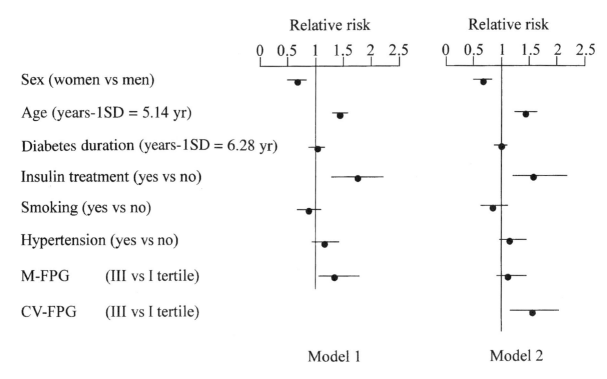

Figure 8.9 Multivariate analysis of mortality from alll causes before (model 1) an after (model 2) controlling for coefficient of variation of FPG (CV-FPG)

There have been few studies investigating this topic in elderly patients. A study of a Swedish diabetic cohort aged 66 ± 12 years showed a 50% higher mortality when fasting glucose level was above 7.8 mM (Andersson and Svardsudd 1995). More interestingly, a Finnish population-based study on 229 Type 2 diabetic patients aged 65–74 years reported HbA_{1c} level to be a predictor of cardiovascular mortality independent of the classical cardiovascular risk factors, such as hypertension or high blood cholesterol (Kuusisto et al 1994). The independent predictive value maintained its strength even when the analysis was restricted to patients without a previous cardiovascular event. In this study, the relationship between HbA_{1c} and the risk of cardiovascular events showed a significant dose–response trend.

Several studies of Type 1 diabetic patients have shown the beneficial effects of tight control of blood glucose on the initiation and progression of diabetic retinopathy, nephropathy, microalbuminuria, and neuropathy. In the Diabetes Control and Complications Trial, cardiovascular events were also reduced, although not significantly, by 41% in the group of

patients aged 13–39 years with good glycaemic control (DCCT 1993). Intensive glucose control in patients with newly diagnosed Type 2 diabetes in the United Kingdom Prospective Diabetes Study (UKPDS 1998), who had a low risk of microvascular complications, had a beneficial effect on aggregate diabetes-related endpoints (i.e. any diabetes-related endpoint, diabetes-related deaths, all-cause mortality, myocardial infarction, stroke, amputation or death from peripheral vascular disease, microvascular complications), and significantly reduced the rate of progression from normoalbuminuria to microalbuminuria. The University Group Diabetes Program (1975), the Kumamoto Study (Shichiri et al 2000), and the Veterans Affairs Cooperative Study (1995) did not show significant beneficial effects due to improved glycaemic control on macrovascular disease and cardiovascular mortality. The UKPDS found a borderline significant reduction in the number of myocardial infarctions with intensive blood glucose control, but significantly fewer diabetes-related deaths and strokes were seen only with tight blood pressure control. A recent study, conducted on microalbuminuric Type 2 diabetic patients aged between 40 and 65 years, showed that nearly 4 years of intensive multifactorial treatment slowed the progression leading to nephropathy, retinopathy and autonomic neuropathy (Gaede et al 1999).

No intervention trial focused on intensive glucose control has been performed in elderly Type 2 diabetic patients. It seems reasonable to recommend tight control in most patients, because it is presumed that the mechanisms by which glucose causes macro- and microvascular complications are the same in both middle-aged and elderly diabetic patients. Nevertheless, the hazard of hypoglycaemia should not be underestimated in elderly patients with intensive treatment (Frier 1993). In fact, hypoglycaemia, in subjects who are particularly vulnerable to substrate deficiency, might precipitate a lethal cardiovascular event. In this regard, it is noteworthy that patients with well-documented hypoglycaemic episodes were more represented among subjects of tertile III of CV-FPG in the Verona Diabetes Study.

In conclusion, in elderly diabetic patients it seems crucial to obtain both good metabolic control and stability of glycaemia over time in order to reduce mortality.

Treatment

There is no convincing evidence that pharmacological therapy of diabetes in elderly patients improves survival. Nevertheless, it must be observed that the type of treatment can change over time, and usually the proportion of diet-treated patients declines with increasing age, whereas the proportion of those treated with insulin increases. As previously shown in Figure 8.6, there is a strong association between therapy and mortality risk, but it is difficult to separate the effect of therapy itself from the effect of the severity of diabetes. In everyday clinical practice the approach to therapy of Type 2 diabetes is stepwise, and the decision to treat patients with insulin is based on the level of hyperglycaemia and/or the presence of chronic complication or associated diseases. In multivariate analysis, even accounting for level of glucose control (mean FPG or HbA_{1c}), the association between therapy and mortality is affected by other confounders, such as complications and comorbidities.

Thus, the mode of therapy remains a marker of disease severity and increased mortality risk rather than the cause of them. These changes may reflect a progressive increase of severity of diabetes as well as

the effect of complications and comorbidity over time (Figure 8.7). Several studies have consistently reported an increased mortality rate in diabetic subjects treated with oral agents compared with those on diet (University Group Diabetes Program 1975; Reunanen 1983; Sasaki et al 1983; Rosengren et al 1989; Brun et al 2000; Muggeo et al 2000), and an ever higher increase in patients treated with insulin (Knuiman, Welborn and Whittall 1992; Muggeo et al 1995b). The association between insulin and mortality does not increase with the dose, further supporting the absence of a cause-effect relationship.

The Model of Diabetes Care

The impact of the model of diabetes care on mortality has been attracting more attention in recent years (Griffin 1998). There is some indirect evidence that patients attending a specialized clinic experience lower mortality than those not attending. It has been reported that patients cared for by physicians at a diabetes centre receive better diabetes care than those seen by physicians at a general medicine clinic (Hayes and Harries 1994).

The Verona Diabetes Study compared 4047 Type 2 diabetic patients regularly attending the Verona Diabetes Centre with 3101 who did not (Zoppini et al 1999). The patients were followed for 10 years in order to ascertain life-status and the causes of death. Patients attending the centre were examined periodically by an experienced diabetologist to assess metabolic control, to re-evaluate the ongoing therapy, and to screen for diabetic complications and cardiovascular risk factors. Educational courses concerning diabetes and its complications, as well as the control of cardiovascular risk factors, were organized either for individual patients or for small groups of patients. Moreover, patients attending the centre received advice from a professional dietician. Patients attending the centre experienced a reduction of risk of mortality from all causes of about 15%, independently of the contribution of other variables. This effect was similar in patients aged 56–74 years and in those older than 75 years.

Depression

It has been reported that depression occurs more frequently in people with diabetes, and particularly in those with complications, rather than in non-diabetic people (Gavard, Lustman and Clouse 1993).

Depression score predicts mortality in elderly diabetic patients independently, and outweighs the effect of predictors such as coronary artery disease, retinopathy and hypertension (Rosenthal et al 1998). The most plausible explanation is that depression is a marker rather than a reflection of other factors.

Not all patients experiencing chronic illnesses become depressed, and the ability to use available resources effectively to cope with stressful events may affect a person's reaction to the disease. In fact, the social impact of diabetes relates to mortality and is possibly affected by the depression score. Even if the mortality risk does not increase, elderly diabetic patients are hospitalized more often than elderly patients without diabetes, and the demand made on hospital services is high. Depression needs to be treated aggressively in elderly people with diabetes in order to improve compliance and reduce the risk of suicide (Goodnick, Henry and Buki 1995).

CONCLUSION

Diabetes is an important contributor to mortality and reduces life expectancy in elderly patients. The most frequent cause of death is cardiovascular disease. The risk profile of mortality changes with advancing age in patients with diabetes, as in the general population. Some risk factors express their powerful deleterious effect at an earlier age (Figure 8.10), when the RR of mortality is the greatest (Figure 8.3). During this lifespan the RR of mortality in patients with Type 2 diabetes peaks and some risk factors express their maximal effect (Figure 8.10). These include gender, obesity and mode of treatment. In patients aged 75 years and older, some of these predictors partially lose significance. Among the parameters of long-term glucose control, mean fasting glucose is a predictor of mortality only when in the multivariate analysis the variability (i.e coefficient of variation) is not included in the model. When the long-term glucose instability is considered, in Type 2 diabetic patients the coefficient of variation of FPG becomes the strongest predictor of mortality, especially in patients older than 75 years. The patients with the highest variability also experience the greatest rate of hypoglycaemic events, and this exposes the patients to an adjunctive risk of cardiovascular mortality.

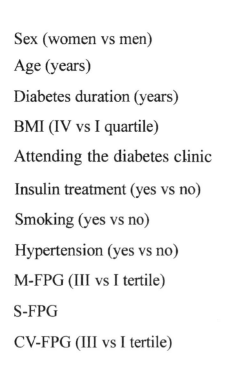 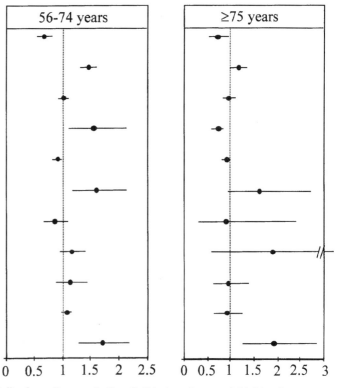

Figure 8.10 Comparison of the main predictors of mortality from all causes in Type 2 diabetic patients aged 56–74 and ≥ 75 years; multivariate analysis carried out with the Cox regression model

Stabilizing glycaemia and body mass index, along with a global control of risk factors, would prevent many deaths. Achievement of those targets requires continuing efforts to educate patients, physicians and the general community.

REFERENCES

Abraira C, Colwell JA, Nuttall FQ et al, for the VA CSDM Group (1995) Veterans Affairs Cooperative Study on Glycemic Control and Complications in Type II Diabetes: results of the feasibility trial. *Diabetes Care*, **8**, 1113–1123.

Andersson DKG, Svardsudd K (1995) Long-term glycemic control relates to mortality in Type II diabetes. *Diabetes Care*, **12**, 1534–1543.

Balkau B, Papoz L (1992) Certification of cause of death in French diabetic patients. *Journal of Epidemiology and Community Health*, **46**, 63–65.

Balkau B, Shipley M, Jarrett RJ, Pyorala K, Pyorala M, Forhan A, Eschwege E (1998) High blood glucose concentration is a risk factor for mortality in middle-aged nondiabetic men: 20-year follow-up in the Whitehall Study, The Paris Prospective Study, and the Helsinky Policeman Study. *Diabetes Care*, **21**, 360–367.

Barrett-Connor E (1997) Sex differences in coronary heart disease. *Circulation*, **95**, 252–264.

Barrett-Connor E, Wingard DL (1983) Sex differential in ischemic heart disease mortality in diabetics: a prospective population-based study. *American Journal of Epidemiology*, **118**, 489–496.

Basu A, Close CF, Jenkins D, Krentz AJ Nattrass M, Wright AD (1993) Persisting mortality in diabetic ketoacidosis. *Diabetic Medicine*, **10**, 282–284.

Beaglehole R (1991) Coronary heart disease and elderly people: no mass treatment of risk factor yet. *British Medical Journal*, **303**, 69–70.

Brun E, Nelson RG, Bennett PH, Imperatore G, Zoppini G, Verlato G, Muggeo M (2000) Diabetes duration and cause specific mortality in the Verona Diabetes Study. *Diabetes Care*, **23**, 1119–1123.

Bruno G, Merlatti F, Boffetta P. Cavallo-Perin P, Barbero G, Gallone G, Pagano G (1999) Impact of glycaemic control, hypertension and insulin treatment on general and cause-specific mortality: an Italian population-based cohort of Type II (non-insulin-dependent) diabetes mellitus. *Diabetologia*, **42**, 297–301.

Cacciatori V, Bonora E, Travia D, Zenere M, Tosi F, Branzi P, Marini F, Poli M, Raffaelli A, Zenari L, Moghetti P, Muggeo M (1991) Comparison of elderly diabetes and mature age diabetes: similarities and differences. *Archives of Gerontology and Geriatrics*, (Suppl. 2), 223–226.

Castelli WP, Wilson PW, Levy D, Anderson K (1989) Cardiovascular risk factors in the elderly. *American Journal of Cardiology*, **63**, 12H–19H.

Ceriello A (1998) The emerging role of post-prandial hyperglicemic spikes in the pathogenesis of diabetic complications. *Diabetic Medicine*, **15**, 188–193.

Ceriello A (2000) The post-prandial state and cardiovascular disease: relevance to diabetes mellitus. *Diabetes and Metabolism Research Review*, **16**, 125–132.

Cook JT, Page RC, Levy JC, Hammersley MS, Walravens EK, Turner RC (1996) Hyperglycaemic progression in subjects with impaired glucose tolerance: association with decline in beta cell function. *Diabetic Medicine*, **13**, 953–959.

Croxson SCM, Price DE, Burden, Jagger C, Burden AC (1994) The mortality of elderly people with diabetes. *Diabetic Medicine*, **11**, 250–252.

DCCT (Diabetes Control and Complications Trial) Research Group (1993) The effect of intensive treatment of diabetes on the development and progression of long-term complications in insulin-dependent diabetes mellitus. *New England Journal of Medicine*, **329**, 977–986.

De Fronzo RA (1992) Pathogenesis of Type 2 (non-insulin dependent) diabetes mellitus: a balanced overview. *Diabetologia*, **35**, 389–397.

De Marco R, Locatelli F, Zoppini G, Verlato G, Bonora E, Muggeo M (1999) Cause-specific mortality in Type 2 diabetes: the Verona diabetes study. *Diabetes Care*, **22**, 756–761.

DECODE Study Group (1999) Glucose tolerance and mortality: comparison of WHO and American diabetes Association diagnostic criteria. *Lancet*, **354**, 617–621.

Ford ES, DeStefano F (1991) Risk factors for mortality from all causes and from coronary heart disease among persons with diabetes: findings from the National Health and Nutrition Examination Survey 1, Epidemiologic Follow-up Study. *American Journal of Epidemiology*, **133**, 1220–1230.

Frier BM (1993) Hypoglycemia in the diabetic adult. *Clinics in Endocrinology and Metabolism*, **7**, 757–777.

Frost PH, Davis Br, Burlando AJ, Curb JD, Guthrie GP, Isacsohn JL, Wassertheil-Smoller S, Wilson AC, Stamler J, for the Systolic Hypertension in the Elderly Research Group (1996) Coronary heart disease risk factors in men and women aged 60 years and older. *Circulation*, **94**, 26–34.

Fuller JH (1994) Mortality from diabetes In: Williams R, Papoz L, Fuller J (eds) *Diabetes in Europe*. London: John Libbey, 108–116.

Fuller JH, Elford J, Goldblatt P, Aldestein M (1983) Diabetes mortality: new light on an understimeted public health problem. *Diabetologia*, **24**, 336–341.

Gaede P, Vedel P, Parving HH, Pedersen O (1999) Intensified multifactorial intervention in patients with Type 2 diabetes mellitus and microalbuminuria: the Steno Type 2 randomised study. *Lancet*, **353**, 617–622.

Gall MA, Borch-Johsen K, Houggard P, Nielsen FS, Parving HH (1995) Albuminuria and poor glycemic control predict mortality in NIDDM. *Diabetes*, **44**, 1303–1309.

Gavard JA, Lustman PJ, Clouse RE (1993) Prevalence of depression in adults with diabetes: an epidemiological evaluation. *Diabetes Care*, **16**, 1167–1178.

Giuliano D, Marfella R, Coppola L, Verrazzo G, Acampora R, Giunta R, Lucarelli C, D'Onofrio F (1997) Vascular effects of acute hyperglycemia in humans are reserved by L-arginine: evidence for reduced availability of nitric oxide during hyperglycemia. *Circulation*, **95**, 1783–1790.

Goodnick PJ, Henry JH, Buki VMV (1995) Treatment of depression in patients with diabetes mellitus. *Journal of Clinical Psychiatry*, **56**, 128–136.

Griffin S (1998) Diabetes care in general practice: meta-analysis of randomized controlled trials. *British Medical Journal*, **317**, 390–395.

Grundy SC, Benjamin IJ, Burke GL, Chait A, Eckel RH, Howard BV, Mitch W, Smith SC, Sowers JR (1999) Diabetes and cardiovascular disease, a statement for healthcare professionals from the Heart Association. *Circulation*, **100**, 1134–1146.

Gu K, Cowie CC, Harris MI (1998) Mortality in adults with and without diabetes in a National Cohort of the US population, 1971–1993. *Diabetes Care*, **21**, 1138–1145.

Haffner SM, Stern MP, Hazuda HP, Mitchell BD, Patterson JK (1990) Cardiovascular risk factors in confirmed prediabetic individuals: does the clock for coronary disease start ticking before the onset of clinical diabetes? *JAMA*, **263**, 2893–2898.

Hanefeld M, Fisher S, Julius U, Schulze J, Schwanenbeck U, Schmechel H, Ziegelash HJ, Lindner J (1996) Risk factors for myocardial infarction and death in newly detected NIDDM: the Diabetes Interventions Study, 11-year follow-up. *Diabetologia*, **39**, 1577–1583.

Harris MI (1992) Undiagnosed NIDDM: clinical and public health issue. *Diabetes Care*, **15**, 815–819.

Harris MI, Hadden WC, Knowler WC, Bennet PH (1987) Prevalance of diabetes and impaired glucose tolerance and plasma glucose levels in US population aged 20–74 y. *Diabetes*, **36**, 523–534.

Harris MI, Klein R, Welborn TA, Knuiman MV (1993) Onset of NIDDM occurs at least 4–7 y before clinical diagnosis. *Diabetes Care*, **16**, 815–819.

Hayes TM, Harries J (1994) Randomized controlled trial of routine hospital clinic care versus routine general practice care of Type 2 diabetics. *British Medical Journal*, **289**, 728–730.

Kannel WB, McGee DL (1979) Diabetes and glucose tolerance as risk factors for cardivascular disease: the Framingham study. *Diabetes Care*, **2**, 120–126.

Knuiman MW, Welborn TA, Whittall DE (1992) An analysis of excess mortality rates for person with Type 2 diabetes mellitus in Western Australia using the Cox proportional hazards regression model. *American Journal of Epidemiology*, **135**, 638–648.

Krumbolz HM, Seeman TE, Merill SS, de Leon M, Vaccarino V, Silverman DL, Tsukahara R, Ostfeld AM, Berkman LF (1994) Lack of association between cholesterol and coronary heart disease mortality and morbidity and all-cause mortality in persons older than 70 years. *JAMA*, **272**, 1335–1340.

Kuusisto J, Mykkaken L, Pyorala K, Laasko MK (1994) NIDDM and its metabolic control predict coronary heart disease in elderly subjects. *Diabetes*, **43**, 960–967.

Laakso M (1996) Glycemic control and the risk of coronary heart disease in patients with non-insulin-dependent diabetes mellitus. *Annals of Internal Medicine*, **124**, 127–130.

Lehto S, Ronnemaa TA, Pyorala K, Laakso M (1996) Risk factors predicting lower extremity amputations in patients with NIDDM. *Diabetes Care*, **19**, 607–612.

Lehto S, Ronnemaa TA, Pyorala K, Laakso M (2000) Cardiovascular risk factors clustering with endogenous hyperinsulinaemia predict death from coronary heart disease in patients with Type 2 diabetes. *Diabetologia*, **43**, 148–155.

Lowel H, Koening W, Engel S, Hormann A, Keil U (2000) The impact of diabetes mellitus on survival after myocardial infarction: can it be modified by drug treatment? Results of a population-based myocardial infarction register follow-up study. *Diabetologia*, **43**, 218–226.

Marfella R, Rossi F, Giuliano D (1999) QTc dispersion, hyperglycemia and hyperinsulinemia. *Circulation*, **100**, 149.

Marfella R, Esposito K, Giunta R, Coppola G, De Angelis L, Farzati B, Paolisso G, Giuliano D (2000) Circulating adhesion molecules in humans: role of hyperglycemia and hyperinsulinemia. *Circulation*, **101**, 2247–2251.

Morley JE (1998) The elderly Type 2 diabetic patients: special considerations. *Diabetic Medicine*, **15**, S41–S46.

Moss SE, Klein R, Klein BEK, Meuer SM (1994) The association of glycemic control and cause-specific mortality in a diabetic population. *Archives of Internal Medicine*, **154**, 2473–2479.

Muggeo M (1998) Accelerated complications in Type 2 diabetes mellitus: the need for greater awareness and earlier detection. *Diabetic Medicine*, **15** (Suppl. 4), 560–62.

Muggeo M, Verlato G, Bonora E, Bressan F, Girotto S, Corbellini M, Gemma ML, Moghetti P, Zenere M, Cacciatori V, Zoppini G, R deMarco (1995a) The Verona Diabetes Study: a population-based survey on known diabetes mellitus prevalence and 5-year all-cause mortality. *Diabetologia*, **38**, 318–325.

Muggeo M, Verlato G, Bonora E, Ciani F, Moghetti P, Eastman R, Crepaldi G, de Marco R (1995b) Long-term instability of fasting plasma glucose predicts mortality in elderly NIDDM patients: the Verona Diabetes Study. *Diabetologia*, **38**, 672–679.

Muggeo M, Verlato G, Bonora E, Zoppini G, Corbellini M, de Marco R (1997) Long-term instability of fasting plasma glucose, a novel predictor of cardiovascular mortality in elderly patients with non-insulin-dependent diabetes mellitus: the Verona Diabetes Study. *Circulation*, **961**, 1750–1754.

Muggeo M, Zoppini G, Bonora E, Burn E, Bonodonna RC, Moghetti P, Verlato G (2000) Fasting plasma glucose variability predicts 10-year survival of Type 2 diabetic patients. *Diabetes Care*, **23**, 45–50.

Pyorala K, Laakso M, Uusitupa M (1987) Diabetes and atherosclerosis: an epidemiological view. *Diabetes and Metabolism Review*, **3**, 463–524.

Reunanen A (1983) Mortality in Type 2 diabetes. *Annals of Clinical Research*, **15**, (Suppl. 37), 26–28.

Rosengren A, Welin L, Tsipogianni A, Wilhelmsen L (1989) Impact of cardiovasucular risk factors on coronary heart disease and mortality among middle aged diabetic men: a general population study. *British Medical Journal*, **299**, 1127–1131.

Rosenthal MJ, Fajardo M, Gilmore S, Morley JE, Naliboff BD (1998) Hospitalization and mortality of diabetes in older adults. *Diabetes Care*, **21**, 231–235.

Rossing P, Hougaard P, Borch-Jonsen K, Parving HH (1996) Predictors of mortality in insulin dependent diabetes: 10-year observation follow up study. *British Medical Journal*, **313**, 779–784.

Sasaki A, Uehara M, Horiuchi N, Hasagawa K (1983) A long-term follow-up study of Japanese diabetic patients: mortality and causes of death. *Diabetologia*, **25**, 309–312.

Shichiri M, Kishikawa H, Ohkubo Y, Nakayasu W (2000) Long term results of the Kumamoto Study on optimal diabetes control in Type 2 diabetic patients. *Diabetes Care*, **23**, B21–B29.

Sievers ML, Bennett PH, Nelson RG (1999) Effect of glycemia on mortality in Pima Indians with Type 2 diabetes. *Diabetes*, **48**, 896–902.

Sinclair J, Robert IE, Croxson SCM (1997) Mortality in older people with diabetes mellitus. *Diabetic Medicine*, **14**, 639–647.

Stamler J, Vaccaro O, Neaton JD, Wentworth D (1993) Diabetes, other risk factors, and 12-year cardiovascular mortality for men screen in the Multiple Risk Factor Intervention Trial (MRFIT). *Diabetes Care*, **16**, 434–444.

Travia D, Bonora E, Cacciatori V, Zenere M, Tosi F, Branzi P, Moghetti P, Raffaelli A, Marini F, Poli M, Zenari L, Muggeo M (1991) Study of some putative pathogenetic factors of diabetes mellitus in the elderly. *Archives of Gerontology and Geriatrics*, (Suppl. 2), 219–222.

UK Prospective Diabetes Study (UKPDS) Group (1998) Intensive blood-glucose control with sulphonylureas or insulin compared with conventional treatment and risk of complications in patients with Type 2 diabetes. *Lancet*, **352**, 837–853.

University Group Diabetes Program (1975) A study of the effects of hypoglycemic agents on vascular complications in patients with adult-onset diabetes. *Diabetes*, **25**, 1129–1253.

Uusitupa MIJ, Niskanen LK, Siitonen O, Voutilainen E, Pyorala K (1993) Ten-year cardiovascular mortality in relation to risk factors and abnormalities in lipoprotein composition in Type 2 (non-insulin dependent) diabetic and non-diabetic subjects. *Diabetologia*, **36**, 1175–1184.

Waugh NR, Dallas JH, Jung RT, Newton RW (1989) Mortality in a cohort of diabetic patients: causes and relatives risks. *Diabetologia*, **32**, 103–104.

Wienberger M, Cowper PA, Kirkman MS, Vinicor F (1990) Economic impact of diabetes mellitus in the elderly. *Clinics in Geriatric Medicine*, **6**, 959–970.

Wilson PW (1998) Diabetes mellitus and coronary heart disease. *American Journal of Kidney Disease*, **32**, S89–S100.

Wingard DLW, Barrett-Connor E (1995) Hearth disease and diabetes. In: *Diabetes in America*, 2nd edn. Bethesda, MD: National Institutes of Health, National Institute of Diabetes and Digestive and Kidney Disease, 423–440.

Wong JSK, Pearson DWM, Murchison LE, Williams MJ, Narayan V (1991) Mortality in diabetes mellitus: experience of a geographically defined population. *Diabetic Medicine*, **8**, 135–139.

Zoppini G, Verlato G, Bonora E, Muggeo M (1999) Attending the diabetes center is associated with reduced cardiovascular mortality in Type 2 diabetic patients: the Verona Diabetes Study. *Diabetes and Metabolism Research Review*, **15**, 170–174.

Zwaag RV, Runyan JW, Davidson JK, Delcher HK, Mainzer I, Bagget HW (1983) A cohort study of mortality of two clinic populations of patients with diabetes mellitus. *Diabetes Care*, **6**, 341–146.

9

Visual Loss

Amanda Butcher, Paul Dodson

Birmingham Heartlands Hospital, Birmingham

INTRODUCTION

Those caring for the elderly diabetic population need to be aware of the threat to sight posed by diabetic retinopathy (DR) and other ocular conditions that increase in frequency in old age. This chapter reviews diabetic retinopathy from the standpoint of the older patient with diabetes. It also outlines some other common causes of visual loss in the general elderly population—of which diabetes, its management and consequent cardiovascular status, may have an important, though indirect bearing.

The elderly diabetic population is a heterogeneous group consisting of Type 1 and 2 diabetic patients. Patients may have longstanding or recently diagnosed diabetes and will have different histories in terms of control of their diabetes, with many Type 2 patients on insulin treatment. They will also differ in terms of hypertension and lipid status. These differences, along with an as yet poorly understood genetic component, mean that within the diabetic population a full spectrum of diabetic eye disease will occur in the elderly group.

It is clear that the risk of diabetic complications is related to the duration of the disease. The Wisconsin epidemiological studies showed that the prevalence of DR is greater than 95% after 15 years of disease in patients diagnosed as diabetic before the age of 30 (Klein, Klein and Meis 1984a). For those diagnosed after that age, 30% have signs of retinopathy at diagnosis, rising to 60% after 15 years of diabetes (Klein, Klein and Moss 1984b). The United Kingdom Prospective Diabetes Study (UKPDS) of Type 2 patients found a similar rate of 38% prevalence of DR at diagnosis. The same study further established that in Type 2 patients the prevalence of maculopathy requiring treatment was 10% and proliferative diabetic retinopathy (PDR) 4% (Kohner, Stratton and Aldington 1993).

A recent survey of patients in a general diabetic clinic revealed the following causes of severe visual impairment (SVI, defined as Snellen visual acuity 6/36 or less). From a total of 309 notes surveyed, 89 patients had SVI; however in 49 of these patients (55%) the SVI was due to causes other than DR. Of these, 10 patients had amblyopia, which is a visual developmental problem and would not be amenable to treatment. In five patients SVI related to cataract, four patients had age-related macula degeneration, and 18 patients had retinovascular disease (Nithyananthan 2000). The presence of any of these conditions could lead to diagnostic difficulties for screening personnel.

From the above figures it can be concluded that:

1. The majority of elderly diabetic patients will have DR of some description.
2. The 'general rule' that Type 1 patients suffer with PDR and Type 2 patients with maculopathy is not strictly true. All grades of DR are apparent in the elderly diabetic group.
3. All Type 2 patients must have proper screening, with mydriasis, for retinopathy at diagnosis of diabetes, followed by annual screening.
4. Five percent of patients, despite having diabetes for 15 years, do not have DR.
5. Causes of visual loss other than DR are important in the elderly diabetic patient group.

CAUSES OF DIABETIC RETINOPATHY

Diabetic retinopathy is a microvascular complication of diabetes. It occurs with increasing frequency in both types of diabetes with time from onset of the diabetes.

Diabetes in Old Age. Second Edition. Edited by A. J. Sinclair and P. Finucane. © 2001 John Wiley & Sons Ltd.

Type 2 diabetes is more frequently, but not exclusively, associated with maculopathy.

High blood glucose affects retinal blood flow and metabolism and has direct effects on the cells associated with retinal blood vessels, endothelial cells and pericytes. More recently it has become apparent that levels of blood pressure associated with diabetes have effects on the development and progression of diabetic retinopathy.

High blood glucose increases the blood flow in the retina owing to an increase in metabolic demand. High blood glucose results in the activation of an alternative metabolic pathway resulting in the production of lactic acid, a potent vasodilator. Blood flow through the vessels also increases owing to the loss of pericytes around the vessels, which in the normal retina play a role in autoregulation. The resulting uncontrolled blood flow affects the capillary wall by increasing production of vasoactive substances and increasing endothelial cell proliferation, eventually resulting in the closure of capillaries. This leads to a state of chronic hypoxia in the retina, stimulating the production of a number of growth factors, including vascular endothelial growth factor (VEGF). VEGF acts via the beta isoform of protein kinase C to stimulate endothelial cell growth (leading to the development of retinal new vessels), but it also results in increased vascular permeability (resulting in exudative complications) (Frank 1991; Clermont et al 1997).

TYPES OF RETINOPATHY

Clinically, retinopathy is best considered divided into categories which enable the clinician to plan management and explain prognosis. The four major subdivisions are:

- background diabetic retinopathy
- preproliferative retinopathy
- proliferative retinopathy
- maculopathy.

Background and Pre-proliferative Diabetic Retinopathy

Background diabetic retinopathy (BDR) is so called because the lesions associated with it lie within the retina itself and are not sight-threatening (Figure 9.1). Lesions seen in BDR are microaneurysms, blot haemorrhages and exudates.

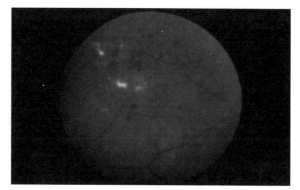

Figure 9.1 *Background diabetic retinopathy.* Typical features of exudation, microaneurysms, and dot haemorrhages are shown in the retinal periphery

Lesions associated with pre-proliferative retinopathy are cottonwool spots (CWS), venous dilatation, beading and looping, and intraretinal microvascular abnormalities (IRMAs).

BDR starts with microaneurysms and proceeds to add blot haemorrages (i.e. ruptured microaneurysms deep within the retina). This leads to the classic picture of 'dots and blots'. Splinter haemorrhages—small haemorrhages in the superficial nerve fibre layer of the retina—may also form part of this picture where there is coexistent hypertension. Exudates are the result of leakage of lipids and proteins from affected vessels. They may form circinate rings where the leakage centres on a leaking microaneurysm. As capillary shutdown progresses and the retina becomes increasingly ischaemic, CWS may appear as these represent actual retinal infarcts. They may also be apparent with uncontrolled hypertension and with periods of changing glucose control.

More serious signs of retinal ischaemia and impending proliferative complications are changes in the venous vasculature. Initially these consist of venous dilatation proceeding to venous 'beading' (the affected vessel looking like a string of sausages), venous looping and reduplication and the appearance of intraretinal microvascular abnormalities, which represent swollen intraretinal capillaries, enlarging to support the failing capillary circulation. These have a characteristic appearance and are always flat on the retina, distinguishing them from neovascularization. The grade of increasing retinal ischaemia as described can be called preproliferative retinopathy and should increase the index of suspicion for the presence of new vessels and also lead to more frequent review of the retinopathy, on the basis that the earlier neovascularization is detected the more responsive it is to treatment.

Proliferative Retinopathy

The discovery of newly diagnosed neovascularization anywhere on the retina is an ophthalmic emergency. The presence of new vessels puts the patient at high risk of vitreous haemorrhage and resultant complications that can lead to permanently and severely impaired vision. The ideal is to lower the patient's risk of reaching this stage by rigorous diabetic and hypertension control; but failing that, detecting and therefore treating retinal new vessels as promptly as possible does reduce the SVI rate. This can be done by responding to signs of increasing retinal ischaemia picked up at routine screening with frequent and thorough retinal examinations and by ready access to laser treatment immediately it becomes indicated. For practical purposes the retinal screener should refer the patient for specialist review at the point where retinal ischaemia becomes established; that is, when pre-proliferative retinopathy is present.

Areas commonly developing new vessels and deserving of special attention during retinal screening are the optic disc (Figure 9.2), the temporal and nasal watershed areas and the vascular arcades. It should be highlighted, however, that any area of the retina can develop new vessels (Figure 9.3). Any quadrant of these retina demonstrating the stigmata of ischaemia highlighted above should be scrupulously examined. The elderly developing retinal new vessels in their 60th decade may be less at risk of the complications of these if they have already sustained a posterior vitreous detachment. This removes the vitreous interface that allows the new vessels to grow forwards into the

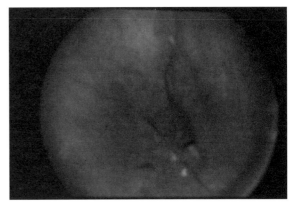

Figure 9.3 *New Vessels in the Retinal Periphery. (NVC).* New vessels arise from the venous side of the retinal circulation and may occur in the periphery of the retina. These are termed NVE. There is a high risk of pre-retinal haemorrhage which has already occurred in this example

intraocular space, placing traction on the retina and leading to retinal detachment. The risk of vitreous haemorrhage is also reduced as the new vessels tend to lie flat on the retinal surface and are therefore not susceptible to sheering stress that may cause them to rupture (Figure 9.4).

Maculopathy

Maculopathy refers to any retinopathy occurring in the macula area of the retina. For purposes of screening this is taken as the area confined within one disc diameter of the fovea. It is subdivided into exudative (diffuse or focal), ischaemic or mixed.

The ophthalmologist may need to use fundus fluorescein angiography (FFA) to aid with accurate

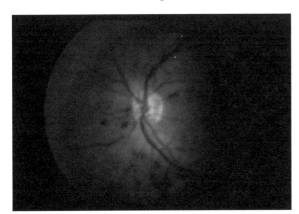

Figure 9.2 *New vessels on the optic disc (NVD).* New vessels (angiogenesis), termed neovascularisation, are shown on the optic disc resulting from retinal ischaemia. These vessels are fine and friable, and there is a high risk of subsequent haemorrhage. This finding as a new diagnosis should prompt urgent referral to an ophthalmologist

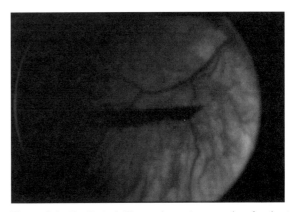

Figure 9.4 *Pre-Retinal Haemorrhage.* An example of a boat shaped haemorrhage which is pre-retinal which has arisen from peripheral new vessels (NVE). These may give rise to symptoms of floaters or spiders in the field of vision

diagnosis and management. This is a technique to allow direct visualization of the retinal circulation, highlighting areas of capillary leakage and closure. Following mydriasis, an injection of fluorescein dye is administered via a peripheral cannula. Fundal photography is then carried out using special filters.

The mechanism of visual loss in exudative maculopathy is the development of oedema destroying the delicate structure of the retina within the macula and especially the fovea, resulting in the loss of central vision and acuity. Macula oedema can be seen stereoscopically with the slit lamp as a thickening of the retina. Sometimes it takes on a cystic appearance and is termed 'cystoid macula oedema'. Macula oedema is difficult to assess with direct methods of retinal examination as they are not stereoscopic. For the screening, using other features of macula oedema (i.e. microanuerysms and exudates within the temporal arcades (Figure 9.5) or a reduction in visual acuity) should prompt referral to the ophthalmologist.

Focal maculopathy is so called as in this group the area of macula oedema is well defined, sometimes clearly focused around a leaking microaneurysm. Where the oedema is less clearly defined and there is no one site of leakage, the maculopathy is termed diffuse in nature. The differences between these two groups have clear implications for treatment and outcome. The threshold for treatment has been clearly defined by large studies using the concept of 'clinically significant oedema', defined as that which is sight-threatening. Any macula with clinically significant oedema should be assessed with a view to treatment. Where an area of focal leakage is not obvious, an FFA

may be appropriate to define the areas of leakage and thus highlight areas for laser treatment. An FFA may also be deemed appropriate to demonstrate the presence of macula ischaemia.

Ischaemic maculopathy occurs due to capillary shutdown occurring directly within the macula area. It is often clinically difficult to identify as the macula has a greyish and rather featureless appearance. It is heralded firstly by a reduction in visual acuity, with few retinal signs. An FFA may be necessary for diagnosis (Figure 9.6). Unfortunately there is no effective laser treatment for this type of maculopathy, and indeed laser therapy may be deleterious. In addition, significant retinal ischaemia predisposes to proliferative complications, and so these patients still require regular review to assess for development of PDR.

Mixed maculopathy is sometimes seen where there are areas of both exudation and ischaemia. The FFA forms the basis for treating areas of leakage in patients with mixed maculopathy with a view to limiting the area of macula treated with laser. However, if the fovea itself is ischaemic or the ischaemia is predominant, laser treatment would not be recommended as it may extend the area of ischaemia and be hazardous to sight (Easty and Sparrow 1999; Dodson, Gibson and Kritzunger 1994).

Neovascular glaucoma. Untreated proliferative diabetic retinopathy may progress with neovascular-

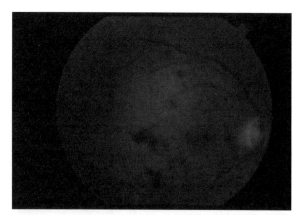

Figure 9.6 *Ischaemic Maculopathy.* This diagnosis and retinal appearance often leads to difficulties in diagnosis with direct ophthalmoscopy. The retinal appearance of ischaemic maculopathy is of a pale, featureless macula region with deep intraretinal haemorrhages indicating retinal ischaemia. Examination by stereo-biomicroscopy demonstrated the presence of macula oedema and vision was compromised at $^6/_{18}$. Subsequent fluorescein angiogram demonstrated significant ischaemia in the macula region with areas of capillary non perfusion

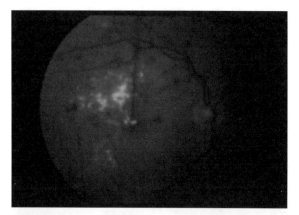

Figure 9.5 *Exudative Maculpathy.* Leakage and exudation occurs in the macula region leading to macula oedema and deterioation in visual activity. This example shows exudation encroaching on the forea and focal laser was subsequently performed

ization of the iris and the drainage angle of the eye. This may be accompanied by a fibrosing process, which progressively prevents aqueous fluid circulating and drainage from the angle, allowing the development of an extremely high intraocular pressure (IOP). This in turn causes the cornea to decompensate and become oedematous. The optic nerve rapidly atrophies under such high IOP. The eye may become intensely painful owing to the combination of high pressure and the development of corneal erosions. If iris rubeosis is seen at an early stage, progression may be halted by aggressive laser treatment. However, once the cornea becomes oedematous there is no possibility of laser treatment as the laser can no longer focus on the retina. If the eye becomes painful and the pain cannot be controlled by topical steroid and atropine drops, cryotherapy, applied to the ciliary body via the sclera, may halt production of aqueous to allow the intraocular pressure to reduce to a more comfortable level. Rarely the only option for pain control is to eviscerate the ocular contents.

LASER TREATMENT OF DIABETIC RETINOPATHY

Laser treatment is carried out through a dilated pupil using a contact lens applied to the cornea anaesthetized by topical anaesthetic drops (Figure 9.7). There are a number of lasers that may be used, such as Argon or diode lasers. The wavelength chosen ranges from 488 to 577 nm. Operators avoid the shorter blue end of the spectrum as this can lead to effects not only on the blue

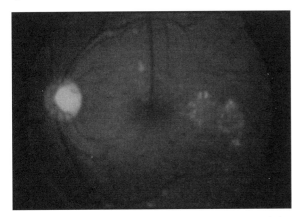

Figure 9.7 *Focal Laser Treatment for Maculopathy.* Exudative maculopathy is demonstrated. Within the rings of exudate (circinates), fluffy white areas are shown which are focal laser treatments. This will result in resolution of macula oedema and resorption of the exudates over many months

vision of the patient but also to cumulative effects on the operator's own blue perception. The effect of the laser is a result of thermal damage caused by absorption of the light energy into pigmented retinal tissues.

Treatment of Proliferative DR

Newly diagnosed new vessels on the disc should be treated as an emergency. Treatment of this condition with the laser is a particularly invasive procedure, termed 'pan-retinal photocoagulation' (PRP). It may be uncomfortable for some patients, particularly if the treatment needs repeating on a number of occasions. If necessary this can be alleviated by carrying out treatment under an orbital anaesthetic block; it is very rare to require a general anaesthetic. Without laser intervention however the risk of severe visual loss in these patients is 50–70% at 2 and 5 years (Diabetic Retinopathy Research Group 1978).

There are several possible complications of pan-retinal photocoagulation. First, as the abnormal, new retinal vessels involute they may bleed, giving rise to a vitreous haemorrhage which will reduce vision for the patient and prevent further assessment of retinopathy until it clears. Usually resolution of the haemorrhage occurs spontaneously over some months. If the haemorrhage is slow to resolve or retinal assessment felt essential, an operation to remove the vitreous and clear the haemorrhage may be carried out (vitrectomy). The timing of this is judged on the individual case. Especially in the elderly, the neovascular process can be slow and vitrectomy carries the risk of introducing infection to the eye as well as causing retinal detachment.

A further possible complication is loss of peripheral vision. This is a direct effect of the treatment itself, which is effectively ablation of healthy retinal tissue by placing spaced burns in the periphery of the retina (Figure 9.8). This results in loss of visual field (peripheral vision). After a full treatment the field is reduced by 40–50%. If the treatment involves both eyes this may affect the fitness to drive.

There may be exacerbation of coexisting macula oedema. Wherever possible macula oedema should be treated before PRP. There may also be other side-effects such as reduction in night vision and contrast sensitivity.

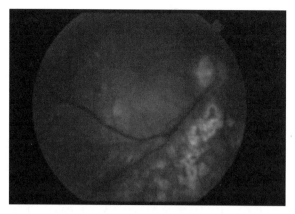

Figure 9.8 *Pan retinal photocoagulation (PRP).* This example shows the result of PRP with retinal atrophy and pigmentation in discrete round treatment areas. Laser treatments are undertaken in the laser periphery, usually requiring at least 3,000 treatments, performed over 2–3 treatment sessions

Treatment of Maculopathy

The rationale for the laser treatment of maculopathy is to 'dry up' patches of oedema before they encroach on the fovea and reduce vision (see Fig. 9.7). The exact mechanism of the benefit of the laser is still unclear. Some authors believe it may result from stimulation of the retinal pigment epithelium (RPE) underlying the retina to 'pump' the fluid away. Others suggest that the closure of microaneurysms is crucial. The resolution of the signs of the maculopathy may take some months to occur. Where sight-threatening macula oedema exists, laser treatment will reduce the risk of visual deterioration in 50% of patients (ETDRS 1987).

There is no benefit of laser treatment in ischaemic retinopathy.

Foveal involvement of the laser treatment results in severe loss of acuity. It may result from error of judgement by the operator or from inadvertent extension of an area of ischaemia into the fovea.

PREVENTION OF DIABETIC RETINOPATHY

The UKPDS and DCCT trials have provided sound clinical evidence that tight control of hyperglycaemia is a major factor in the prevention of all diabetic complications, including retinopathy. The DCCT demonstrated that for Type 1 diabetics maintaining an HbA_{1c} of 7% or less resulted in a reduced risk of developing retinopathy of 76% and a reduction in mean risk of retinopathy progression of 54%, when compared with a parallel group with poorer glycaemic control ($HbA_{1c} < 9\%$). This reduction in retinopathy

risk was seen in all sub-groups of the study and in all centres participating (DCCT Research Group 1993). The UKPDS has also demonstrated a reduction of risk of retinopathy with tight glycaemic control in Type 2 patients ($HbA_{1c} < 7\%$) giving a 25% risk reduction for retinal photocoagulation (UKPDS 1998a). It was also instrumental in highlighting the vital role that the control of hypertension has to play in reducing complication rates in Type 2 patients. Both clinical and economic data support the rigorous control of blood pressure to study defined levels, often necessitating multiple antihypertensive agents to achieve a target blood pressure of $< 140\,\text{mmHg}$ (UKPDS 1998b). Using these targets, the UKPDS demonstrated a 37% reduced rate of progression of retinopathy and a 47% reduced risk of loosing more than three lines of visual acuity as measured by the ETDRS chart (ETDRS 1987).

The UKPDS did not show any particular advantage of ACE inhibitors over other antihypertensive therapies, in contrast to some studies (Chaturvedi et al 1998; HOPE 2000) which have suggested beneficial effects on retinopathy. Experimentally it has been shown that retinal vessel autoregulation is impaired in the presence of diabetes, suggesting that hyperglycaemia and hypertension may work together to promote diabetic retinopathy. Raised levels of angiotensin and renin, that may be seen in Type 1 diabetics, and ACE produced locally in the eye, have also been implicated as aggravating factors. Subsequently evidence has emerged in Type 1 diabetes that the ACE inhibitors, serving to block these pathways, may have specific effects retarding progression of diabetic retinopathy.

The EUCLID study was a double-blind, randomized parallel clinical trial of lisinopril and placebo. Five hundred and thirty Type 1 diabetics with blood pressures $<155\,\text{mmHg}$ systolic and $75\text{–}90\,\text{mmHg}$ diastolic and who were norm- or microalbuminuric or less, were studied. Retinal photographs were graded and progression and regression of the retinopathy between grades was noted. The results were adjusted for many possible confounding factors, including HbA_{1c}, baseline blood pressure, albumin excretion rate, duration of diabetes etc., and demonstrated beneficial effects with a halving of the progression of retinopathy both between nonproliferative grades and between nonproliferative and proliferative (halved from 25% to 12%). This study supports the concept that patients with diabetes and hypertension should receive an ACE-I as first-line treatment whenever possible. In Type 2 patients with diabetes, the MICRO-HOPE study supported the substantial benefit of ACE inhibition with regard to cardiovascular outcome and a trend to reduction in microvascular disease.

Implementing Targets

The benefit in terms of visual outcome for patients with tight control of all risk factors would be substantial. The UKPDS (1998a) estimated a 25% reduction in mainly focal laser treatment requirement, which should have a significant impact on ophthalmology practice. There is also no lack of data setting effective targets for treatment (HbA$_{1c}$ < 7%, BP < 140/85 mmHg DCCT Research Group 1993; UKPDS 1998a; Hansson et al 1997), but the implementation of targets is difficult in view of drug requirements, compliance, supervision and cost. The diabetic patient may attend a number of different specialty outpatient clinics, and responsibility for the control of risk factors may become muddled. This may be particularly important in ophthalmology as up to 20% of Type 2 patients can have retinopathy at diagnosis and patients may be referred directly to the eye clinic via optometrists and community retinopathy screening programs with no input from hospital diabetologists.

Recently controversy has been raised in the literature about the role, if any, the ophthalmologist should play in the management of risk factors (Silvestri 1999). Many eye units will not have access to a medical ophthalmologist, and diabetic eye care is therefore provided by a general ophthalmologist. General ophthalmologists are not trained to initiate medical therapies for diabetic retinopathy, the emphasis remaining firmly on laser treatment. Laser intervention for exudative maculopathy will reduce the risk of sight loss but a timely intervention to tighten control of risk factors should reduce the patient's risk of developing sight-threatening DR.

Ischaemic maculopathy is a particularly difficult problem for ophthalmologists. There is currently no beneficial ophthalmic intervention. A recent study comparing exudative and ischaemic retinopathy has shown uncontrolled hypertension to be the most statistically significant factor differentiating patients with ischaemic and exudative maculopathy and also differentiating those diabetics with maculopathy from those without (Dale 2000).

Although this does not prove cause, taken alongside the UKPDS data (most maculopathy occurs in Type 2 diabetics) it is suggestive that lowering BP to study defined levels could significantly impact on this untreatable cause of blindness.

Screening

Screening for diabetic retinopathy is essential. It is accepted that, at the present time, despite improved understanding of the need to improve control of underlying risk factors, DR cannot be completely prevented; 20 years after diagnosis almost all of those with Type 1 diabetes and 60% with Type 2 will have some degree of retinopathy. Sight-threatening retinopathy should be diagnosed when an effective assessment method is used, and treatment is generally effective if given early enough (laser treatment prevents further visual loss rather than improving visual acuity), making retinal screening of the older diabetic age group a very worthwhile use of resources and mandatory. Screening is particularly important in the elderly as deteriorating vision may sometimes be tolerated by this group as 'to be expected at my age'.

It is equally important to screen elderly patients presenting to the ophthalmologist with retinovascular disease for diabetes as retinopathy may be the presenting feature (Table 9.1). Nationally approved pro-

Table 9.1 Indications for referral to an ophthalmologist

Urgent referral
Same day ophthalmology review

- preretinal and/or vitreous haemorrhage
- retinal detachment

Ophthalmology review within 2–3 days

- new vessels on the disc
- new vessels elsewhere
- rubeosis iridis

Early referral
Ophthalmology review within 3–4 weeks

- preproliferative retinopathy
- nonproliferative retinopathy with macula involvement
- haemorrhage and/or hard exudates within one disc diameter from the centre of the fovea

Routine referral:

- nonproliferative retinopathy with large circinate or plaque within the major temporal arcade but not threatening the macula
- retinal findings not characteristic of diabetic retinopathy
- background retinopathy with reduced vision but without maculopathy to determine cause of visual loss
- reduced visual acuity not corrected by pinhole, suggestive of macula oedema (Royal College of Opthalmologists, Guidelines for Diabetic Retionpathy 1999)
- inadequate retinal view or imaging (e.g. cataract or vitreous haemorrhage)

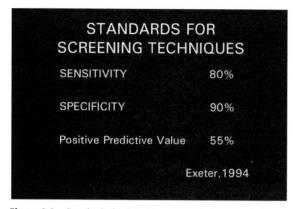

Figure 9.9 *Standards for Screening for Diabetic Retinopathy*

tocols for screening will be the way forward to ensure good quality of screening for all patients.

The quality of the screening method used in the elderly is an important issue as the existence of age-related comorbidity increases. The screening method used should be specific enough to exclude age-related macula degeneration and drusen, for example, but sensitive enough to allow treatment of the retina before it causes sight-threatening retinal damage (Figure 9.9). Digital fundus photography is likely to be the method of choice for a national screening program as it fulfils sensitivity and specificity requirements and provides hard copy to allow for external quality assurance (Gillow 2000).

WHAT HOPE FOR THE FUTURE?

The search continues for a pharmacological agent to prevent or halt the progression of diabetic retinopathy. Many factors have been found associated with this process in the retina and a number of abnormal metabolic pathways have been identified. It seems unlikely that one single factor will hold all the therapeutic answers; but there is hope that, by unravelling the complex interplay between glycaemic control, blood pressure and angiogenic factors, effective treatments for prevention or retarding the pathological process will emerge.

Chronic hyperglycaemia is a major factor in the development of diabetic retinopathy. Possible mechanisms by which hyperglycaemia is thought to induce retinal complications have already been discussed. Although inhibiting these pathways in animals has been promising, unfortunately no phar-

macological agent has yet successfully reduced retinopathy in man.

A more recent promising development in this area has been the selective inhibition of the beta isoform of protein kinase C which is the main mediator for the retinal effects of VEGF. Animal experiments have been completed and human trials of protein kinase C inhibition are currently underway (Koya and Kind 1998).

Another approach has centred on the effects of other known angiogenic growth factors such as growth hormone and IGF-1. Initial data have suggested the potential for growth hormone antagonist therapy (long-acting octreotide by injection) in ameliorating progression of DR, and controlled trials are being undertaken (Grant et al 2000). In the last few years, data have confirmed that increasing serum cholesterol levels are a risk factor for diabetic retinopathy. With the advent of 'statin' therapy, small studies have suggested potential benefit of this therapy in patients with diabetic maculopathy (Gordon et al 1991).

Unlike with diabetic nephropathy, there is no familial predisposition to retinopathy and there has been no link found with differing ACE genotype or other mutations. Continued study of these variants or other genetic susceptibility factors may one day open up new therapeutic avenues.

NON-DR CAUSES OF DECREASED VISION IN OLDER DIABETICS

Cataract

Cataract is the most common cause of deteriorating vision in the elderly population. The lens thickens and opacifies with age and the lens opacities seen in the diabetic population are usually consistent with these changes, although the increased metabolic insult to the lens in diabetic patients causes these changes to accelerate and occur prematurely (Figure 9.10). A rarer form of cataract seen only in the diabetic population and as a direct result of poor diabetic control in Type 1 patients may occur. This is termed the 'snow-flake' cataract which resembles white flakes occurring in the lens just under the lens capsule. Usually they do not affect vision but tend to make fundal examination difficult.

Type 2 diabetics may present with blurring of vision due to increased myopia resulting from overhydration and swelling of the lens secondary to prolonged high blood glucose. These refractive effects reverse as the

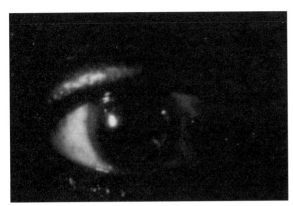

Figure 9.10 *Cataract.* This finding is the most common occular abnormality in diabetic patient. The example shows peripheral spoke lens opacities

blood glucose level normalizes. It is prudent, however, to delay prescription of glasses for these patients by about 3 months to ensure the metabolic lens effects are fully resolved. Similar temporary refractive changes may also be seen in Type 1 patients who are undergoing rapid swings in blood glucose

The label 'cataract' should be reserved to classify permanent lens opacities that affect vision. They result from three main pathogenic mechanisms.

1. The polyol pathway results in increased glucose (entering the lens from an aqueous humor with an abnormally high glucose level) conversion by aldose reductase to sorbitol. Sorbitol does not readily diffuse from the lens. This sets up an osmotic gradient moving water into lens cells, which swell and rupture, resulting in opacity formation. Although aldose reductase inhibitors have been shown to inhibit this process in animal studies, unfortunately this has not proved to be the case in human trials.
2. Excess sugars also directly cause increased glycation of lens proteins. This results in protein aggregation within the lens, leading to a reduction in lens transparency.
3. Increased glucose levels also results in an excess of free radical formation (oxidative stress). In the normal lens free radicals are detoxified by a number of enzymatic processes, but in the diabetic patient these clearance mechanisms may be insufficient, allowing free radicals to cause irreversible lens cell damage.

Referral to an ophthalmologist for assessment of the lens opacities should be delayed until affects on vision

become symptomatic, or the lens opacity prevents screening for, or treatment of, diabetic retinopathy. This second criterion often leads to surgery to remove cataract sooner in diabetic patients than in non-diabetic patients, particularly if there is significant diabetic retinopathy that cannot be visualized and therefore the patient's retina is thought to be at risk.

Once cataract formation fulfilling the above criteria has occurred, surgical treatment is indicated. Cataracts are easily treated surgically. The visual outcome of the surgery should be the same as for non-diabetic patients where there is no retinopathy. However, if the patient has already developed DR the visual outcome will depend on the level of remaining macula function. A technically perfect surgical procedure will not restore normal visual acuity if the macula has sustained permanent damage. Given the difficulty of assessing the macula through a cataractous lens, visual prognosis can be hard to predict in some cases and a guarded visual prognosis should be given. The surgery can usually be carried out under local anaesthetic as a daycase, with no modification but with some increased risk of postoperative complications such as inflammation, infection and posterior capsular thickening. Most units have their own protocol for the management of oral hypoglycaemics and insulin perioperatively according to anaesthetist preference. The aim of perioperative management is to prevent hypoglycaemia during the procedure. It is generally accepted, however, that during the preoperative weeks diabetic control should be optimized. Diabetic patients with poorly controlled glucose levels are prone to slower wound healing and have an increased risk of postoperative inflammation.

All diabetic patients are at risk from progression of DR after cataract surgery. The progression of proliferative retinopathy and the development of rubeosis iridis can to some extent be mitigated by adequate preoperative pan-retinal photocoagulation. By definition, however, the presence of a cataract may make this impossible, in which case consideration should be given to intraoperative laser therapy. It should be noted that the postoperative period is associated in all patients with a risk of cystoid macula oedema, which usually spontaneously resolves. It is vital in the diabetic patient to distinguish this from deterioration in diabetic maculopathy, which may be difficult clinically and FFA may be necessary.

A reduction in vision commencing a few weeks postoperatively, associated with opacification seen with the direct ophthalmoscope, may signify posterior lens capsule thickening behind the new lens implant. This complication can be more severe in the diabetic patient but may be successfully treated with a laser capsulotomy (Easty and Sparrow 1999).

Age related Macula Degeneration

There are a number of prevalence studies of this condition, but unfortunately they vary in their definition of what constitutes ARMD. It is a poorly understood degenerative retinal condition which occurs as a spectrum, but can basically be divided into two main types:

- dry ARMD, where there is slow degeneration of the retinal pigment epithelium, vital for nourishment and function of the retina (Figure 9.11)
- choroidal neovascularization, leading to a rapid loss of central vision resulting from growth of abnormal choroidal vessels (unknown stimulus) into the retina, resulting in haemorrhage, exudation oedema and destruction of the RPE.

In spite of this diagnostic confusion, all agree that the prevalence of ARMD increases with age and that the dry type is more prevalent than the neovascular type. Age-related macula degeneration is an increasingly important cause of loss of central vision as the diabetic population ages. There is no increased risk for the diabetic patient; but although the cause is unclear a number of risk factors have been elucidated, some of which occur with high frequency in the diabetic

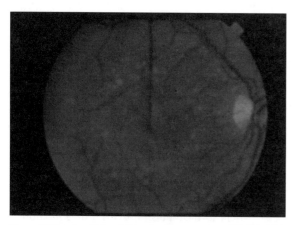

Figure 9.11 *Age Related Macular Degeneration (ARMD).* This example demonstrates Drusen encircling the macular, but no charges of diabetic retinopathy, and visual acuity was normal. This dry form of ARMD in after mistaken for exudative diabetic maculopathy and may lead to unnecessary diabetic eye clinic referral

population. They are atherosclerosis, cerebrovascular disease, diastolic blood pressure >95 mmHg, antihypertensive medication, and elevated serum cholesterol. Some stages of ARMD can easily be mistaken for DR; in particular, macular drusen can be mistaken for macular exudates which do not in themselves pose a significant risk to vision. The presence of exudates and haemorrhage in the macula would warrant specialist opinion whether due to DR or choroidal neovascularization as rarely ARMD of this type may be amenable to laser therapy to minimize its effect on vision.

Retinal Vein Occlusion

The aetiology of retinal vein occlusion (RVO) is multifactorial, but pathologically the primary event for its development is damage to the wall of the venous vasculature. Risk factors include the major risk factors for cardiovascular disease, and therefore diabetic patients are clearly at increased risk, particularly those with concomitant hypertension and hyperlipidaemia.

RVO can occur in two main forms: branch retinal vein occlusion (BRVO) and central retinal vein occlusion (CRVO). Both need ophthalmic review, to assess ocular risk factors such as raised intraocular pressure and to assess the risk of developing ischaemic sequelae.

BRVO and CRVO have characteristic appearances including haemorrhages, exudates and macula oedema, but could easily be mistaken for DR. BRVO can be differentiated by its sectorial nature (Figure 9.12). A CRVO may appear as an uncharacteristically unilaterally florid DR (Figure 9.13). The sequlae of RVO could also be confused as progression of DR. If the RVO causes sufficient ischaemia the development of new vessels will ensue. Laser treatment may be beneficial and follows the same guiding principles as for PDR; i.e. pan- or sector retinal photocoagulation (BRVOS 1986). With a BRVO causing macula oedema resulting in a visual acuity of less than 6/12 six months after the initial event, laser treatment of the oedema has been shown to be of visual benefit. Macula oedema is invariably present with an ischaemic CRVO but this has been shown to be not amenable to laser treatment (BRVOS 1984).

The risk of a recurrence of retinal vein occlusion in the other eye has been shown to be 15% after 5 years of follow-up. The risk of recurrence can be modified by tight control of medical risk factors (Dodson 1985).

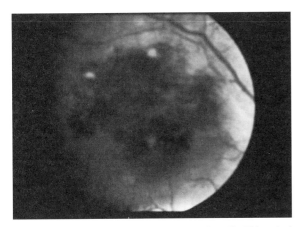

Figure 9.12 *Braach Retinal Vein Occlusion (BRVO)*. This retinal photograph shows an occlusion of a branch retinal vein at an arterio-venous crossing, leading to retinal haemorrhage and retinal thickening and oedema. In this case, hypertension, and hypercholesterolaemia were underlying, and visual outcome was poor ($^6/_{60}$) in this type II diabetic

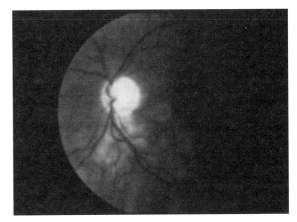

Figure 9.14 *Glaucomatous Optic Disc*. Examination of this optic disc shows an increased cup to disc ratio, with the optic cup close is the optic disc rim. This finding was associated with raised intra-ocular pressure and visual field loss, due to chronic simple glaucoma (open angle)

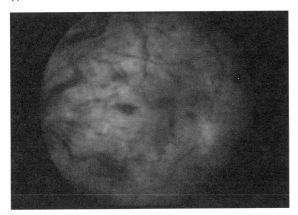

Figure 9.13 *Central Retinal Vein Occlusion (CRVO)*. This retinal photographs demonstrates the typical features of a CRVO, with multiple retinal haemorrhage, dilated tortuous retinal veins, swelling of the optic disc, and in this case, significant visual loss due to macula oedema (6/36). This condition is usually unilateral and is a common non diabetic retinopathic cause of visual loss in diabetic subjects

also a higher incidence of both POAG and normal tension glaucoma in this group (Dielmans et al 1994; Mitchell and Smith 1997). Glaucoma is a form of optic neuropathy (Figure 9.14) with two main hypotheses of underlying cause. The first or 'mechanical' hypothesis explains the progressive loss of optic nerve fibres in terms of direct injury to the optic nerve head caused by an abnormally high intraocular pressure. The second theory explains the neuropathy in terms of poor microcirculation in the optic nerve head itself leading to progressive infarction of optic nerve fibres. The second theory is supported by the existence of 'normal-tension glaucoma'. This disease is similar to the more common primary open-angle glaucoma with progressive loss of optic nerve fibres leading to visual field defects—but in contrast there is no evidence of raised intraocular pressure.

Diabetic patients should have intraocular pressures checked regularly. This can be carried out at routine optometry checks. Later-stage glaucoma may be detected clinically during retinal screening by the presence of optic disc cupping, with a cup disc ratio >0.5. There is a range of medical and surgical therapeutic options to control intraocular pressure and slow the rate of visual field loss.

For the diabetic patient this is in agreement with the targets for prevention of cardiovascular disease in diabetic clinical practice.

Glaucoma

Primary open-angle glaucoma (POAG) is a condition which has increasing incidence with age. It has a high prevalence in the general population and increased prevalence with diabetes. Two studies have confirmed higher intraocular pressures in diabetic patients and

Non-arteritic Anterior Ischaemic Optic Neuropathy

Damage and occlusion of the posterior ciliary artery supply of the optic nerve results in sudden, painless visual loss in the form of an altitudinal field defect or central scotoma. In patients who do not have an underlying inflammatory giant cell arteritis, the risk factors are predominantly those of atherosclerotic disease. A proportion of cases are idiopathic (around 50%), the remaining having an increased prevalence of hypertension, hypercholesterolemia and elevated fibrinogen levels. At the time of the onset of the visual loss the patient may develop optic disc swelling, representing ischemia of the optic nerve head. Vision often improves spontaneously over time, although it may not reach premorbid levels of acuity. There is no treatment to speed or improve prognosis. There is a risk of recurrence affecting the other eye of 24% over 5 years; and although it is unclear yet whether there is any modifiable risk factor associated with this (Beri et al 1987), early data suggests aspirin therapy may be protective against recurrence in the fellow eye.

ADAPTATION TO LIFE WITH REDUCED VISION

For the elderly patient, adapting to life with reduced vision is an immense challenge. It is important that, where appropriate the individual be registered either partially sighted or blind according to national guidelines so that local social services can assess the need for involvement of the support agencies. There is a wide spectrum of visual impairment: very few patients loose all sight and each case needs to be assessed individually. The patient should be referred to a low visual aid (LVA) clinic (usually run by an optometrist with a special interest in LVA) to try various aids to maximize residual sight. These aids cannot restore normal vision but may help the patient to carry out daily tasks such as reading small amounts of type or signing a cheque.

As the diabetic patient approaches old age strenuous efforts must continue to prevent DR by a concerted effort to maintain diabetic, hypertensive and lipid control. This will also benefit general health and reduce the incidence of other retinovascular diseases. The elderly must have fundal screening both at presentation with diabetes and annually thereafter, and should have appropriate and timely referral to an ophthalmologist. They should clearly understand the link between their diabetic management and risks to sight. Should severe visual impairment occur, assessment is appropriate to maximize remaining sight and to provide necessary social support.

ACKNOWLEDGEMENT

The figures in this chapter were originally published in Dodson, Gibson and Kritzinger (Chapman & Hall, 1994) and are reproduced here by permission of Arnold Publishers.

REFERENCES

Beri MR, Klugman et al (1987) Anterior ischaemic optic neuropathy: incidence of bilaterality and various influencing factors. *Journal of Ophthalmology*, **94**, 1020–1028.

Branch Retinal Vein Occlusion Study Group (1984) Argon laser photocoagulation for macula oedema in branch vein occlusion. *American Journal of Ophthalmology*, **98**, 271–282.

BRVOS (Branch Vein Occlusion Study) Group (1986) (ellip) Argon laser scatter photocoagulation for prevention of neovascular and vitreous haemorrhage in branch vein occlusion. *Archives of Ophthalmology*, **104**, 114–109.

Chaturvedi N, Sjolie AK, Stephenson JM, et al (1998) Effect of lisinopril on the progression of retinopathy in normotensive people with Type 1 diabetes: EUCLID study. *Lancet*, **353**, 28–31.

Clermont AC, Aiello LP, Mori F et al (1997) Vascular endothelial growth factor and severity of non-proliferative diabetic retinopathymediate retinal haemodynamics in vivo: a potential role for VEGF in the progression of non-proliferative DR. *American Journal of Ophthalmology*, **124**, 433–446.

Complications of diabetes. *Effective Healthcare*, August 2–11, (1999).

Dale J, Farmer J (2000) Ischaemic and exudative maculopathy: are their risk factors different? *Diabetic Medicine*, **17** (Suppl. 1): 47.

DCCT Research Group (1993) The effect of intensive treatment of diabetes on the development and progression of long-term complications in insulin-dependent diabetes mellitus. *New England Journal of Medicine*, **329**, 977–986.

Diabetic Retinopathy Research Group (1978) Photocoagulation treatment of proliferative diabetic retinopathy: the second report of Diabetic Retinopathy Study findings. *Ophthalmology*, **85**, 82–106.

Dielmans I, Jong PT et al (1994) Primary open angle glaucoma, intraocular pressure and diabetes mellitus in the general elderly population: the Rotterdam study. *Ophthalmology*, **103**, 1271–1275.

Dodson PM, et al (1985) Medical conditions underlying recurrence of RVO. *British Journal of Ophthalmology*, **69**, 493–496.

Dodson PM, Gibson JM, Kritzinger EE (1994) *Clinical Retinopathies*. London: Chapman & Hall.

Easty DL, Sparrow JM (eds) (1999) *Textbook of Ophthalmology*. Oxford: Oxford University Press.

ETDRS (Early Treatment Diabetic Retinopathy Study) Research Group (1987) Treatment techniques and clinical guidelines for photocoagulation of diabetic macular oedema. *Ophthalmology*, **94**, 761–764.

Frank RN (1991) On the pathogenesis of diabetic retinopathy: a 1990 update. *Ophthalmology*, **98**, 586–592.

Gillow T, Garvican L (2000) Diabetic retinopathy screening: edging towards a national programme. *Mod Diabetes Management*, **1**, 2–4.

Gordon B, Chang S, et al (1991) The effects of lipid lowering on diabetic retinopathy. *American Journal of Ophthalmology*, **112**, 385–391.

Grant MB, Mames RN et al (2000) The efficacy of octreotide in the therapy of severe nonproliferative and early proliferative diabetic retinopathy. *Diabetes Care*, **23**, 504–509.

Hansson L, Zanchetti A, Carruthers SG, et al (1997) Effect of intensive blood pressure lowering and low dose aspirin in patients with hypertension: principal results of the hypertension optimum treatment (HOT) randomised trial. *Lancet*, **350**, 1755–1762.

Hope (Heart Outcomes Prevention Evaluation) study investigators (2000) Effects of Ramipril on cardiovascular and microvascular outcomes in people with diabetes mellitus: results of the HOPE and MICRO-HOPE substudy. *Lancet*, **355**, 253–259.

Klein R, Klein BEK, Moss SE (1984a) The Wisconsin Epidemiological Study II: Prevalence and risk of diabetic retinopathy when age of diagnosis is less than thirty years. *Archives of Ophthalmology*, **102**, 520–526.

Klein R, Klein BEK, Moss SE (1984b) The Wisconsin Epidemiological Study II: prevalence and risk of diabetic retinopathy when age of diagnosis is thirty or more years. *Archives of Ophthalmology*, **102**, 527–533.

Kohner EM, Stratton IM, Aldington SJ (1993) Prevalence of diabetic retinopathy at diagnosis of NIDDM in the United Kingdom Prospective Diabetes study. *Investigative Ophthalmology and Visual Science*, **34**, 713 (abstract).

Koya D, Kind G (1998) Protein kinase C activation and the development of diabetic complications. *Diabetes*, **147**, 859–866.

Mitchell P, Smith W (1997) Open angle glaucoma and diabetes: the Blue Mountain Study, Australia. *Ophthalmology*, **104**, 712–718.

Nithyananthan R, Farmer J et al (2000) Can severe visual impairment be reduced by intervention (formal annual review and community retinopathy screening) in a diabetic population? *Diabetes Medicine*, **17** (Suppl.), 49.

Silvestri G (1999) Management of retinopathy in Type II diabetes. The 'bad companions' of diabetes: should the ophthalmologist get involved? *Eye*, **13**, 131–132.

UK Prospective Diabetes Study Group (1998a) Intensive blood-glucose control with sulphonylureas or insulin compared with conventional treatment and risk of complications in patients with type II diabetes. *Lancet*, **352**, 837–853.

UK Prospective Diabetes Study Group (1998b) Tight blood pressure control and risk of macrovascular and microvascular complications in type II diabetes. *British Medical Journal*, **317**, 703–713.

10

Hypoglycaemia

Vincent McAulay, Brian M. Frier

Royal Infirmary of Edinburgh

INTRODUCTION

Hypoglycaemia is the most serious and disruptive side-effect of the treatment of diabetes in the elderly. While it is a recognized clinical consequence of the use of insulin and sulphonylureas in all age groups requiring such therapy, the frequency of hypoglycaemia is underestimated in elderly people with diabetes. This may be because its clinical manifestations are unrecognized or are wrongly attributed to other pathological conditions such as cerebral ischaemia or degenerative disorders.

The effects of hypoglycaemia can be severe in elderly patients, many of whom are physically frail and have coexisting macrovascular disease. They may therefore be at increased risk of suffering a major vascular event such as myocardial infarction and stroke as a consequence of hypoglycaemia. In addition, frequent and unpredictable hypoglycaemia in an old person, causing problems such as dizziness, disturbed balance, weakness, transient loss of consciousness and falls, can undermine their self-confidence and have a destabilizing effect on their independence and ability to live alone. The imposition of the burden of prevention and treatment of hypoglycaemia on relatives and carers, many of whom may also be elderly, may provoke further domestic difficulties, threatening the independence of the affected individual, and possibly precipitating their transfer to residential care. The emergence of hypoglycaemia as a prominent problem in an elderly person with diabetes may influence their management by encouraging health attendants to avoid the risk of exposure to a low blood glucose and to accept poor or suboptimal glycaemic control.

Although most people who develop diabetes later in life have Type 2 diabetes as a consequence of the decline in pancreatic beta-cell function that occurs with progressive duration of diabetes, treatment with insulin is increasing in elderly people with Type 2 diabetes. Some older people have an insulin-deficient form of diabetes, and require insulin from the time of diagnosis. Although hypoglycaemia is considered to be a relatively uncommon side-effect of oral hypoglycaemic agents (UK Prospective Diabetes Study Group 1998), many sulphonylureas promote hypoglycaemia of varying frequency and severity. The expanding practice of combining oral hypoglycaemic agents with insulin in the treatment of Type 2 diabetes may exacerbate this problem, particularly in the elderly patient. The risk of exposure to insulin-induced hypoglycaemia is therefore rising steadily in older people with diabetes.

Before examining epidemiology and morbidity, it is important to ascertain whether age, per se, affects the symptomatic awareness of, and counter-regulatory hormonal response to, acute hypoglycaemia, and how these fundamental responses to a low blood glucose may be modified by the presence of Type 2 diabetes in an ageing population.

PHYSIOLOGICAL RESPONSES TO HYPOGLYCAEMIA

Counter-regulation

The human brain is dependent upon glucose as its principal source of energy and requires a continuous supply of glucose via the cerebral circulation. Depriving the brain of glucose rapidly causes neuroglycopenia, which has various effects, including impairment of cognitive function.

In humans, several mechanisms have evolved to maintain glucose homeostasis and so protect the

---

Diabetes in Old Age. Second Edition. Edited by A. J. Sinclair and P. Finucane. © 2001 John Wiley & Sons Ltd.

integrity and functioning of the brain (Cryer 1993). A decline in blood glucose concentration activates a characteristic hierarchy of responses, commencing with the suppression of endogenous insulin secretion, the release of several counter-regulatory hormones, and the subsequent development of characteristic symptoms (Figure 10.1). These alert the informed individual to the development of hypoglycaemia, so allowing him or her to take early and appropriate action (the ingestion of carbohydrate) to assist recovery. Such protective responses are usually effective in maintaining the arterial blood glucose concentration within a normoglycaemic range (which can be arbitrarily defined as a blood glucose above 3.8 mM), which protects the brain from exposure to neuroglycopenia. Glucose counter-regulation is controlled from centres within the brain (mainly the ventromedial hypothalamus) assisted by activation of hypothalamic autonomic nervous centres with stimulation of the peripheral sympatho-adrenal system. This contributes to glucose counter-regulation through the peripheral actions of catecholamines and by the generation of characteristic autonomic warning symptoms (Figure 10.2). Although glucagon is the most potent counter-regulatory hormone, the role of adrenaline becomes paramount if the secretory response of glucagon is deficient (Gerich 1988). Other counter-regulatory hormones, such as cortisol and growth hormone, have greater importance in promoting recovery from prolonged hypoglycaemia.

Glucagon and adrenaline stimulate hepatic glycogenolysis, releasing glucose from glycogen stored in the liver, and also promote gluconeogenesis from

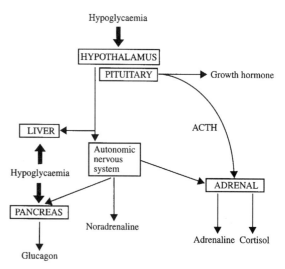

Figure 10.2 Principal components of glucose counter-regulation in humans

three-carbon precursors such as alanine, lactate and glycerol. The energy for this process is provided by the hepatic oxidation of free fatty acids that are released by lipolysis. Catecholamines inhibit insulin secretion, diminish the peripheral uptake of glucose, stimulate lipolysis and proteolysis, and promote glycogenolysis in peripheral muscle to provide lactate, which is utilized for gluconeogenesis in the liver and kidney.

Symptoms

Both the sympathetic and parasympathetic divisions of the autonomic nervous system are activated during hypoglycaemia, leading to the direct neural stimulation of end-organs via peripheral autonomic nerves, and the physiological effects are augmented by the secretion of adrenaline from the adrenal medulla (Cryer et al 1989) (Figure 10.3). Studies in young adults using physiological and pharmacological methods to assess the symptoms of hypoglycaemia have confirmed that the symptoms of pounding heart, tremulousness and feeling nervous or anxious are adrenergic in nature (Towler et al 1993). The sweating response to hypoglycaemia is mediated primarily via sympathetic cholinergic stimulation (Corrall et al 1983; Towler et al 1993), with circulating catecholamines possibly contributing through activation of alpha-adrenoceptors (Macdonald and Maggs 1993).

Deprivation of glucose in the brain leads to rapid interference with information processing, the onset of

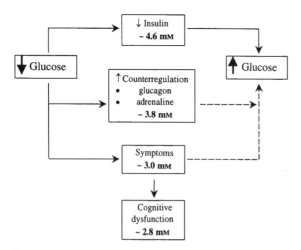

Figure 10.1 Hierarchy of responses to hypoglycaemia in non-diabetic humans

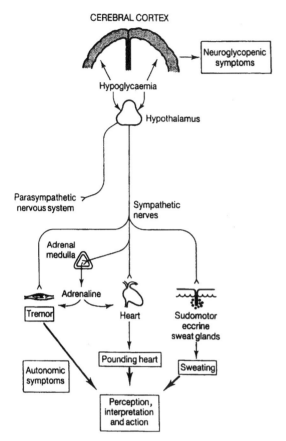

CEREBRAL CORTEX

Neuroglycopenic symptoms

Hypoglycaemia

Hypothalamus

Parasympathetic nervous system

Sympathetic nerves

Adrenal medulla

Adrenaline

Tremor

Heart

Sudomotor eccrine sweat glands

Autonomic symptoms

Pounding heart

Sweating

Perception, interpretation and action

Figure 10.3 Activation of the autonomic nervous system and the sympatho-adrenal system during hypoglycaemia. Reproduced from *Hypoglycaemia and Diabetes* (eds Frier BM, Fisher BM) by permission of Edward Arnold (Publisher) Ltd

Table 10.1 Classification of symptoms of hypoglycaemia in patients with insulin-treated diabetes

Children (pre-pubertal)	Adults	Elderly
Autonomic/ neuroglycopenic Behavioural	Autonomic Neuroglycopenic Nonspecific malaise	Autonomic Neuroglycopenic Neurological

Reproduced from *Hypoglycaemia in Clinical Diabetes* (eds Frier BM, Fisher BM) by permission of John Wiley & Sons Ltd (1999)

idiosyncratic and vary between individuals. They may also differ in intensity in different situations, and their perception can be influenced by distraction or other external influences. In perceiving the onset of hypoglycaemia (often described as subjective 'awareness'), the intensity of a few cardinal symptoms is of importance to the individual, rather than the total number or nature of the symptoms generated. An assessment of the subjective reality of symptoms is therefore essential in attempting any form of measurement or devising a scoring system. Both autonomic and neuroglycopenic symptoms appear to be of equal value in warning people with Type 1 diabetes of the onset of hypoglycaemia, provided that the symptoms peculiar to the individual are identified and interpreted correctly (Deary 1999).

cognitive dysfunction, and the development of neuroglycopenic symptoms such as difficulty concentrating, feelings of tiredness and drowsiness, faintness, dizziness, generalized weakness, confusion, difficulty speaking and blurring of vision.

Statistical techniques have also been used to classify the symptoms of hypoglycaemia. On applying methods such as 'principal components analysis', the symptoms of hypoglycaemia segregate into three distinct factors or groups: *neuroglycopenic, autonomic* and *general malaise* (Deary et al 1993). This 'three factor' validated model containing 11 common symptoms of hypoglycaemia (the Edinburgh Hypoglycaemia Scale), has been used to classify symptoms objectively in various groups of subjects, and has shown age-specific differences in the nature of hypoglycaemic symptoms as classified by this statistical method (Table 10.1). Symptoms of hypoglycaemia are

Glycaemic Thresholds

Different physiological responses occur when the declining blood glucose reaches specific concentrations. Although these glycaemic thresholds are readily reproducible in non-diabetic humans (Vea et al 1992), they are plastic and dynamic and can be modified. In non-diabetic humans the glycaemic threshold at which the secretion of most counter-regulatory hormones is triggered is around 3.8 mM (arterialized blood glucose), so that counter-regulation is usually activated when blood glucose falls below the normal range. Counter-regulation therefore occurs at a higher blood glucose than that at which the symptomatic response to hypoglycaemia occurs (3.0 mM) and before the onset of cognitive dysfunction (2.8 mM) (Figure 10.1). The glycaemic threshold for symptoms coincides with the classical autonomic 'reaction' to hypoglycaemia which can be identified by the sudden development of physiological changes (Frier and Fisher 1999).

In people with diabetes, glycaemic thresholds can be modified by the prevailing glycaemic state, and parti-

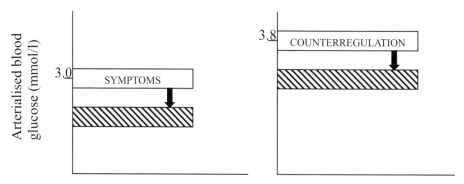

Figure 10.4 Glycaemic thresholds for counter-regulatory hormonal secretion and the onset of symptoms can vary depending on the prevailing level of glycaemic control in people with diabetes. Strict glycaemic control is associated with a higher glycaemic threshold (i.e. a lower blood glucose concentration is required), providing a more intense hypoglycaemic stimulus

cularly by strict control (Figure 10.4), and can also be influenced by metabolic perturbations such as preceding (antecedent) hypoglycaemia. Many studies in people with insulin-treated diabetes who have strict glycaemic control have demonstrated that the counter-regulatory hormonal and symptomatic responses to hypoglycaemia do not occur until a much lower blood glucose concentration is reached, particularly when the glycated haemoglobin concentration is within the non-diabetic range (Amiel 1999). Similarly, antecedent hypoglycaemia lasting for one hour or more has been shown to diminish the magnitude of the symptomatic and neuroendocrine responses to any subsequent episode of hypoglycaemia occurring within the following 24–48 hours (Frier and Fisher 1999) (Figure 10.5). This may be one of the mechanisms that induces

impaired awareness of hypoglycaemia in people with Type 1 diabetes.

ACQUIRED HYPOGLYCAEMIA SYNDROMES IN TYPE 1 DIABETES

Counter-regulatory Deficiencies

In many people with Type 1 diabetes, the glucagon secretory response to hypoglycaemia becomes diminished or absent within a few years of the onset of insulin-deficient diabetes. With glucagon deficiency alone, blood glucose recovery from hypoglycaemia is relatively unaffected because counter-regulation is maintained by the actions of adrenaline. However, in up to 45% of people who have Type 1 diabetes of long duration, dual impairment of the secretion of glucagon and adrenaline is observed (Gerich and Bolli 1993), predisposing them to serious deficiencies of glucose counter-regulation when exposed to hypoglycaemia, delaying the recovery of blood glucose and allowing progression to more severe hypoglycaemia (Table 10.2). People with Type 1 diabetes of long duration are

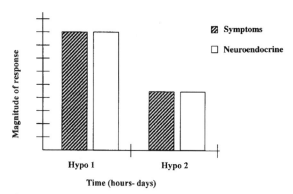

Figure 10.5 Schematic representation of the effect of antecedent hypoglycaemia on the neuroendocrine and symptomatic responses to subsequent hypoglycaemia. Reproduced from *Hypoglycaemia in Clinical Practice* (eds Frier BM, Fisher BM) by permission of John Wiley & Sons Ltd (1999)

Table 10.2 Frequency of abnormal counter-regulatory responses to hypoglycaemia in patients with Type 1 diabetes

Duration of diabetes	Glucagon (%)	Adrenaline (%)	Cortisol (%)	Growth hormone (%)
< 1 y	27	9	0	0
1–5 years	75	25	0	0
5–10 years	100	44	11	11
> 10 years	92	66	25	25

Reproduced from *Hypoglycaemia and Diabetes* (eds Frier BM, Fisher BM) by permission of Edward Arnold (Publisher) Ltd

Table 10.3 Factors influencing normal awareness of hypoglycaemia

Internal	External
Physiological	*Drugs*
Recent glycaemic control	Beta-adrenoceptor blockers (non-selective)
Degree of neuroglycopenia	Hypnotics, tranquillizers
Symptom intensity/sensitivity	Alcohol
Psychological	*Environmental*
Arousal	Sleep
Focused attention	Posture
Congruence; denial	Distraction
Competing explanations	
Education	
Knowledge	
Symptom belief	

Reproduced from *Hypoglycaemia in Clinical Diabetes* (eds Frier BM, Fisher BM) by permission of John Wiley & Sons Ltd (1999)

therefore at increased risk of developing severe and prolonged hypoglycaemia, particularly when intensive insulin therapy is used (White et al 1983). These counter-regulatory deficiencies co-segregate with impaired awareness of hypoglycaemia in people with Type 1 diabetes (Ryder et al 1990), suggesting a common pathogenetic mechanism within the brain.

Impaired Awareness of Hypoglycaemia

Many factors can influence the awareness of hypoglycaemia (Table 10.3). When the symptomatic warning is diminished or inadequate in people with diabetes, this is described as *impaired awareness of hypoglycaemia* or *hypoglycaemia unawareness*. Impaired awareness is not an 'all or none' phenomenon. 'Partial' impairment of awareness may develop, with the individual being aware of some episodes of hypoglycaemia but not others. Alternatively, he or she may experience a reduction in the intensity or number of symptoms which varies between hypoglycaemic events, and progress to 'absent' awareness where the patient is no longer aware of the onset of hypoglycaemia. Several mechanisms underlying this problem have been proposed (Table 10.4).

Impaired awareness of hypoglycaemia is common, affecting around one-quarter of all insulin-treated patients, becomes more prevalent with increasing duration of diabetes, and predisposes the patient to a high risk of developing severe hypoglycaemia (Frier and Fisher 1999). In some patients, impaired awareness may be reversible, being attributable to an elevated glycaemic threshold during intensive insulin therapy or has followed recurrent severe hypoglycaemia (Cryer et al 1994); but in patients with Type 1 diabetes of long duration it may be a permanent defect.

Central Autonomic Failure

Because hormonal counter-regulatory deficiencies and impaired awareness of hypoglycaemia co-segregate and are associated with an increased frequency of severe hypoglycaemia, the concept of a 'hypoglycaemia-associated autonomic failure' has been proposed by Cryer (1992). The suggestion is that recurrent severe hypoglycaemia may be the primary problem which causes these abnormalities, and by establishing a vicious circle perpetuates this state.

Table 10.4 Possible mechanisms of impaired awareness of hypoglycaemia

CNS adaptation
Chronic exposure to low blood glucose
Strict glycaemic control in diabetic patients
Insulinoma in non-diabetic patients

Recurrent transient exposure to low blood glucose
Antecedent hypoglycaemia

CNS glucoregulatory failure
Counter-regulatory deficiency (hypothalamic defect?)
Hypoglycaemia-associated central autonomic failure

Reproduced from *Hypoglycaemia in Clinical Diabetes* (eds Frier BM, Fisher BM) by permission of John Wiley & Sons Ltd (1999)

EFFECTS OF AGE ON PHYSIOLOGICAL RESPONSES TO HYPOGLYCAEMIA

Counter-regulatory Mechanisms

Because many physiological processes alter with advancing age in humans, it is important to determine whether the ageing process per se may affect the nature and efficacy of the glucose counter-regulatory response to hypoglycaemia. In non-diabetic elderly subjects, a study of the counter-regulatory hormonal responses to hypoglycaemia induced by an intravenous infusion of insulin suggested that diminished secretion of growth hormone and cortisol is a feature of advanced age (Marker, Cryer and Clutter 1992), and a modest impairment of hormonal counter-regulatory secretion was present with some attenuation of the blood glucose recovery (Marker et al 1992). Insulin clearance was reduced, as was the secretion of glucagon, while the release of adrenaline was delayed, and these changes were unaffected by preceding physical training, suggesting that they were not related to a sedentary lifestyle (Marker et al 1992). However, a study using the hyperinsulinaemic glucose clamp technique has indicated that age per se had no effect (Meneilly et al 1985). Comparative analysis and interpretation of these studies are problematical because of differences between study groups in the speed of onset and duration of hypoglycaemia and of the magnitude of the plasma insulin concentrations achieved, factors which can influence the nature of the counter-regulatory hormonal response.

A study in older non-diabetic subjects (mean age 76 years) by Meneilly, Cheung and Tuokko (1994a), using a stepped glucose clamp technique, demonstrated deficiencies in the secretion of glucagon and adrenaline. Ortiz-Alonso et al (1994) compared counter-regulatory responses in 11 older non-diabetic individuals (mean age 65 years) with 13 young, healthy volunteers (mean age 24 years). Subtle differences were observed in the magnitude of the hormonal counter-regulatory responses in the older group (in whom the adrenaline, glucagon, pancreatic polypeptide and cortisol responses were lower) in response to modest hypoglycaemia (arterialized blood glucose 3.3 mM). However, no such differences were demonstrated when the hypoglycaemic stimulus was more profound (arterialized blood glucose 2.8 mM). Two further studies in non-diabetic elderly subjects using similar designs and methodologies have not demonstrated any significant age-related impairments

of the counter-regulatory hormonal responses to hypoglycaemia (Brierley et al 1995; Matyka et al 1997).

Symptomatic Response to Hypoglycaemia

Differences between age groups in the symptom profiles to hypoglycaemia have been demonstrated in children and adults with insulin-treated diabetes (Deary 1999), and older people with diabetes have been observed to experience a cluster of 'neurological' symptoms (unsteadiness, poor coordination, slurring of speech and visual disturbances) (Jaap et al 1998) in addition to the classical autonomic and neuroglycopenic groups of symptoms recognized in young adults (Table 10.5). Age per se may therefore modify the nature and intensity of some symptoms of hypoglycaemia, possibly as a consequence of other age-related changes such as effects on cerebral circulation, and the presence of underlying cerebrovascular disease or degenerative abnormalities of the central nervous system (Table 10.6).

In a small group of non-diabetic subjects in whom hypoglycaemia was induced using a stepped glucose clamp, lower symptom scores were recorded in the seven older subjects (mean age 72 years) than in the six younger subjects (mean age 30 years), and the usual haemodynamic responses to hypoglycaemia (particularly a rise in heart rate) were absent in the older group (Brierley et al 1995). This suggests that symptomatic awareness of hypoglycaemia may be

Table 10.5   Symptoms of hypoglycaemia in the elderly

Neuroglycopenic	Autonomic	Neurological
Weakness	Sweating	Unsteadiness
Drowsiness	Shaking	Poor coordination
Poor concentration	Pounding heart	Double vision
Dizziness	Anxiety	Blurred vision
Confusion		Slurred speech
Lightheadedness		

Table 10.6   Hypoglycaemia in the elderly: effects of age

1. Mild attenuation of blood glucose recovery may occur (hepatic glucose production is diminished)
2. Modest reductions in counter-regulatory hormonal responses are demonstrable (but maximal response to more severe hypoglycaemia)
3. Symptom response is less intense with altered glycaemic threshold and reduced awareness of hypoglycaemia

reduced in the elderly, and is associated with an attenuated end-organ response to sympatho-adrenal stimulation. As this generates many of the autonomic symptoms of hypoglycaemia, perception of hypoglycaemia is affected.

In another study of older non-diabetic subjects, the symptomatic response to hypoglycaemia commenced at a lower blood glucose (mean ± SD: 3.0 ± 0.2 mM) than in a younger group (3.6 ± 0.1 mM), suggesting that the glycaemic threshold for the generation of symptoms is modified by age, with a lower blood glucose being required to initiate a symptomatic response (Matyka et al 1997) (Table 10.7).

Cognitive Function

The hierarchy of the cognitive changes in response to hypoglycaemia may change with age. In the study of non-diabetic subjects by Matyka et al (1997), the responses to moderate hypoglycaemia of seven elderly men were compared with those of seven young men. The four-choice reaction time, a measure of psychomotor coordination, deteriorated in the older men at a mean ± SD plasma glucose of 3.0 ± 0.1 mM compared with 2.6 ± 0.1 mM in the young group, and the abnormality was more profound (Figure 10.6). Because the symptomatic response to hypoglycaemia commenced at a lower blood glucose concentration in the older men than in the young adults (3.0 ± 0.2 versus 3.6 ± 0.1 mM), in the older subjects the glycaemic thresholds for subjective symptomatic awareness of hypoglycaemia and for the onset of cognitive dysfunction were coincidental. A similar problem has been observed in patients with Type 1 diabetes who have developed impaired awareness of hypoglycaemia, in whom the onset of the cognitive dysfunction induced by hypoglycaemia either precedes or is coincidental with the onset of a symptomatic response (Frier and Fisher 1999). This observation suggests that the elderly may be at an intrinsically greater risk of

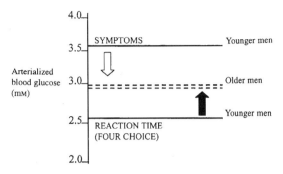

Figure 10.6 The difference between the glycaemic threshold for subjective awareness of hypoglycaemia and that for the onset of cognitive dysfunction may be absent in the elderly. Derived from data in Matyka et al (1997)

developing neuroglycopenia because the onset of warning symptoms and cognitive impairment occur simultaneously, so interfering with their ability to recognize and take action to self-treat a low blood glucose.

EFFECTS OF TYPE 2 DIABETES ON RESPONSES TO HYPOGLYCAEMIA

Counter-regulation

Good glycaemic control in Type 2 diabetes limits the development and severity of vascular complications, but achieving this with insulin and many of the oral hypoglycaemic agents inevitably increases the risk of hypoglycaemia (UK Prospective Diabetes Study Group 1998). The counter-regulatory and symptomatic responses to hypoglycaemia have been studied in patients with Type 2 diabetes, but earlier studies were performed using a variety of techniques and protocols which makes comparisons between studies either difficult or impossible. Problems included the study of heterogeneous groups of subjects with Type 1 and Type 2 diabetes (Reynolds et al 1977), or variation in the magnitude of the hypoglycaemic stimulus between subjects because the blood glucose differed at baseline (Nonaka et al 1977; Polonsky et al 1984). Using the hyperinsulinaemic glucose clamp technique, Heller, Macdonald and Tattersall (1987) induced hypoglycaemia in 10 non-obese subjects with Type 2 diabetes (mean age 42 years) and in 10 non-diabetic controls. No differences were observed between the groups in the *venous* blood glucose nadir (approximately 2.4 mM), the rate of fall, and the rate of recovery of blood glucose. The basal and incremental values of

Table 10.7 Hypoglycaemia in the elderly: symptoms

1. Autonomic symptoms are not selectively diminished
2. Intensity of all symptoms (historical reports and experimental studies) is low
3. Glycaemic threshold for onset of symptoms is altered by age; a lower blood glucose is required to initiate symptoms
4. Cognitive dysfunction induced simultaneously by hypoglycaemia may interfere with perception of symptoms
5. Awareness of hypoglycaemia may be reduced by ageing

glucagon, growth hormone and cortisol were similar. Other studies, using intravenous bolus injection or infusion of insulin to induce hypoglycaemia, demonstrated that the counter-regulatory hormonal responses were normal in people with Type 2 diabetes (Table 10.8).

Meneilly, Cheung and Tuokko (1994b) used a glucose clamp method to lower the blood glucose in a stepwise fashion in older non-obese subjects, 10 having Type 2 diabetes (mean age 74 years) and 10 being healthy non-obese controls (mean age 72 years). At an arterialized blood glucose concentration of 2.8 mM, the subjects with diabetes exhibited lower increments of glucagon and growth hormone, whereas in the non-diabetic subjects the magnitudes of the adrenaline and cortisol secretory responses were higher.

Bolli et al (1984) used the subcutaneous route of administration of insulin to induce mild hypoglycaemia (arterialized plasma glucose nadir 3.4 mM) in 13 relatively young, non-obese subjects with Type 2 diabetes (mean age 46 years) and in 11 matched non-diabetic controls. The diabetic subjects received an intravenous insulin infusion overnight to ensure that their baseline blood glucose at the start of the hypoglycaemia study was comparable with the non-diabetic control group. Over a 12-hour period, the blood glucose recovery was slightly slower in the people with Type 2 diabetes and the maximal responses of glucagon, cortisol and growth hormone were 50% lower than those observed in the controls. By contrast, the adrenaline response was similar in both groups and the noradrenaline response was higher in the subjects with Type 2 diabetes.

Using the glucose clamp procedure to achieve an arterialized blood glucose of 2.7 mM, Landstedt-Hallin, Adamson and Lins (1999a) demonstrated that oral glibenclamide suppressed the glucagon response during acute insulin-induced hypoglycaemia in 13 patients with Type 2 diabetes (mean age 57 years). This is an important observation since many patients with Type 2 diabetes are treated with a combination of sulphonylureas and isophane insulin administered at bedtime.

In conclusion, few counter-regulatory hormonal deficiencies of significance have been observed in people with Type 2 diabetes, in contrast to the pronounced counter-regulatory hormonal deficiencies exhibited by many individuals with Type 1 diabetes (Table 10.9). None of the studies in people with Type 2 diabetes has demonstrated any abnormality of the

Table 10.8 Studies of hormonal counter-regulation to hypoglycaemia in patients with Type 2 diabetes

Study	Number of patients	Method of hypoglycaemia induction	Mean glucose nadir (mM)	Hormonal response
Nonaka et al (1977)	27	IV insulin bolus	2.0	Reduced glucagon
Levitt et al (1979)	10	IV insulin bolus	1.8	No impairment
Boden et al (1983)	10	IV insulin infusion	1.7	No impairment
Polonsky et al (1984)	8	IV insulin infusion	1.9	No impairment
Bolli et al (1984)	13	SC insulin bolus	3.4	Reduced glucagon, cortisol and growth hormone
Heller et al (1987)	10	IV insulin infusion	2.4	No impairment
Meneilly et al (1994b)	10	IV insulin infusion	2.8	Reduced glucagon and growth hormone; increased adrenaline and cortisol
Shamoon et al (1994)	9	IV insulin infusion	3.4	Reduced glucagon and increased adrenaline
Korzon-Burakowska et al (1998)	7	IV insulin infusion	2.4	Glucagon response preserved in 5 patients; magnitude of adrenaline response was increased when glycaemic control was poor
Levy et al (1998)	11	IV insulin infusion	2.2	No impairment

Table 10.9 Combined effects of age and Type 2 diabetes

1. Modest attenuation of blood glucose recovery observed (no rise in hepatic glucose production and decline in peripheral utilization)
2. Some counter-regulatory hormonal responses are reduced (but not adrenaline)
3. Counter-regulatory hormonal response to profound hypoglycaemia is intact; subtle abnormalities are revealed by slow fall in blood glucose
4. Some tests of cognitive function (psychomotor tests) are more abnormal than in controls

adrenaline response to hypoglycaemia. However, this may change when patients with Type 2 diabetes have progressed to pancreatic beta-cell failure, and then behave like people with Type 1 diabetes.

Symptoms of Hypoglycaemia

Allowing for differences in age, the symptoms of hypoglycaemia do not appear to differ between people with Type 1 and Type 2 diabetes, nor does the agent inducing hypoglycaemia influence the nature of the symptoms. People with Type 2 diabetes who were receiving treatment with insulin reported a similar symptom profile associated with hypoglycaemia as did a group with Type 1 diabetes, who were matched for duration of insulin therapy, but not for age or duration of diabetes (Hepburn et al 1993). Using the hyperinsulinaemic glucose-clamp technique, Levy et al (1998) showed that the hypoglycaemic symptoms experienced by subjects with Type 2 and Type 1 diabetes, who had a similar quality of glycaemic control, were identical. In a different study, the nature of the symptomatic response to a similar degree of hypoglycaemia, induced either by insulin or with tolbutamide, was compared in a group of non-diabetic subjects, and no differences were observed either in the nature or intensity of symptoms (Peacey et al 1996). The agent inducing the hypoglycaemia does not therefore appear to be important, as identical symptoms were produced when blood glucose was lowered in the same individual, although interindividual differences were evident because of the idiosyncratic nature of hypoglycaemic symptoms.

Symptoms in Elderly People with Type 2 Diabetes

Older people with Type 2 diabetes have been shown to have a lower intensity, and more limited perception, of autonomic symptoms of hypoglycaemia than age-matched non-diabetic elderly subjects (Meneilly et al 1994b). In a descriptive study of 45 elderly patients with Type 2 diabetes who were receiving treatment either with insulin or a sulphonylurea, the symptoms of hypoglycaemia that were recognized most commonly were nonspecific in nature and included weakness, unsteadiness, sleepiness and faintness (Thomson et al 1991). In a retrospective study of people with Type 2 diabetes treated with insulin (Jaap et al 1998), the hypoglycaemia symptoms that were reported with the greatest frequency and intensity were mainly 'neuro-

logical' in nature and included unsteadiness, light-headedness and poor concentration (Table 10.5). Trembling (71.2%) and sweating (75%) also featured prominently, contrasting with a Canadian study in which it was claimed that the autonomic symptoms of hypoglycaemia in the elderly were attenuated (Meneilly et al 1994a). However, the latter study did not use an age-specific symptom questionnaire, and differences in symptom questionnaires and in scoring methods of inducing hypoglycaemia may account for the differences in symptom profiles that have been described.

Using the statistical technique of principal components analysis, the hypoglycaemia symptoms of elderly people with Type 2 diabetes could be separated into neuroglycopenic and autonomic groups, but the typical symptoms of a 'general malaise' group of symptoms such as headache or nausea were rare (Jaap et al 1998). However, symptoms such as impaired motor coordination and slurring of speech were prominent. In elderly people, these symptoms may be misinterpreted as representing either cerebral ischaemia, intermittent haemodynamic changes associated with cardiac dysrhythmia, or vasovagal and syncopal attacks. Health-care professionals should be aware of the age-specific differences in hypoglycaemic symptoms (Table 10.1), both from the need to identify and treat hypoglycaemia, and for educational purposes.

EPIDEMIOLOGY OF HYPOGLYCAEMIA IN ELDERLY PEOPLE WITH DIABETES

Incidence

The frequency of hypoglycaemia in people with diabetes is difficult to determine with accuracy and most clinical studies have probably underestimated the total number of hypoglycaemic events.

In subjects with Type 1 diabetes, retrospective recall of mild (self-treated) episodes of hypoglycaemia is inaccurate beyond a period of one week, and prospective recording of hypoglycaemia is essential to obtain a precise measure (Pramming et al 1991). Recall of severe hypoglycaemia may be affected by amnesia of the event, so that confirmation by observers and relatives is desirable to verify the accuracy of self-reporting.

The frequency of hypoglycaemia among people with Type 2 diabetes may be even more difficult to ascertain and is prone to underestimation, partly because many are old, their memory may be impaired, their knowledge of symptoms is often very limited, and symptoms of hypoglycaemia may be attributed incorrectly to other conditions.

Sulphonylurea-induced Hypoglycaemia in Type 2 Diabetes

One Swedish report of the annual incidence of sulphonylurea-induced hypoglycaemia of sufficient severity to require hospital treatment recorded a rate of 4.2 per 1000 patients (Dahlen et al 1984), but other European surveys have estimated this to be much lower at 0.19–0.25 per 1000 patient-years (Berger 1985; Campbell 1985). This contrasts with the much higher incidence of *insulin-induced* hypoglycaemic coma which has been estimated conservatively at 100 per 1000 patient-years (Gerich 1989), and severe hypoglycaemia—defined as an episode requiring external assistance for recovery—is probably three times more frequent than coma (Tattersall 1999). A 2-year prospective trial that involved 321 subjects with Type 2 diabetes receiving treatment with either chlorpropamide or glibenclamide recorded an incidence of *symptomatic* hypoglycaemia of 19 per 1000 patient-years (Clarke and Campbell 1975). Around one-fifth of a relatively young group of 203 patients with Type 2 diabetes who were receiving treatment with oral sulphonylureas had experienced symptoms suggestive of hypoglycaemia on at least one occasion during the previous 6 months (Jennings, Wilson and Ward 1989). Symptoms were reported most frequently with long-acting preparations such as glibenclamide, and in association with other medications recognized to potentiate their hypoglycaemic effect. Several studies have attempted to explain the differential risk of hypoglycaemia with sulphonylureas by examining the sensitivity of different types of K_{ATP} channels in the pancreatic β-cell to sulphonylureas (Ashcroft and Gribble 2000; Gribble and Ashcroft 1999). Gliclazide was found to have a high affinity and strong selectivity for the beta-cell type of K_{ATP} channel and this was reversible. It is speculated that these observations may part explain why gliclazide may have less potential to hypoglycaemia than glibenclamide which has an irreversible binding to the β-cell K_{ATP} channel.

In the USA, Shorr et al (1997) undertook a retrospective cohort study of almost 20 000 elderly people with diabetes receiving treatment with either insulin or sulphonylureas, who were enrolling for health insurance. The incidence of fatal hypoglycaemia and of serious hypoglycaemia (defined as an emergency admission to hospital with a documented blood glucose concentration <2.8 mM) was approximately 2 per 100 patient-years. People treated with insulin had a higher incidence of serious hypoglycaemia than those treated with sulphonylureas (3 per 100 patient-years, versus 1 per 100 patient-years).

Insulin-induced Hypoglycaemia in Type 2 Diabetes

Few large-scale studies have recorded the frequency of hypoglycaemic episodes in people with Type 2 diabetes treated with insulin over a protracted period. The proportion of patients experiencing hypoglycaemia during the first 10 years of the UKPDS is shown in Table 10.10. People in the intensively treated group of the UKPDS experienced significantly more episodes of hypoglycaemia than did those in the conventionally treated group (UK Prospective Diabetes Study Group 1998); but this was still much lower than estimated frequencies of severe hypoglycaemia, ranging from 1.1 to 1.6 episodes per patient per year, in unselected cohorts of people with Type 1 diabetes in specialist centres in Denmark (Pramming et al 1991) and in Scotland (MacLeod, Hepburn and Frier 1993) in whom strict glycaemic control was not an objective. In a smaller study, the prevalence of severe hypoglycaemia was estimated retrospectively in 104 people with Type 2 diabetes of long duration who had progressed to pancreatic beta-cell failure and required insulin, and was not much lower than that of a group of patients with Type 1 diabetes who were matched for duration of insulin therapy but not for age or duration of diabetes (Hepburn et al 1993). However, in a pilot study in the USA of 14 people with Type 2 diabetes on maximal

Table 10.10 Proportion of patients with Type 2 diabetes experiencing hypoglycaemia per year in UK Prospective Diabetes Study over 10 years of the study by principal treatment regimen (mean figures are shown)

	One or more episodes of hypoglycaemia (%)	Any episode of hypoglycaemia (%)
Diet	0.1	1.2
Chlorpropamide	0.4	11.0
Glibenclamide	0.6	17.7
Insulin	2.3	36.5

Source: Derived from UKPDS (1998).

doses of oral hypoglycaemic agents, the use of insulin therapy for 6 months not only lowered mean HbA_{1c} from 7.7% to 5.1%, but the hypoglycaemia that occurred was mild, infrequent and declined in frequency from an initial level of 4.1 to 1.3 episodes per patient per month at the end of the study (Henry et al 1993).

The incidence of hypoglycaemia is generally low in patients with Type 2 diabetes who are treated with insulin before the development of severe insulin deficiency, probably because many are overweight and have insulin resistance. Hypoglycaemia may be much less of a problem in people with insulin-treated Type 2 diabetes because their counter-regulatory hormonal responses are not compromised, the plasma free insulin profile is more stable, and glycaemic targets are often less strict in older people than in young people with Type 1 diabetes.

ADVERSE EFFECTS OF HYPOGLYCAEMIA

Mortality

Mortality associated with sulphonylurea-induced hypoglycaemia has been calculated to be 0.014 to 0.033 per 1000 patient-years (Berger 1985; Campbell 1985), contrasting with an estimated mortality from insulin-induced hypoglycaemia in the UK for diabetic patients under 50 years of age of approximately 0.2 per 1000 patient-years (Tunbridge 1981). In one series, 10% of patients with severe sulphonylurea-induced hypoglycaemia who were admitted to hospital subsequently died (Seltzer 1972). Other reviews of the outcome of severe hypoglycaemia associated with sulphonylurea therapy cite a mortality rate of approximately 10% (Campbell 1993).

Morbidity

The morbidity associated with hypoglycaemia in people with diabetes has been reviewed by Frier (1992), Fisher and Heller (1999) and Perros and Deary (1999). Because of increasing physical frailty and concomitant diseases such as osteoporosis, the elderly may be more susceptible to physical injury during hypoglycaemia, with fractures of long bones, joint dislocations, soft tissue injuries, head injuries and occasionally burns being described as a direct consequence of accidents associated with hypoglycaemia. Hypothermia may also be a direct consequence of hypoglycaemic coma, and the fall in skin temperature

during experimentally induced hypoglycaemia is significantly greater in the presence of the nonselective beta adrenoceptor-blocker propranolol (Macdonald et al 1982).

Acute hypoglycaemia provokes a profound haemodynamic response secondary to sympatho-adrenal activation and the secretion of adrenaline, causing an increase in the workload of the heart and a widening of pulse pressure (Fisher and Heller 1999). Although this degree of haemodynamic stress seldom causes any pathophysiological problem to the young person with normal cardiac function, in the older individual with diabetes (who may have underlying macrovascular disease) hypoglycaemia may have serious or even fatal consequences. In diabetic patients who have coronary heart disease, cardiac arrhythmias may be induced. These have been described during experimentally induced hypoglycaemia and in anecdotal case reports, with atrial fibrillation, nodal rhythms, and premature atrial and ventricular contractions all being observed during hypoglycaemia in diabetic patients who had no overt clinical evidence of heart disease (Lindström et al 1992; Fisher and Heller 1999). Sudden death during hypoglycaemia-induced cardiac arrhythmia has been described in individual case reports (Frier et al 1995; Burke and Kearney 1999). Transient ventricular tachycardia has been observed during experimental hypoglycaemia in a non-diabetic subject with coronary heart disease, and acute myocardial infarction has also been reported in association with acute hypoglycaemia (Fisher and Heller 1999). Acute hypoglycaemia can lengthen the QT interval on the electrocardiogram in both non-diabetic and diabetic subjects (Marques et al 1997). QT dispersion is a marker of spatial difference in myocardial recovery time that, when increased, indicates an increased risk of ventricular arrhythmias and sudden death. This was significantly higher during acute insulin-induced hypoglycaemia in 13 patients with Type 2 diabetes aged 48–63 years (Landstedt-Hallin et al 1999b). When combined with the effects of catecholamine-mediated hypokalaemia and the profound haemodynamic changes associated with acute hypoglycaemia, the potential for inducing a serious cardiac arrhythmia is enhanced in elderly people who may have coronary heart disease (Table 10.11).

Various psychological and neurological manifestations of acute hypoglycaemia can cause variable loss of sensory and motor functions (Table 10.12). Transient ischaemic attacks and transient hemiplegia may be a feature of neuroglycopenia, and less commonly, permanent neurological deficits have been described,

Table 10.11 Potential cardiac sequelae of acute hypoglycaemia

Frequent ventricular and atrial ectopics
Prolongation of QT-interval
Atrial fibrillation
Non-sustained ventricular tachycardia
Silent myocardial ischaemia
Angina
Myocardial infarction

Table 10.12 Neuropsychological manifestations of severe hypoglycaemia

Neurological
Focal or generalized convulsions
Coma
Hemiparesis; TIAs
Ataxia; choreoathetosis
Focal neurological deficits
Decortication
Psychological
Cognitive impairment
Behavioural/personality changes
Automatism or aggressive behaviour; psychosis

especially in elderly patients. These are presumably caused by mechanisms such as direct focal cerebral damage from glucopenia, acute thrombotic occlusion secondary to the haemodynamic, haemostatic and haemorrheological effects of hypoglycaemia, or by cerebral ischaemia provoked by changes in regional blood flow in the brain (Perros and Deary 1999). Elderly people who experience intermittent hypoglycaemia, particularly from the effect of long-acting oral hypoglycaemic agents, may be misdiagnosed as having transient ischaemic attacks. In a retrospective review of 778 cases of drug-induced hypoglycaemia, permanent neurological deficit was described in 5% of the survivors (Seltzer 1979). In a report of 102 cases of hypoglycaemic coma induced either by insulin or by glibenclamide, physical injury was reported in seven patients, myocardial ischaemia in two and stroke in one (Ben-Ami et al 1999).

RISK FACTORS

Retrospective studies have identified advanced age and fasting as the two major risk factors associated with sulphonylurea-induced hypoglycaemia (Asplund et al

1983, 1991; Seltzer 1989; Shorr et al 1997; Stahl and Berger 1999). The principal risk factors are shown in Table 10.13, and are most pertinent to the elderly. Surveys in Sweden (Asplund et al 1983, 1991) of fatal and severe cases of hypoglycaemia revealed that severe hypoglycaemia was common in the first month of treatment and was not related to the dose of the drug used; coma and serious morbidity were common sequelae. A frequent problem in the elderly is intercurrent illness during which caloric intake is reduced substantially, but the dose of sulphonylurea is maintained, so provoking severe hypoglycaemia. However, adherence to therapy is a common problem, particularly with increasing frequency of administration and number of drugs prescribed (Paes, Bakker and Soe-Angie 1997; Donnan et al 2000). Sometimes hypoglycaemia is induced when older people with diabetes are admitted to hospital and their prescribed dose of oral hypoglycaemic medication is now administered accurately. This may be compounded by modification of diet in hospital with reduction in carbohydrate consumption in the hospital diet or through loss of appetite associated with illness. Shorr et al (1997) identified admission to hospital in the preceding 30 days as the strongest predictor of severe hypoglycaemia in their cohort of 20 000 elderly Americans. In persons aged 80 years or older, the risk of serious hypoglycaemia was increased further within 30 days of discharge from hospital.

More recently, the importance of some of these 'conventional' risk factors has been challenged, with randomized controlled trials suggesting that fasting can be well-tolerated in healthy elderly people with Type 2 diabetes who are taking maximal doses of sulphonylureas once daily (Burge et al 1998). Similarly, moderate exercise during fasting has been shown to be well-tolerated among elderly people with Type 2 diabetes treated with oral sulphonylureas (Riddle, McDaniel and Tive 1997). This suggests that, with

Table 10.13 Risk factors for sulphonylurea-induced hypoglycaemia

Age (not dose of drug)
Impaired renal function
Previous history of cardiovascular disease or stroke
Reduced food intake; diarrhoea
Alcohol ingestion
Adverse drug interactions
Use of long-acting sulphonylureas
Recent hospital admission

more careful clinical selection of people who are suitable for treatment with sulphonylureas, the risk of hypoglycaemia can be minimized.

Fasting and Exercise

In a randomized study of the effect of a 23-hour fast, 52 subjects with Type 2 diabetes (mean age 65 years) received either glibenclamide, a sustained-release formulation of glipizide, or a placebo; none of the participants experienced hypoglycaemia during each study arm (Burge et al 1998). In a study of 25 obese subjects with Type 2 diabetes (age 33–80 years) who had received 9 weeks' treatment with sustained-release glipizide or placebo, no hypoglycaemia was experienced when overnight fasting was followed by 90 minutes of standardized exercise. Furthermore, the blood glucose decrement from the fasting baseline concentration was modest and equal in both groups, although not all of the subjects in this study were taking the same dose of medication and many probably had insulin resistance (Riddle et al 1997).

Alcohol

Alcohol inhibits hepatic gluconeogenesis even at blood concentrations that are not usually associated with intoxication. In subjects with Type 1 diabetes, it impairs the ability to perceive and interpret the symptoms of hypoglycaemia (Kerr et al 1990). Burge et al (1999) performed a prospective, double-blind, placebo-controlled trial in 10 older subjects with Type 2 diabetes (mean age 68 y) to assess the effects of combining alcohol ingestion with fasting. After a 14-hour fast, the administration of glibenclamide and intravenous alcohol (equivalent to drinking one or two alcoholic beverages) resulted in a lower blood glucose nadir (4.3 ± 1.2 mM) than in the group who did not receive alcohol (5.0 ± 1.4 mM). In a subject who developed hypoglycaemia (defined as blood glucose <2.8 mM with typical symptoms or any blood glucose concentration <2.2 mM) during both arms of the study, hypoglycaemia occurred earlier (at 5 hours) in the ethanol study compared with the placebo arm (8.5 hours). This observation is of practical importance since the quantity of alcohol administered in the study was of a similar amount to that consumed on a regular basis by many people with Type 2 diabetes.

Long-acting Sulphonylurea Agents

Many studies have recorded higher rates of hypoglycaemia with long-acting sulphonylureas such as chlorpropamide and glibenclamide. A community-based study over a 12-year period in Basle in Switzerland demonstrated that treatment of elderly subjects with Type 2 diabetes with longer-acting sulphonylureas was three times more likely to precipitate admission to hospital with severe hypoglycaemia than the use of short-acting agents (Stahl and Berger 1999). Tessier et al (1994) studied a cohort of 22 subjects with Type 2 diabetes who were older than 70 years. The subjects were treated for 6 months with either glibenclamide or gliclazide in a randomized, double-blind fashion and the treatment groups were matched for age, BMI and dose of medication. At one month the mean glycated haemoglobin values were similar in the two groups. The majority of hypoglycaemic events occurred in the month after the initiation of therapy, with a greater frequency observed in those treated with glibenclamide (13 episodes) compared with gliclazide (4 episodes) (Figure 10.7).

In a different randomized, crossover trial of glipizide and glibenclamide in 21 subjects with Type 2 diabetes, aged 60–80 years, all of whom performed regular blood glucose monitoring, Brodows (1992) observed that asymptomatic biochemical hypoglycaemia occurred in 11% of the group treated with glibenclamide compared with 7% of those treated with glipizide (Figure 10.8). However, not all long-acting sulphonylureas provoke hypoglycaemia. Glimepiride is administered once daily and stimulates insulin production primarily in response to meals, but the in-

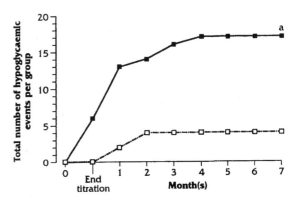

Figure 10.7 Frequency of hypoglycaemic events: ■ glibenclamide, □ gliclazide; [a]$p < 0.01$ between groups. Reproduced from Tessier et al (1994) with permission of the American Diabetes Association

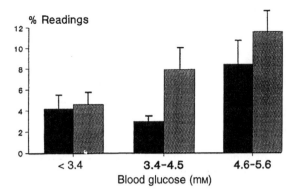

Figure 10.8 Prevalence of home blood glucose readings <5.6 mM during glipizide (solid bars) and glibenclamide (hatched bars) treatment. Values are means ± standard error. Reproduced from Brodows (1992) with permission of John Wiley & Sons Ltd

cidence of reported hypoglycaemia is low (Campbell 1998). In randomized studies comparing glimepiride with glibenclamide and gliclazide, the incidence of symptomatic hypoglycaemia was lower in the glimepiride-treated patients (Schneider 1996). This contrasts with the results of an earlier double-blind comparative study of glimepiride and gliclazide in patients with Type 2 diabetes in Japan which demonstrated lower hypoglycaemic rates in the gliclazide-treated group (2.6%) compared with the glimepiride group (4.8%) (Kaneko et al 1993).

Almost all sulphonylurea drugs are metabolized in the liver to metabolites that are subsequently excreted in the urine. While most of these metabolites either have minimal or no metabolic activity, the two major hepatic metabolites of chlorpropamide do possess hypoglycaemic activity. In combination with its long half-life of approximately 36 hours, chlorpropamide is more likely to induce prolonged hypoglycaemia in elderly people because of the normal age-related decline in the glomerular filtration rate. In general the use of long-acting sulphonylureas should be avoided in elderly patients with Type 2 diabetes and in those with renal impairment. Renal impairment prolongs the biological activity of sulphonylurea agents that are cleared primarily through the kidneys, and in this situation treatment should be either with a sulphonylurea that is metabolized mainly in the liver, such as gliclazide, or with insulin.

In Germany, it is estimated that more than 50% of all patients with Type 2 diabetes are treated with sulphonylurea drugs, mostly with the long-acting glibenclamide (Lorenz and Hillenbrand 1993), use of which has declined considerably in the UK. Glibenclamide-induced hypoglycaemia may be more pronounced because the drug accumulates within pancreatic beta cells and its metabolites retain some hypoglycaemic activity. Despite this, many elderly patients with Type 2 diabetes who have accompanying risk factors for hypoglycaemia are still being prescribed these agents (Yap et al 1998; Ben-Ami et al 1999). In a review of 150 elderly people with Type 2 diabetes, 40 of the 45 who were taking glibenclamide had one or more identifiable risk factors for hypoglycaemia (Yap et al 1998). Although most sulphonylureas can cause fatal hypoglycaemia, this has been associated most frequently with chlorpropamide and glibenclamide (Ferner and Neil 1988).

Adverse Drug Interactions

Several adverse drug interactions between sulphonylureas and other commonly prescribed medications are recognized that increase the risk of sulphonylurea-induced hypoglycaemia. In a comprehensive review, 15% of patients with sulphonylurea-induced hypoglycaemia were simultaneously taking medications known to increase the risk of hypoglycaemia (Seltzer 1989). Many drugs can potentiate the effects of sulphonylurea agents via a variety of mechanisms, and the important drug interactions promoting hypoglycaemia are summarized in Table 10.14.

Table 10.14 Drug interactions with sulphonylureas leading to hypoglycaemia

Interaction	Drug
Displacement from albumin binding sites	Aspirin, fibrates, sulphonamides, warfarin, trimethoprim
Decreased renal excretion	Probenecid, aspirin, allopurinol
Decreased hepatic metabolism	Warfarin, monoamine oxidase inhibitors
Insulin secretagogues	Nonsteroidal antiinflammatory drugs, low-dose aspirin
Inhibition of gluconeogenesis	Alcohol
Increased peripheral glucose uptake	Aspirin

TREATMENT

Hypoglycaemia is only one of a number of differential diagnoses in the elderly diabetic patient presenting in a comatose state. Although manifestations of cerebrovascular disease may be suspected, hypoglycaemia should be excluded by blood glucose testing. However, even when the blood glucose is low, other common causes such as stroke, intracerebral or subarachnoid haemorrhage, head injury and deliberate or accidental drug or alcohol overdose must not be overlooked. A failure to respond either rapidly or at all to treatment with parenteral glucose should raise suspicion of other causes of coma. Failure to recover consciousness following an episode of severe hypoglycaemia may be associated with cerebral oedema, which has a poor prognosis. Affected patients require management in hospital in an intensive care unit with the use of agents such as mannitol, steroids and high-flow oxygen. This suspected diagnosis should be confirmed, and other causes of coma excluded, by neuroimaging of the brain. Although most patients recover rapidly from an episode of hypoglycaemia, it can take as long as 40–90

minutes after blood glucose returns to normal for cognitive function to be fully restored (Blackman et al 1992; Lindgren et al 1996).

The treatment of hypoglycaemia in people with Type 2 diabetes follows the same basic principles as in Type 1 diabetes, but important differences are present between those treated with insulin and those treated with sulphonylureas (Figure 10.9). In the conscious individual, acute hypoglycaemia is treated with rapid-acting oral carbohydrate, usually in the form of glucose tablets or confectionery such as sweets or chocolate. Beverages with a high glucose content are also suitable, such as fresh orange juice. Following this, some form of long-acting carbohydrate should be ingested to prevent recurrence of the hypoglycaemia. In the drowsy or unconscious patient who cannot swallow, an intravenous injection of dextrose (20–50 mL of a 50% solution) will reverse neuroglycopenia rapidly. Glucagon is very effective if administered to people treated with insulin who are semi-conscious or in hypoglycaemic coma. Glucagon (1 mg by intramuscular injection) can be administered by a friend or relative familiar with the technique or by paramedical staff, but

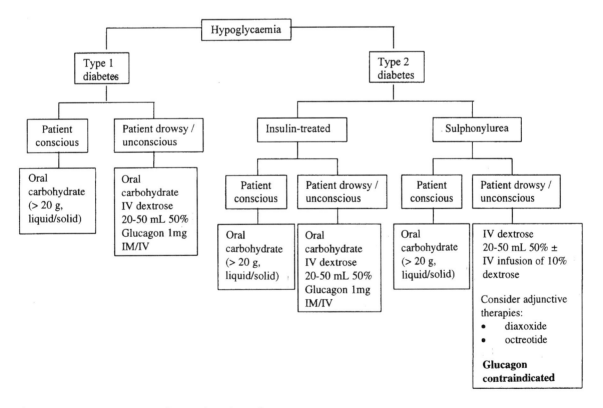

Figure 10.9 Treatment measures for acute hypoglycaemia

can induce nausea and/or vomiting. It acts through promoting hepatic glycogenolysis to stimulate hepatic glucose output, so is sometimes ineffective in patients with protracted hypoglycaemia whose stores of glycogen are exhausted, in people with advanced liver disease or alcohol abuse, and in those with malnutrition or inanition.

Sulphonylurea-induced Hypoglycaemia

Mild sulphonylurea-induced hypoglycaemia is treated in a similar fashion to insulin-induced hypoglycaemia by the ingestion of rapid-acting glucose followed by longer-acting carbohydrate as food (bread, biscuits, cereal or other alternatives). Sulphonylurea-induced hypoglycaemic coma requires inpatient management, and following administration of intravenous dextrose the patient should not be discharged immediately from hospital despite apparent recovery, as hypoglycaemia from this cause is often prolonged with frequent relapses (Gale 1980; Marks 1981; Ferner and Neil 1988). Glucagon can stimulate insulin secretion in people with Type 2 diabetes who have residual pancreatic beta-cell function (Marri, Cozzolino and Palumbo 1968) and therefore may be contraindicated in the treatment of sulphonylurea-induced hypoglycaemia. Following a bolus intravenous injection of 20–50 mL of 50% dextrose, many patients require prolonged intravenous infusion of 10% (or even 20%) dextrose to maintain a blood glucose concentration above 5.0 mM. The duration of the intravenous infusion will depend upon the half-life of the sulphonylurea ingested, and in cases of overdose it may be necessary to continue the dextrose infusion for several days.

Adjunctive Therapies

Diazoxide has a direct inhibitory effect on insulin secretion and has been used as an adjunct to dextrose infusion in the treatment of sulphonylurea-induced hypoglycaemia (Johnson, Schade and Peake 1977; Palatnick, Meatherall and Tenenbein 1991). In the unconscious patient, diazoxide can be infused intravenously (300 mg over 30 minutes and repeated every 4 hours if necessary), or in the conscious patient can be administered orally (300 mg every 4 hours). Octreotide, a long-acting synthetic analogue of somatostatin, was used to treat sulphonylurea-induced hypoglycaemia successfully in a non-diabetic patient

who had taken an overdose of tolbutamide (Krentz et al 1993). Octreotide reverses the hyperinsulinaemia induced by excessive administration of a sulphonylurea, and, in contrast to diazoxide, reduces the amount of dextrose required to maintain euglycaemia (Boyle et al 1993).

KNOWLEDGE OF SYMPTOMS

Many patients and their relatives are remarkably uninformed about the symptoms of hypoglycaemia (Mutch and Dingwall-Fordyce 1985; Thomson et al 1991) and its emergency treatment. In one study, 9% of elderly people who were taking sulphonylureas or insulin were unable to state any of the symptoms associated with hypoglycaemia. Only 20% of the group said that they had been told about the symptoms of hypoglycaemia. Of particular concern, people who were living alone had no better knowledge of symptoms despite being at greater risk (Mutch and Dingwall-Fordyce 1985). Knowledge of the symptoms of hypoglycaemia was unrelated to the duration of diabetes and living alone, and did not differ between men and women. However, older people knew even less about hypoglycaemia than did younger individuals with diabetes. Many people with diabetes taking sulphonylureas did not know about the potential risk of developing hypoglycaemia, whereas people treated with insulin were more knowledgeable on this subject. These findings were confirmed by a different study in which 88% of elderly people taking sulphonylureas did not know about the potential risk of hypoglycaemia, whereas only 32% of those treated with insulin denied any knowledge of hypoglycaemia (Thomson et al 1991). This lack of knowledge extends to the treatment of hypoglycaemia, with around 20% of elderly people with insulin-treated diabetes being unfamiliar with the appropriate measures required to treat symptomatic hypoglycaemia (Pegg et al 1991). This reflects the problems of providing information about side-effects of therapy, and the putative deficiencies of the education for an elderly group with Type 2 diabetes, some of whom have impaired verbal memory, who may have difficulty retaining information about the risk of drug-induced hypoglycaemia, and who require regular reinforcement about possible symptoms and their treatment (Strachan et al 1997). Many elderly patients with Type 2 diabetes are treated in primary care, and education about therapeutic side-effects must not be overlooked.

PREVENTION OF HYPOGLYCAEMIA

All patients taking insulin or sulphonylureas should receive education about the symptoms of hypoglycaemia, the most appropriate form of self-management, and should be advised to take regular meals to ensure an adequate intake of carbohydrate. All patients taking insulin should carry a card or other form of identification stating that they have diabetes and what treatment they are taking. People who are self-administering insulin should carry a source of rapid-acting carbohydrate. Individuals at increased risk of hypoglycaemia should be identified, such as those older than 70 years and people with renal impairment. In elderly people with Type 2 diabetes, the longer-acting sulphonylurea agents such as chlorpropamide and glibenclamide (but not glimepiride) should be avoided, and short-acting sulphonylureas such as glipizide, gliclazide, or even the more old-fashioned tolbutamide, should be used and commenced at the lowest dose; this can be titrated against the patient's fasting or post-prandial blood glucose. Persistently low blood glucose values will require a reduction in dose. Consideration should also be given to the use of alternative oral hypoglycaemic agents that either do not cause or have a lower risk of hypoglycaemia, such as metformin, acarbose or miglitol, and the thiazolidinediones. Utilization of fast-acting insulin analogues and fixed mixtures containing these insulin preparations may also be of value in elderly people treated with insulin, particularly to avoid nocturnal hypoglycaemia.

To improve adherence to prescribed oral hypoglycaemic therapy, a dosette box can be used in an attempt to reduce the risk of overdose due to forgetfulness and to the difficulties of coping with polypharmacy. Clinicians must be particularly aware of drug interactions with sulphonylureas and anticipate and modify their prescribing patterns accordingly (Table 10.14). It is important to provide adequate information to relatives and other carers who may be administering medications and monitoring blood glucose at home, because they may lack knowledge of the symptoms and consequences of hypoglycaemia (Table 10.15).

SUMMARY AND CONCLUSIONS

1. Hypoglycaemia in the elderly person with Type 2 diabetes is a potentially serious and underestimated clinical problem that has a significant morbidity and mortality.
2. Many symptoms of hypoglycaemia in the elderly are 'neurological' in type, the cause of which may be misinterpreted as representing a cerebrovascular event or cardiac arrhythmia.
3. The effects of ageing and of Type 2 diabetes on hormonal counter-regulation, symptoms and awareness of hypoglycaemia should be considered when deciding upon targets for glycaemic control in elderly people with diabetes.
4. Although most elderly people have Type 2 diabetes, insulin therapy is increasingly being used. At present, the counter-regulatory hormonal deficiencies and impaired awareness of hypoglycaemia that are common in people with Type 1 diabetes are seldom observed in elderly patients with diabetes, but these may increase in prevalence.
5. Although hypoglycaemia is a common side-effect of insulin therapy, it occasionally may be a life-threatening problem in people taking long-acting sulphonylureas, especially those of advanced years who have concomitant renal impairment and/or inadequate caloric intake.
6. Long-acting sulphonylureas such as glibenclamide and chlorpropamide should be avoided in the elderly. Adverse drug interactions with sulphonylurea agents can cause profound hypoglycaemia.
7. Important differences exist in the immediate treatment of hypoglycaemia whether induced by insulin or sulphonylureas; the use of glucagon may be contraindicated in sulphonylurea-induced hypoglycaemia.
8. People with diabetes who are treated with sulphonylureas or insulin, and their relatives or carers, must be fully informed about the symptoms and effects of hypoglycaemia and its emergency management, and this should be reinforced with appropriate education at intervals.

Table 10.15 Prevention of hypoglycaemia

1. Identify high risk patients: advanced age, renal impairment
2. Avoid long-acting sulphonylurea preparations
3. Use short-acting sulphonylurea (e.g. gliclazide)
4. Be aware of drug interactions
5. Educate patients and relatives/carers about hypoglycaemia
6. Consider agents that do not cause hypoglycaemia

REFERENCES

Amiel SA (1999) Risks of strict glycaemic control. In: Frier BM, Fisher BM (eds) *Hypoglycaemia in Clinical Diabetes*. Chichester: John Wiley, 147–166.

Ashcroft FM, Gribble FM (2000) Tissue-specific effects of sulfonylureas. Lessons from studies of cloned K_{ATP} channels. *Journal of Diabetes Complications*, **14**, 192–196.

Asplund K, Wilholm BE, Lithner F (1983) Glibenclamide associated hypoglycaemia: a report on 57 cases. *Diabetologia*, **24**, 412–417.

Asplund K, Wilholm BE, Lundman B (1991) Severe hypoglycaemia during treatment with glipizide. *Diabetic Medicine*, **8**, 726–731.

Ben-Ami H, Nagachandran P, Mendelson A, Edoute Y (1999) Drug-induced hypoglycemic coma in 102 diabetic patients. *Archives of Internal Medicine*, **159**, 281–284.

Berger W (1985) Incidence of severe side-effects during therapy with sulfonylureas and biguanides. *Hormone and Metabolic Research*, **15** (Suppl.), 111–115.

Blackman JD, Towle VL, Sturis J, Lewis GF, Spire JP, Polonsky KS (1992) Hypoglycemic thresholds for cognitive dysfunction in IDDM. *Diabetes*, **41**, 392–399.

Boden G, Soriano M, Hoeldtke RD, Owen OE (1983) Counter-regulatory hormone release and glucose recovery after hypoglycemia in non-insulin-dependent diabetic patients. *Diabetes*, **32**, 1055–1059.

Bolli GB, Tsalikian E, Haymond MW, Cryer PE, Gerich JE (1984) Defective glucose counter-regulation after subcutaneous insulin in non-insulin-dependent diabetes mellitus. *Journal of Clinical Investigation*, **73**, 1532–1541.

Boyle PJ, Justice K, Krentz AJ, Nagy RJ, Schade DS (1993) Octreotide reverses hyperinsulinemia and prevents hypoglycemia induced by sulfonylurea overdoses. *Journal of Clinical Endocrinology and Metabolism*, **76**, 752–756.

Brierley EJ, Broughton DL, James OWF, Alberti KGMM (1995) Reduced awareness of hypoglycaemia in the elderly despite an intact counter-regulatory response. *Quarterly Journal of Medicine*, **88**, 439–445.

Brodows RG (1992) Benefits and risks with glyburide and glipizide in elderly NIDDM patients. *Diabetes Care*, **15**, 75–80.

Burge MR, Schmitz-Fiorentino K, Fischette C, Qualls CR, Schade DS (1998) A prospective trial of risk factors for sulfonylurea-induced hypoglycemia in Type 2 diabetes mellitus. *JAMA*, **14**, 137–143.

Burge MR, Zeise TM, Sobhy TA, Rassam AG, Schade DS (1999) Low-dose ethanol predisposes elderly fasted patients with Type 2 diabetes to sulfonylurea-induced low blood glucose. *Diabetes Care*, **22**, 2037–2043.

Burke BJ, Kearney TK (1999) Hypoglycaemia and cardiac arrest. *Practical Diabetes International*, **16**, 189–190.

Campbell IW (1985) Metformin and the sulphonylureas: the comparative risk. *Hormone and Metabolic Research*, **15** (Suppl.), 105–111.

Campbell IW (1993) Hypoglycaemia and Type 2 diabetes: sulphonylureas. In: Frier BM, Fisher BM (eds) *Hypoglycaemia and Diabetes. Clinical and Physiological Aspects*. London: Edward Arnold, 387–392.

Campbell RK (1998) Glimepiride: role of a new sulfonylurea in the treatment of Type 2 diabetes mellitus. *Annals of Pharmacotherapy*, **32**, 1044–1052.

Clarke BF, Campbell IW (1975) Long-term comparative trial of glibenclamide and chlorpropamide in diet-failed, maturity onset diabetics. *Lancet*, **1**, 246–248.

Corrall RJM, Frier BM, Davidson NMcD, Hopkins WM, French EB (1983) Cholinergic manifestations of the acute autonomic reaction to hypoglycaemia in man. *Clinical Science*, **64**, 49–53.

Cryer PE (1992) Iatrogenic hypoglycemia as a cause of hypoglycemia-associated autonomic failure in IDDM: a vicious cycle. *Diabetes*, **41**, 255–260.

Cryer PE (1993) Glucose counter-regulation: prevention and correction of hypoglycemia in humans. *American Journal of Physiology*, **264**, E149–E155.

Cryer PE, Binder C, Bolli GB, Cherrington AD, Gale EAM, Gerich JE, Sherwin RS (1989) Hypoglycemia in IDDM. *Diabetes*, **38**, 1193–1199.

Cryer PE, Fisher JN, Shamoon H (1994) Hypoglycemia. *Diabetes Care*, **17**, 734–755.

Dahlen M, Bergman U, Idman L, Martinsson L, Karlsson G (1984) Epidemiology of hypoglycaemia in patients on oral antidiabetic drugs in the island of Gotland, Sweden. *Acta Endocrinologica*, **263** (Suppl.), 21 (abstract).

Deary IJ (1999) Symptoms of hypoglycamia and effects on mental performance and emotions. In: Frier BM, Fisher BM (eds) *Hypoglycaemia in Clinical Diabetes*. Chichester: John Wiley, 29–54.

Deary IJ, Hepburn DA, MacLeod KM, Frier BM (1993) Partitioning the symptoms of hypoglycaemia using multi-sample confirmatory factor analysis. *Diabetologia*, **36**, 771–777.

Donnan PT, Brennan GM, Macdonald TM, Morris AD (2000) Population-based adherence to prescribed medication in Type 2 diabetes: cause for concern. *Diabetic Medicine*, **17** (Suppl. 1),

Ferner RE, Neil HA (1988) Sulphonylureas and hypoglycaemia. *British Medical Journal*, **296**, 949–950.

Fisher BM, Heller SR (1999) Mortality, cardiovascular morbidity and possible effects of hypoglycaemia on diabetic complications. In: Frier BM, Fisher BM (eds) *Hypoglycaemia in Clinical Diabetes*. Chichester: John Wiley 167–186.

Frier BM (1992) Hypoglycaemia: how much harm? *Hospital Update*, **18**, 876–884.

Frier BM, Fisher BM (1999) Impaired hypoglycaemia awareness. In: Frier BM, Fisher BM (eds) *Hypoglycaemia in Clinical Diabetes*. Chichester: John Wiley 111–146.

Frier BM, Barr StCG, Walker JD (1995) Fatal cardiac arrest following acute hypoglycaemia in a diabetic patient. *Practical Diabetes International* **12**, 284.

Gale EAM (1980) Hypoglycaemia. *Clinics in Endocrinology and Metabolism*, **9**, 461–475.

Gerich JE (1988) Glucose counter-regulation and its impact on diabetes mellitus. *Diabetes*, **37**, 1608–1617.

Gerich JE (1989) Oral hypoglycemic agents. *New England Journal of Medicine*, **321**, 1231–1245.

Gerich JE, Bolli GB (1993) Counter-regulatory failure. In: Frier BM, Fisher BM (eds) *Hypoglycaemia and Diabetes: Clinical and Physiological Aspects*. London: Edward Arnold, 253–267.

Gribble FM, Ashcroft FM (1999) Differential sensitivity of beta-cell and extrapancreatic K_{ATP} channels to gliclazide. *Diabetologia*, **42**, 845–848.

Heller SR, Macdonald IA, Tattersall RB (1987) Counter-regulation in Type 2 (non-insulin-dependent) diabetes mellitus: normal endocrine and glycaemic responses, up to ten years after diagnosis. *Diabetologia*, **30**, 924–929.

Henry RR, Gumbiner B, Ditzler T, Wallace P, Lyon R, Glauber HS (1993) Intensive conventional insulin therapy for Type II diabetes: metabolic effects during a 6-mo outpatient trial. *Diabetes Care*, **16**, 21–31.

Hepburn DA, MacLeod KM, Pell ACH, Scougal IJ, Frier BM (1993) Frequency and symptoms of hypoglycaemia experienced by patients with Type 2 diabetes treated with insulin. *Diabetic Medicine*, **10**, 231–237.

Jaap AJ, Jones GC, McCrimmon RJ, Deary IJ, Frier BM (1998) Perceived symptoms of hypoglycaemia in elderly Type 2 diabetic patients treated with insulin. *Diabetic Medicine*, **15**, 398–401.

Jennings AM, Wilson RM, Ward JD (1989) Symptomatic hypoglycemia in NIDDM patients treated with oral hypoglycemic agents. *Diabetes Care*, **12**, 203–208.

Johnson SF, Schade DS, Peake GT (1977) Chlorpropamide-induced hypoglycemia: successful treatment with diazoxide. *American Journal of Medicine*, **63**, 799–804.

Kerr D, Macdonald IA, Heller SR, Tattersall RB (1990) Alcohol causes hypoglycaemic unawareness in healthy volunteers and patients with Type I (insulin-dependent) diabetes. *Diabetologia*, **33**, 216–221.

Korzon-Burakowska A, Hopkins D, Matyka K, Lomas J, Pernet A, Macdonald I, Amiel S (1998) Effects of glycemic control on protective responses against hypoglycemia in Type 2 diabetes. *Diabetes Care*, **21**, 283–290.

Krentz AJ, Boyle PJ, Justice KM, Wright AD, Schade DS (1993) Successful treatment of severe refractory sulfonylurea-induced hypoglycemia with octreotide. *Diabetes Care*, **16**, 184–186.

Landstedt-Hallin L, Adamson U, Lins PE (1999a) Oral glibenclamide suppresses glucagon secretion during insulin-induced hypoglycaemia in patients with Type 2 diabetes. *Journal of Clinical Endocrinology and Metabolism*, **84**: 3140–3145.

Landstedt-Hallin L, Englund A, Adamson U, Lins PE (1999b) Increased QT dispersion during hypoglycaemia in patients with Type 2 diabetes. *Journal of Internal Medicine*, **246**: 299–307.

Levitt NS, Vinik AI, Sive AA, Child P, Jackson WPU (1979) Studies on plasma glucagon concentration in maturity-onset diabetics with autonomic neuropathy. *Diabetes*, **28**, 1015–1021.

Levy CJ, Kinsley BT, Bajaj M, Simonson DC (1998) Effect of glycemic control on glucose counter-regulation during hypoglycemia in NIDDM. *Diabetes Care*, **21**, 1330–1338.

Lindgren M, Eckert B, Stenberg G, Agardh CD (1996) Restitution of neurophysiological functions, performance, and subjective symptoms after moderate insulin-induced hypoglycaemia in non-diabetic men. *Diabetic Medicine*, **13**, 218–225.

Lindström T, Jorfeldt L, Tegler L, Arnqvist HJ (1992) Hypoglycaemia and cardiac arrhythmias in patients with Type 2 diabetes mellitus. *Diabetic Medicine*, **9**, 536–541.

Lorenz N, Hillenbrand H (1993) Wieviel Diabetiker gibt es in Deutschland? *Diabetres Journal*, **11**, 4–8.

Macdonald IA, Maggs DA (1993) Cutaneous blood flow, sweating, tremor and temperature regulation in hypoglycaemia. In: Frier BM, Fisher BM (eds) *Hypoglycaemia and Diabetes: Clinical and Physiological Aspects*. London: Edward Arnold, 132–143.

Macdonald IA, Bennett T, Gale EAM, Green JH, Walford S (1982) The effect of propranolol or metoprolol on thermoregulation during insulin-induced hypoglycaemia in man. *Clinical Science*, **63**, 301–310.

MacLeod KM, Hepburn DA, Frier BM (1993) Frequency and morbidity of severe hypoglycaemia in insulin-treated diabetic patients. *Diabetic Medicine*, **10**, 238–245.

Marker JC, Cryer PE, Clutter WE (1992) Attenuated glucose recovery from hypoglycemia in the elderly. *Diabetes*, **41**, 671–678.

Marks V (1981) Drug-induced hypoglycaemia. In: Marks V, Rose FC (eds) *Hypoglycaemia*, 2nd edn. Oxford: Blackwell Scientific, 357–386.

Marri G, Cozzolino G, Palumbo R (1968) Glucagon in sulphonylurea hypoglycaemia? *Lancet*, **i**, 303–304.

Marques JLB, George E, Peacey SR, Harris ND, Macdonald IA, Cochrane T, Heller SR (1997) Altered ventricular repolarisation during hypoglycaemia in patients with diabetes. *Diabetic Medicine*, **14**, 648–654.

Matyka K, Evans M, Lomas J, Cranston I, Macdonald I, Amiel SA (1997) Altered hierarchy of protective responses against severe hypoglycemia in normal aging in healthy men. *Diabetes Care*, **20**, 135–141.

Meneilly GS, Minaker KL, Young JB, Landsberg L, Rowe JW (1985) Counter-regulatory responses to insulin-induced glucose reduction in the elderly. *Journal of Clinical Endocrinology and Metabolism*, **61**, 178–182.

Meneilly GS, Cheung E, Tuokko H (1994a) Altered responses to hypoglycemia of healthy elderly people. *Journal of Clinical Endocrinology and Metabolism*, **78**, 1341–1348.

Meneilly GS, Cheung E, Tuokko H (1994b) Counter-regulatory hormone responses to hypoglycemia in the elderly patient with diabetes. *Diabetes*, **43**, 403–410.

Mutch WJ, Dingwall-Fordyce I (1985) Is it a hypo? Knowledge of symptoms of hypoglycaemia in elderly diabetic patients. *Diabetic Medicine*, **2**, 54–56.

Nonaka K, Toyoshima T, Yoshida T, Matsuyama T, Trarni S, Nishikawa M (1977) The nature of hyperglucagonaemia in diabetes mellitus. In: Foa TP, Jajos JS, Foa NL (eds) *Glucagon: Its Role in Physiology and Clinical Medicine*. New York: Springer-Verlag, 662–677.

Ortiz-Alonso FJ, Galecki A, Herman WH, Smith MJ, Jacquez JA, Halter JB (1994) Hypoglycemia counter-regulation in elderly humans: relationship to glucose levels. *American Journal of Physiology*, **267**, E497–E506.

Paes AHP, Bakker A, Soe-Agnie CJ (1997) Impact of dosage frequency on patient compliance. *Diabetes Care*, **20**, 1512–1517.

Reynolds C, Molnar GD, Horwitz DL, Rubenstein AH, Taylor WF, Jiang NS (1977) Abnormalities of endogenous glucagon and insulin in unstable diabetes. *Diabetes*, **26**, 36–45.

Riddle MC, McDaniel PA, Tive LA (1997) Glipizide-GITS does not increase the hypoglycemic effect of mild exercise during fasting in NIDDM. *Diabetes Care*, **20**, 992–994.

Ryder RE, Owens DR, Hayes TM, Ghatei MA, Bloom SR (1990) Unawareness of hypoglycaemia and inadequate hypoglycaemic counter-regulation: no causal relation with diabetic autonomic neuropathy. *British Medical Journal*, **301**, 783–787.

Schneider, J (1996) An overview of the safety and tolerance of glimepiride. *Hormone and Metabolic Research* **28**, 413–418.

Seltzer HS (1972) Drug-induced hypoglycemia: a review based on 473 cases. *Diabetes*, **21**, 955–966.

Seltzer HS (1979) Severe drug-induced hypoglycemia: a review. *Comprehensive Therapy*, **5**, 21–29.

Seltzer HS (1989) Drug-induced hypoglycemia: a review of 1418 cases. *Endocrinology and Metabolism Clinics of North America*, **18**, 163–183.

Shamoon H, Friedman S, Canton C, Zacharowicz L, Hu M, Rossetti L (1994) Increased epinephrine and skeletal muscle responses to hypoglycemia in non-insulin-dependent diabetes mellitus. *Journal of Clinical Investigation*, **93**, 2562–2571.

Shorr RI, Ray WA, Daugherty JR, Griffin MR (1997) Incidence and risk factors for serious hypoglycemia in older persons using insulin or sulfonylureas. *Archives of Internal Medicine*, **157**, 1681–1686.

Stahl M, Berger W (1999) Higher incidence of severe hypoglycaemia leading to hospital admission in Type 2 diabetic patients treated with long-acting versus short-acting sulphonylureas. *Diabetic Medicine*. **16**, 586–590.

Strachan MWJ, Deary IJ, Ewing FME, Frier BM (1997) Is Type II diabetes associated with an increased risk of cognitive dysfunction? A critical review of published studies. *Diabetes Care*, **20**, 438–445.

Tattersall RB (1999) Frequency, causes and treatment of hypoglycaemia. In: Frier BM, Fisher BM (eds). *Hypoglycaemia in Clinical Diabetes*, Chichester: John Wiley, 55–87.

Tessier D, Dawson K, Tetrault JP, Bravo G, Meneilly GS (1994) Glibenclamide vs gliclazide in Type 2 diabetes of the elderly. *Diabetic Medicine*, **11**, 974–980.

Thomson FJ, Masson EA, Leeming JT, Boulton AJM (1991) Lack of knowledge of symptoms of hypoglycaemia by elderly diabetic patients. *Age and Ageing*, **20**, 404–406.

Towler DA, Havlin CE, Craft S, Cryer P (1993) Mechanism of awareness of hypoglycemia: perception of neurogenic (predominantly cholinergic) rather than neuroglycopenic symptoms. *Diabetes*, **42**, 1792–1798.

Tunbridge WMG (1981) Factors contributing to deaths of diabetics under fifty years of age. *Lancet*, **ii**, 569–572.

UK Prospective Diabetes Study Group (1998) Intensive blood-glucose control with sulphonylureas or insulin compared with conventional treatment and risk of complications in patients with Type 2 diabetes. *Lancet*, **352**, 837–853.

Vea H, Jorde R, Sager G, Vaaaler S, Sundsfjord J (1992) Reproducibility of glycaemic thresholds for activation of counter-regulatory hormones and hypoglycaemic symptoms in healthy subjects. *Diabetologia*, **35**, 958–961.

White NH, Skor DA, Cryer PE, Levandoski LA, Bier DM, Santiago JV (1983) Identification of Type 1 diabetic patients at increased risk for hypoglycemia during intensive therapy. *New England Journal of Medicine*, **308**, 485–491.

Yap WS, Peterson GM, Vial JH, Randall CT, Greenaway TM (1998) Review of management of Type 2 diabetes mellitus. *Journal of Clinical Pharmacology & Therapeutics*, **23**, 457–465.

Section III

Treatment and Care Issues

11

Issues in the Initial Management of Type 2 Diabetes

Alan J. Sinclair
University of Birmingham, UK

INTRODUCTION

Diabetes mellitus is the commonest disabling metabolic disorder we encounter in everyday clinical practice and considerable evidence of its economic, social and health burden exists (Harrower 1980; Tattersall 1984; Neil et al 1989; Damsgaard 1990). Interventional strategies likely to reduce this burden must be initiated at an early stage and include aiming for individual and realistic levels of glycaemic control, screening for complications, and involving patients and carers in educational programmes (Sinclair and Barnett 1993).

The present state of diabetic care for older patients varies throughout Europe and North America, but in general there appears to be little indication of geriatric diabetes as a subspeciality interest and relatively no specific provision for those who may be housebound or in institutional care. In the United Kingdom, diabetes care for older people has been accused of being essentially unstructured, poorly coordinated, often inappropriate, suggesting a need for reorganization (Sinclair and Barnett 1993). However, during the last decade, with the increasing recognition that older patients have additional if not unique characteristics Sinclair 1998, 1999), diabetes care for this rather vulnerable population may be improving (Hendra and Sinclair 1997). These characteristics are shown in Table 11.1.

RATIONALE FOR GOOD-QUALITY CARE

Type 2 (non-insulin-dependent) diabetes (NIDDM) accounts for 95% of cases of diabetes in old age (Laakso and Pyorala 1985). Type 1 (insulin-dependent) diabetes (IDDM) can occur *de novo* (Kilvert et al 1986), but its true incidence is unknown (but probably underestimated) and is often diagnosed late (Sturrock et al 1995). The presentation of diabetes in the older patient is varied (Table 11.2). Many cases are detected by noting hyperglycaemia during hospital admissions for other morbidities or acute illnesses, although with detailed enquiry, symptoms of diabetes can be confirmed in a large number. Some patients do not have the classic features of either diabetic ketoacidosis (DKA) or hyperosmolar non-ketotic (HONK) coma but present with a 'mixed' disturbance of hyperglycaemia (blood glucose levels 15–25 mM, arterial blood pH of 7.2 or 7.3 (that is, not particularly acidotic), and without marked dehydration or change in level of consciousness.

The insidious presentation may delay diagnosis and partially account for the high prevalence rate of diabetic complications at the time of diagnosis. Better screening for complications at the time of diagnosis is, therefore, part of the rationale for promoting quality diabetic care for older patients with diabetes (Table 11.3).

Studies described in Chapters 4, 5, 8 and 14 demonstrate that metabolic control (including glycaemic and control of blood pressure) may have benefits in reducing both vascular complication rate in diabetes but may also have an influence on observed survival. Few long-term studies have specifically involved older patients (e.g. aged greater than 75) and none have attempted to assess the benefits of intervention in frail subjects. A brief synopsis of the evidence base for metabolic interventions in geriatric diabetes can be summarized as in Table 11.4. The potential benefits of

Table 11.1 Characteristics of older subjects with diabetes

High levels of comorbidities
Age-related impairment of functional ability
Increased vulnerability to hypoglycaemia
Overlapping and often limited medical follow-up by primary-care
   physicians, diabetic specialists, and geriatricians
A different management system which involves spouses and
   informal carers to a greater extent

Table 11.2 Presentation of diabetes in the elderly

Asymptomatic
Insulin deficiency
Spectrum of vague symptoms:
   Depressed mood
   Apathy
   Mental confusion
Unexplained weight loss/incontinence
Coexisting illness
Diabetic ketoacidosis
Hyperosmolar non-ketotic coma
'Mixed' metabolic disturbance

Table 11.3 Rationale for good-quality care of older diabetics

Early diagnosis may prevent progression of undetected
   complications
Better glycaemic control may reduce incidence of complications
Better screening for maculopathy and cataracts will reduce number
   of blind registrations
Better management and prevention of peripheral vascular disease
   and foot problems will reduce amputation rates
Prevents escalating costs and use of health service resources

Table 11.4 Evidence Base: metabolic interventions in geriatric diabetes

Few published studies
Good evidence for blood pressure lowering
No large trial data for microvascular disease
Good evidence for aspirin in vascular risk reduction
Emerging evidence of benefit for lipid lowering

Table 11.5 Potential benefits of achieving good metabolic control in diabetic elders

Symptom control and reduced fatigue
Reduced risk of metabolic decompensation
Reduced hospitalization
Reduced need for caregiver support
Maintain optimal visual acuity
Maintain optimal cognitive function
? Reduce vascular risk

population of all ages (Rohan et al 1989). Delay in diagnosis of this condition results from lack of awareness of its importance, lack of testing for visual acuity, and failure to use mydriasis. This combined with inexperience at fundal examination, even by medically qualified health professionals, creates an unfortunate situation since more than 70% of patients are likely to benefit from laser photocoagulation Rohan et al 1989).

Elderly patients comprise the majority of diabetic amputees, and the high level of resulting disability is discussed in more detail in Chapter 16. Screening for early signs of skin damage, such as ischaemia or ulceration, is a fundamental requirement to lessen the burden of this complication, which results in fewer than one in 10 patients regaining independent mobility (Houghton et al 1992).

The high cost of diabetic care in Western societies is discussed in detail in Chapter 1. Since the elderly comprise the majority of patients with diabetes, and elderly diabetic patients have a high usage of hospital services (Damsgaard et al 1987), it is clear that health strategies which result in fewer complications and decreased disability will also lead to a fall in diabetes-related costs.

AIMS IN THE EARLY MANAGEMENT

Until fairly recently it was generally accepted that the main aims of treating elderly diabetics were two-fold: (i) to provide relief from symptoms of hyperglycaemia, and (ii) to avoid troubling (and often dangerous) hypoglycaemia in those taking oral hypoglycaemic drugs or insulin. This approach, however, is now inadequate. Increased life expectancy means that many aged diabetics live long enough to suffer from disabling (but potentially preventable) complications such as blindness, lower limb amputation and foot ulceration. Furthermore, some complications are predominantly a

achieving good metabolic control in diabetic elders are listed in Table 11.5, with each item being worthy of research.

Diabetic maculopathy is one of several age-specific complications of diabetes and is an important cause of blindness in older diabetic patients. It is 2.6 times more common that proliferative retinopathy as a cause of diabetic blind registrations among the UK diabetic

Table 11.6 Age-specific complications in diabetes in old age

Diabetic maculopathy
Diabetic amyotrophy
Hyperosmolar non-ketotic coma
Diabetic ophthalmoplegia
Malignant otitis externa
Necrotizing fasciitis

Source: Adapted from Tattersall (1984).

Table 11.7 Aims in managing diabetes in the elderly

Medical
To promote freedom from symptoms of hyperglycaemia
To assess the impact of coexisting disease (e.g. ischaemic heart disease)
To prevent undesirable weight loss
Avoid hypoglycaemia and other adverse drug reactions
To screen for and prevent complications
To achieve a normal life expectancy for patients where possible

Patient-orientated
To maintain general well-being and good quality of life
To acquire skills and knowledge and understanding to adapt to changing requirements in their life-style

feature of the aged (Table 11.6). The essential aims in managing elderly patients with diabetes are listed in Table 11.7. The relative priority of each needs to be established at an early stage in the management.

Acute Presentation

Diabetes in elderly patients with Type 2 diabetes may present acutely in several ways: in diabetic ketoacidosis (DKA) or as hyperosmolar non-ketotic (HONK) coma, or more commonly as hyperglycaemia without significant ketosis or increased osmolality with or without coexisting acute illness; e.g. acute cerebrovascular accident (a mixed metabolic disturbance). Both DKA and HONK coma are covered in more detail in Chapter 5. Various precipitating factors for HONK coma have been identified (Table 11.8). Seriously ill patients require insulin therapy (especially those with ketones) given either as an intravenous infusion or by regular subcutaneous injections of short-acting insulin. In all severe cases, arterial blood gases should be measured to assess acid–base balance.

Table 11.8 Hyperosmolar non-ketotic coma: precipitating factors

50% unknown
Infection
Operation (surgery)
Myocardial infarction
Stroke
Drugs: propanolol, thiazides
Steroids, dialysis, (glucose drinks)

Non-acute Presentation

The majority of elderly Type 2 diabetic patients are not severely unwell at presentation and the majority should ideally be managed in the community by the general practitioner. At this stage there are four important objectives: (i) satisfy yourself that the patient has diabetes, (ii) screen for complications, (iii) identify who will be responsible for diabetic care, i.e. the patient or someone else; and (iv) initiate treatment.

Making the Diagnosis

A detailed discussion of the criteria used to make a diagnosis of diabetes can be found in Chapter 3. It should be appreciated, however, that many patients may not be able to give an accurate history of symptoms; 'classic' symptoms of polyuria and polydipsia due to excessive glycosuria may be absent owing to the raised renal threshold found in elderly subjects. A true fasted blood sample is often difficult to obtain and may be normal in any case (DECODE Study Group 1999), and an oral glucose tolerance test (OGTT) may be thought of as time-consuming and inconvenient.

In addition, many patients have elevated plasma glucose levels which are secondary to acute illness, diabetogenic drug therapy, or other stress-inducing disorders. If the physician has any doubt about the diagnosis of diabetes, it is wise not to treat but to retest later and use an OGTT if necessary.

Screening for Complications at Diagnosis

A detailed history may reveal symptoms of a distal sensory diabeticneuropathy such as numbness, paraesthesiae, burning pains, and hyperaesthesiae from bedclothes at night-time. Symptoms of postural hypotension (especially after treatment for coexisting hypertension with vasodilators has been started), diarrhoea or constipation, and impotence should alert you to the possibility autonomic neuropathy (see Chapter 7). Symptoms of claudication should be inquired about. Physical examination requires measurement of lying and standing blood pressure and assessment of peripheral blood vessels. Visual acuity (VA) can be checked using a 3 m Snellen chart. Patients whose VA is worse than 6/6 in either eye should be examined using the pinhole test which will partially correct a refractive error. Alternatively, they may use their distance glasses if worn. In patients with poor VA which remains unaltered or worsens in the pinhole test, the retina should be closely inspected for lesions, particularly those of maculopathy.

Direct ophthalmoscopy should start with the lens at zero and a red reflex obtained. When present, this indicates that there is no significant evidence of a cataract, vitreous haemorrhage, or retinal detachment. By setting the lens at +10 initially, and using a succession of less powerful lenses, a direct inspection of the cornea, anterior chamber and lens is possible. Diabetic retinopathy should be looked for after pupillary dilation using 0.5–1.0% tropicamide eye-drops. Relative contraindications for this include those with previous eye surgery, lens implants, or history of narrow-angle glaucoma. The precipitation of previously undiagnosed acute glaucoma, although distressing at the time, may be a service to the patient in the long run since treatment may prevent further visual loss. Patients with scattered microaneurysms and blot haemorrhages require review at 6 months. Diabetic maculopathy can be sight-threatening and requires urgent referral to the ophthalmologist. Other reasons for referral include the presence of yellow, waxy hard exudates, proliferative retinopathy, severe cataract formation, or rapid decrease in VA, for example within the previous 3 months (noticed by the patient—subjective; or evidence of a two-line deterioration in VA using a Snellen chart—objective).

Examination of the limbs for sensory neuropathy should include an assessment of knee and ankle reflexes, sensation by testing with a nylon monofilament, pin-prick and cotton wool, vibration sense by 128 Hz tuning fork (bearing in mind the age-associated loss of vibration sense), and proprioception.

Infection, foot ulceration, presence of pressure areas and the presence of sharp, poorly cut nails requires referral to the chiropodist. Management may also include radiology, antibiotic therapy, rest, use of pressure-relieving devices, and even surgery. Effective education including advice about suitable footwear

dramatically reduces the risk of new foot lesions Boulton 1992).

Other investigations include: serum creatinine, glycosylated haemoglobin (HbA$_{1c}$), lipid profile (triglycerides, total and high-density lipoprotein (HDL) cholesterol) in those aged less than 75 years, especially those with coronary artery disease. In patients who may have had undiagnosed diabetes for some time with marked hyperglycaemia, hyperlipidaemia may be present. In these cases, it is worth rechecking their lipids after 6 months to see whether treatment has reversed the abnormality. An electrocardiogram looking for ischaemia, arrhythmias and ventricular hypertrophy is useful. Urinalysis (in the absence of infection) may demonstrate proteinuria, although this is not particularly common at diagnosis in the elderly. Microalbuminuria is also common at diagnosis, but this may secondary to hypertension or congestive heart failure; it is routinely screened for in the author's diabetic clinic when the dipstick test is negative for protein. A Barthel scale and mini-mental state examination to assess both physical disability and mental function should be completed (Sinclair et al 1996). Brain failure may make the patient totally dependent on others (spouse, other relative or district nurse) for both treatment and monitoring.

Patient and Informal Carer Responsibilities

In most situations an individual care plan must be adopted and agreed by all concerned. This may be organized by the primary care physician (general practitioner), although diabetes specialist nurses can play an important role in this decision-making. This will consist of identifying the principal informal carer, setting realistic glycaemic goals, planning the timing and frequency of visits, and being aware of the indications for hospital referral to a specialist (Table 11.9) or admission. Ideally, the healthcare team should aim to provide written information about diabetes for each newly diagnosed patient (and informal carer where appropriate) and organize several educational tutorials over the next 6–12 months.

Wherever possible, a multidisciplinary approach and philosophy shared with the patient (or informal carer) is recommended, with the promotion of self-advocacy being an important goal. With diabetic elders from ethnic minority backgrounds who may pose special problems of language and communication, access and availability of services, cultural and dietary

Table 11.9 Indications for referral to hospital specialist for elderly patients with diabetes

Patients with severe complications (e.g. maculopathy, foot ulceration, peripheral vascular disease)
Patients whose metabolic/symptom control is suboptimal irrespective of treatment (e.g. oral agents or insulin)
Complex management problems in those with coexisting disease (e.g. patients with chronic pulmonary disease taking steroids)
Patients with increasing dependency and immobility (e.g. post-stroke)
Patients not adequately cared for in primary care

differences, it is important to tailor the educational package to meet their needs and provide information about any regional or national societies/organizations involved in diabetes care.

INITIAL TREATMENT

Initial steps in the treatment of older patients with diabetes are discussed in Chapter 15. In patients whose glucose values lie between 8 and 17 mM and who are not troubled by symptoms, an initial 6–12 week course of dietary instruction only is warranted. The main elements of a suitable dietary plan include consuming 50–55% of total energy intake as carbohydrate (including a fibre intake of at least 30 g/day), 30–35% fat intake (< 10% saturated fat), and 10–15% protein.

Dietetic treatment will depend on several factors but must include the patient's ability to cooperate, physical and mental well-being, and the patient's natural desire to be independent. This process is a form of negotiation and some dietitians are now developing a 'Getting Started' diet sheet for initial management. There is a shift away from traditional 'food exchanges' towards a more generalized plan of healthy eating (provision of 'healthy eating messages'). In those patients who are

Table 11.10 Treatment options for diet failures

Further period of intense dietary therapy requiring inputs from both physician and dietician
Specified and appropriate exercise program
Guar gum: little used in UK clinical practice
Acarbose: alpha-glucosidase inhibitor
Oral hypoglycaemic agents: sulphonylureas, metformin, rapaglinide, thiazolidinediones (where license permits)
Insulin therapy: usually considered on a temporary basis in well-defined circumstances only, such as acute illness

overweight, a plan of fat restriction may be beneficial. Other practical advice including alcohol consumption and benefits of exercise are often given at this time.

When dietary advice fails to reduce levels of glycaemia or improve patient well-being, or when initial random glucose levels are greater than 17 mM and patients feel unwell, several treatment options are available (Table 11.10), although in most cases, oral agents are then prescribed.

Physical Activity and Exercise

The contribution of physical inactivity to the development of Type 2 diabetes is discussed in Chapter 2. Structured physical activity (exercise) should be recommended as an adjunct to proper diet and weight control and may even be protective against the development of Type 2 diabetes (Helmrich et al 1991). Brisk walking for 30 minutes each day or swimming for 45–60 minutes up to three times per week are appropriate for older people. Prolonged or unusual exercise may be harmful, however, especially in those with underlying cardiovascular disease, those on insulin therapy (because of delayed hypoglycaemia), and those with sensory loss in their feet where tissue damage may be sustained.

In general, exercise has several beneficial actions: lowering of hyperinsulinaemia and an improvement in glucose tolerance occurs probably secondary to a reduction in insulin resistance (Koivisto 1991). The lipid profile becomes less atherogenic with a reduction in total plasma cholesterol and triglycerides while increasing HDL-cholesterol. A fall in blood pressure may take place as a direct result of exercise as well as the effect of weight loss. Some patients (especially older patients) are unable to participate in exercise programs because of decreased joint mobility due to diabetes-related joint stiffness and/or osteoarthritis, or because of a previous stroke. Limited exercise only is possible in those with poor metabolic control and ketosis or those with ischaemic heart disease, advanced retinal or renal disease.

The importance of promoting weight loss in overweight patients cannot be overemphasized since obese patients with Type 2 diabetes pose several unique problems in diabetic management. First, increasing bodyweight makes the attainment of normoglycaemia by dietary manipulation exceedingly difficult. Second, there is clinical and epidemiological evidence linking obesity, and its consequent insulin resistance and hyperinsulinaemia, with the development of, and exacerbation of, Type 2 diabetes (Ferrari and Weidmann 1990). Furthermore, there is evidence to suggest that insulin resistance and hyperinsulinaemia promote the development of hypertension and dyslipidaemia, which in turn increases the risk of cardiovascular disease (Niskanen, Uusitupa and Pyos 1991). The term 'syndrome X' or metabolic syndrome has been applied to the clinical association of insulin resistance, hypertension, and increased very-low-density lipoprotein and decreased HDL (dyslipidaemia) (Reaven 1988). Third, treatment with sulphonylureas, rapaglinide or insulin is associated with hyperinsulinaemia, which may promote both weight gain and paradoxically increase insulin resistance. These factors are important and should be considered when antidiabetic therapy is instituted.

Oral Agents

Newer oral hypoglycaemic therapies are being evaluated and are discussed in detail in Chapter 15. In choosing a specific drug several factors need to be considered, including renal and hepatic function, co-existing disease, possible drug interactions, and the likelihood of producing significant hypoglycaemia. For this reason, glibenclamide (glyburide) and chlorpropamide, which have prolonged durations of action, can accumulate in renal dysfunction, and have a high associated risk of hypoglycaemia, sometimes with fatal consequences (Asplund, Wilholm and Lithner 1983; Frey and Rosenlund 1970), should not be prescribed for diabetic subjects aged 60 or older. Patients should be warned of the possibility of hypoglycaemia developing and educated with practical advice on how to both avoid and prevent this potentially serious situation developing. In relatively newly diagnosed patients, failure to achieve acceptable glycaemic targets with diet and a single antidiabetic agent (e.g. a sulphonylurea) after 6 months should lead to a further review of treatment.

Specific guidelines relating to the drug treatment of diabetes mellitus in older patients have been published (Sinclair et al 1996). These were based on treatment with four main agents/classes: sulphonylureas, metformin, alpha-glucosidase inhibitors, and insulin. In normal-weight individuals (BMI $> 20\,kg/m^2$ and $< 26\,kg/m^2$), sulphonylureas or alpha-glucosidase inhibitors were recommended with metformin being added to those patients with suboptimal control

on sulphonylureas. In overweight patients (BMI $> 26\,kg/m^2$), metformin was recommended (assuming no contraindications were present) with a sulphonylurea added if control remains unsatisfactory.

More recently, the International Diabetes Federation (European region) has published guidelines of diabetes care for Type 2 diabetes (European Diabetes Policy group 1999). No specific stepwise algorithm has been adopted for drug treatment, leaving the choice to the individual practitioner. One of the important messages from this timely document is that regular review of treatment is essential, since a deterioration in glucose control over time should be expected and this will require an increase in therapy, with insulin likely to be needed in many patients after a variable period of time after diagnosis.

Insulin Therapy

Few newly diagnosed elderly diabetic subjects require insulin therapy to sustain life and prevent DKA, although some patients may have a slowly developing form of Type 1 diabetes and will inevitably require insulin in the future. In everyday clinical practice, the usual indications to start insulin are: (i) persisting symptoms with poor patient well-being, (ii) continued weight loss, and (iii) failure to achieve satisfactory glycaemic control with diet and oral agents. Other indications and detailed aspects relating to this therapy can be found in Chapter 12.

A common error in managing elderly Type 2 diabetics is undue reluctance to start insulin therapy. This view is often shared by patients until they try insulin. Underlying reasons for patient's attitudes include horror of injections, awful stories of 'hypos', fear of further hospitalization, and the belief that taking insulin will change their lives for the worse (Taylor 1992). It is imperative that the decision to start insulin be taken after full discussion with the patient (and carers, as appropriate); and although there are no time limits for when this decision should be taken, the author suggest a maximum of 6 months' perseverance with diet and oral agents before insulin is initiated. In practice, this decision may have been delayed already for several years. Able patients can begin insulin at home like their younger counterparts, with treatment organized by a diabetes specialist nurse (whose professional roles are increasing—see Table 11.11), in cooperation with the general practitioner. Patients who are unwell, or have other severe medical problems, or

Table 11.11 Roles of a diabetes specialist nurse for older adults with diabetes

Teaching, advising and counselling patients and carers, both in the clinic and in the patient's home
Educating patients to achieve self-care where possible
Teaching self-monitoring of blood glucose (or urinalysis, if appr priate): use of special techniques for patients with physical disability or visual loss
Instructing patients and informal carers about insulin administration
Commencement of insulin in the patient's home
Liaising with other health professionals to ensure optimal treatment of the patient
Advising residential care home staff about care of diabetic residents
Providing continuing support and advice to patients and carers

Table 11.12 Components of an initial diabetes care plan

1. Establish realistic glycaemic and blood pressure targets
2. Ensure that all parties are agreed on principal aspects of diabetes care: patient, spouse or family, GP, informal carer, community nurse or hospital specialist, where appropriate
3. Define the frequency and nature of diabetes follow-up
4. Organize glycaemic monitoring by patient or carer
5. Refer to social or community services as necessary
6. Provide advice on stopping smoking, exercise, and alcohol intake

where community support is lacking, need to be admitted. Usually, treatment can start with about 12–16 units of insulin per day and adjusted thereafter. In certain cases, however, such as those with confusion, visual loss, or arthritis, the technique of insulin administration should be taught to the spouse or to another relative or friend.

The success of insulin may be objectively evaluated by factors such as glycaemic control, patient well-being, episodes of hypoglycaemia, or frequency of hospital admissions due to diabetes.

Combination Therapy

It remains controversial whether combining insulin with oral agents has any significant advantages in terms of improved metabolic control or beneficial effects on long-term complications (Raskin 1992). This is discussed in more detail in Chapter 12. However, there is an increasing recognition that combining oral agents with insulin may be appropriate in certain circumstances, and in fact may be the only option in patients where addition of further insulin is not allowed by the patient or not thought to be clinically feasible. Further studies in this area are required to clarify the role of combination therapy in the treatment of Type 2 diabetes.

ESTABLISHING AN INDIVIDUAL DIABETES CARE PLAN

The elements of an initial care plan for diabetic elders are listed in Table 11.12. This is usually applicable during the first 3–6 months after diagnosis (Sinclair et al 1996). The care plan should state precisely what the

roles of the involved individuals are and where boundaries of responsibility lie. The timing and components of the follow-up can be predetermined, as can the date and format of the annual review process which is a mandatory requirement for all diabetic elders.

Effective self-monitoring of glycaemic control is a worthwhile objective for most patients with Type 2 diabetes, especially for those on insulin or who have frequent acute illnesses or hypoglycaemic episodes. In some cases, with the appropriate level of education, patients learn the effects of dietary changes and exercise on blood glucose levels, by frequent use of self-monitoring.

Urine testing for glucose remains a common practice but is inconvenient, messy, and often misleading because of the raised renal threshold of the elderly. Also, both patients and physicians are often uncertain about the significance of glycosuria, and the author no longer advises its routine use. Testing for the presence of ketones (when poor control is present—persistent values of blood glucose >17 mM or during severe acute illness) is worth carrying out if patients and informal carers have been suitably educated about its significance.

Blood glucose monitoring (e.g. using BM reagent strip measurements) should be encouraged in all those able to cooperate. Measurements can be taken twice weekly. Pre-meal and before-bedtime estimations are ideal but few patients are this compliant. In other cases, spouses, district nurses or diabetes specialist nurses may monitor control.

Guidelines for reasonable diabetic control in the elderly are as follows: a fasting glucose of 6–8 mM, and a random level of 7–10 mM. These limits should allow patients to remain well and be relatively free of symptoms of hyperglycaemia, and avoid the risk of hypoglycaemia. It should be remembered that even glucose levels of 11 mM can make some patients feel lethargic and these require lowering. A HbA$_{1c}$ value less than 2% above the upper range of normal for the laboratory should also be aimed for. However, in many patients, stricter control is feasible and should be aimed for.

Metabolic Targeting

Whilst few clinicians would institute aggressive metabolic control in patients aged greater than 75 years, there is increasing evidence of benefit from glucose lowering, blood pressure reduction, and lipid lowering in older populations. Metabolic targeting in geriatric diabetes has a partial evidence base and this has been represented as a series of targets provided in Table 11.13. This assumes a single-disease model and needs to be interpreted on an individual basis. Patients in this category have no evidence of other serious comorbidities, no cognitive impairment, and are generally self-caring. Unfortunately, only about one-third of patients fall into this latter category (Table 11.14), according to the results of a large community-based sample of people aged greater than 65 with diabetes where objective measures of dependency were based

Table 11.13 Metabolic targets for diabetic elders: a single-disease model

---

Glycaemic levels
No specific studies in older people with diabetes
UKPDS: HbA$_{1c}$ < 7%; fasting blood glucose < 7 mM

Blood pressure levels
UKPDS: <140/80 mmHg (not based on older subjects)
HOT study: diastolic lowering to < 83 mmHg
SHEP study: systolic BP < 150 mmHg
Syst-Eur study: systolic BP < 160 mmHg

Lipid levels
No specific studies in older people with diabetes
LIPID,CARE, 4S, VA-HIT studies:
  total cholesterol < 5 mM
  HDL cholesterol > 1.0 mM
  triglycerides < 2.0 mM

Aspirin use
Increasing evidence of benefit
ATS study
HOT study: using 75 mg/day, reduced major cardiovascular
  events by 15% and myocardial infarction by 36%

Abbreviations (studies referenced in Sinclair 2000): ATS, Antiplatelet Trialists Study; CARE, Cholesterol and Recurrent Events Study; HDL, high-density lipoprotein; HOT, Hypertension Optimal Treatment study; LIPID, Long-term Intervention with Pravastatin in Ischaemic Disease; 4S, Swedish Simvastatin Survival Study; SHEP, Systolic Hypertension in the Elderly Program (US); Syst-Eur, Systolic Hypertension in Europe Trial; UKPDS, United Kingdom Prospective Diabetes Study; VA-HIT, Veterans Affairs High-Density Lipoprotein Cholesterol Intervention Trial.

Table 11.14 Metabolic targeting in geriatric diabetes

---

1. Independent in self-care, mobile and mentally alert/single medical disorder:
   Aim Strict glycaemic and blood pressure control; positive decision not to undertake lipid lowering only

2. Relatively independent with some evidence of functional decline and several comorbidities:
   Aim: Optimize glucose and blood pressure control; consider lowering lipids

3. High dependency and frailty; may be a resident of a nursing home and/or cognitively impaired:
   Aim: Symptom control; avoid hypoglycaemia and intrusive monitoring

---

on the Barthel ADL score, Extended ADL score, and the Minimental State Examination score (Sinclair and Bayer 1998).

Prioritizing Diabetes Care for Diabetic Elders

Diabetes care in older adults requires prioritizing and a five-step approach is recommended to provide a framework to develop individual intervention program (Table 11.15). These interventions may include, for example, aggressive treatment of blood glucose and blood pressure, specific rehabilitation programmes for older people with diabetes, or fast-track vascular work-up and early surgical referral (Sinclair 2000). Patients with established cardiovascular disease (or micro-albuminuria) should be actively considered for treatment with ramipril (HOPE Study Investigators 2000), bearing in mind the criteria for metabolic targeting discussed above.

Charts such as those of Yudkin and Chaturvedi (1999) permit an estimate of the overall level of vascular risk to be derived which can be used to inform the physician about which thresholds apply for therapeutic

Table 11.15 Prioritizing diabetes care in older adults: a five-step approach

---

1. Functional assessment including cognitive testing and screening for depression
2. Vascular risk assessment with advice on lifestyle modification and vascular prophylaxis
3. Metabolic targeting (individualized): single-disease model versus frailty model
4. Consider specific interventions for diabetes-related disabilities
5. Assess suitability for self-care versus carer assistance

---

intervention. However, it is important to individualize these estimates very carefully in diabetic elders, since it is likely that they will have several other co-morbidities which may influence the decision to treat. In addition, applying the standard threshold for intervention based on a 10-year risk of coronary heart disease event of 20%, few only of the older patients with diabetes we encounter in every clinical practice would not require intervention.

CONCLUSIONS

The management of the older diabetic patient represents a major challenge to any physician, whether based in the community or in a hospital setting. Hospital physicians without specialist training in diabetes should seek the advice of a consultant diabetologist for patients whose glycaemic control is persistently unacceptable or those with severe diabetic complications; for example, extensive foot ulceration, autonomic neuropathy or painful neuropathy. Patients with significant diabetic eye disease, such as proliferative or preproliferative retinopathy or maculopathy, require prompt referral to a consultant ophthalmologist. A detailed assessment of other cardiovascular risk factors is beyond the scope of this chapter, but the presence of hypertension, ischaemic heart disease or hyperlipidaemia may warrant further attention and interventions. The development of local specifications for diabetic care, agreed by all health professionals involved, helps this process of referral to take place efficiently and with the most benefit for each patient.

REFERENCES

Asplund K, Wilholm BE, Lithner F (1983) Glibenclamide-associated hypoglycaemia: a report of 57 cases. *Diabetologia*, **24**, 412–417.

Boulton AJ (1992) Update on long-term diabetic complications. In: Lewin IG, Seymour CA (eds) *Current Themes in Diabetic Care*. London: Royal College of Physicians of London, 45–53.

Damsgaard EM, Froland A, Green A (1987) Use of hospital services by elderly diabetics: the Frederica Study of diabetic and fasting hyperglycaemic patients aged 60–74 years. *Diabetic Medicine*, **4**, 317–322.

Damsgaard EM (1990) Known diabetes and fasting hyperglycaemia in the elderly. Prevalence and economic impact on health services. *Danish Medical Bulletin*, **37**, 530–546.

DECODE Study (Diabetes Epidemiology: Collaborative Diagnostic Criteria in Europe) (1999) Consequences of the new diagnostic criteria for diabetes in older men and women. *Diabetes Care*, **22**,1667–1671.

European Diabetes Policy Group (1999) *A Desktop Guide to Type 2 Diabetes Mellitus*. International Diabetes Federation (European Region), Brussels, Belgium.

Ferrari P, Weidmann (1990) Insulin, insulin sensitivity and hypertension. *Journal of Human Hypertension*, **8**, 491–450.

Frey HMMM, Rosenlund B (1970) Studies in patients with chlorpropamide-induced hypoglycaemia. *Diabetes*, **19**, 930–937.

Harrower ADB (1980) Prevalence of elderly patients in a hospital population. *British Journal of Clinical Practice*, **34**, 131–133.

HOPE (Heart Outcomes Prevention Evaluation) Study Investigators (2000) Effects of ramipril on cardiovascular and microvascular outcomes in people with diabetes mellitus: results of the HOPE study and MICRO-HOPE substudy. *Lancet*, **355**, 253–259.

Helmrich SP, Ragland DR, Leung RW, Paffenbarger RS (1991) Physical activity and reduced occurrence of non-insulin-dependent diabetes mellitus. *New England Journal Medicine*, **325**, 147–152.

Hendra TJ, Sinclair AJ (1997) Improving the care of elderly diabetic patients: the final report of the St Vincent Joint Task Force for Diabetes. *Age and Ageing*, **26**, 3–6.

Houghton AD, Taylor PR, Thurlow S, Rootes E, McColl I (1992) Success rates for rehabilitation of vascular amputees. *British Journal of Surgery*, **79**, 753–755.

Kilvert A, Fitzgerald MG, Wright AD, Natrass M (1986) Clinical characteristics and aetiological classification of insulin-dependent diabetes in the elderly. *Quarterly Journal of Medicine*, **60**, 865–872.

Koivisto VA (1991) Exercise and diabetes mellitus. In: Pickup JC, Williams G (eds) *Textbook of Diabetes*. Oxford: Blackwell Scientific, 795–802.

Laakso M, Pyorala K (1985) Age of onset and type of diabetes. *Diabetes Care*, **8**, 114–117.

Neil HAW, Thompson AV, Thorogood M, Fowler GH, Mann JL (1989) Diabetes in the elderly: the Oxford community diabetes study. *Diabetic Medicine*, **6**, 608–613.

Niskanen LK, Uusitupa MI, Pyorala K (1991) The relationship of hyperinsulinaemia to the development of hypertension in Type 2 diabetic patients and in non-diabetic subjects. *Journal of Human Hypertension*, **5**, 155–159.

Raskin P (1992) Combination therapy in NIDDM. *New England Journal of Medicine*, **327**, 1453–1454.

Reaven GM (1988) Role of insulin resistance in human disease. *Diabetes*, **37**, 1595–1607.

Rohan TE, Frost CD, Wald NJ (1989) Prevention of blindness by screening for diabetic retinopathy: a quantitative assessment. *British Medical Journal*, **299**, 1198–1201.

Sinclair AJ (1998) Diabetes mellitus. In: Pathy MSJ (ed) *Principles and Practice of Geriatric Medicine*, 3rd edn. Chichester: John Wiley, 1321–1340.

Sinclair AJ (1999) Diabetes in the elderly: a perspective from the United Kingdom. *Clinics in Geriatric Medicine*, **15**, 225–237.

Sinclair AJ (2000) Diabetes in old age: changing concepts in the secondary care arena. *Journal of Royal College of Physical of London*, **34**, 240–244.

Sinclair AJ, Barnett AH (1993) Special needs of elderly diabetic patients. *British Medical Journal*, **306**, 1142–1143.

Sinclair AJ, Bayer AJ (1998) *All Wales Research in Elderly (AWARE) Diabetes Study*. Department of Health Report (UK Government), 121/3040, London.

Sinclair AJ, Turnbull CJ, Croxson SCM (1996) Document of care for older people with diabetes. *Postgraduate Medical Journal*, **72**, 334–338.

Sturrock NDC, Page SR, Clarke P, Tattersall RB (1995) Insulin dependent diabetes in nonagenerians. *British Medical Journal*, **310**, 1117–1118.

Tattersall RB (1984) Diabetes in the elderly: a neglected area? *Diabetologia*, **27**, 167–173.

Taylor R (1992) Use of insulin in non-insulin-dependent diabetes. *Diabetes Review*, **1**, 9–11.

Yudkin JS and Chaturvedi N (1999) Developing risk startification charts for diabetic and nondiabetic subjects. *Diabetic Medicine*, **16**, 219–227.

12

Insulin Therapy

Tim Hendra
Royal Hallamshire Hospital, Sheffield

INTRODUCTION

Elderly people with diabetes are a heterogeneous population who need integrated care centred around their family doctor but with ready access to hospital services and diabetes specialist nurses. The severity of their vascular complications, comorbidities, cognitive impairment, and caregiver support need to be taken into account when considering diabetes treatment. The challenge for health professionals is to identify appropriate goals of treatment for each patient, to provide patient-focused care which recognizes the patient's physical and cognitive abilities, and to have systems in place to adapt this model of care as the patient ages.

Insulin has an important and increasing role. The indications for its use are summarized in Table 12.1. Recent improvements in the organization of care between hospital and primary care, together with the evolving roles of diabetes specialist nurses and practice nurses in educating formal and informal caregivers, monitoring glycaemic control, and setting goals, have made insulin a safe option for many elderly diabetic subjects. Recent studies, in particular the Diabetes Control and Complications Trial (DCCT 1993) and the United Kingdom Prospective Diabetes Study (UKPDS 1998), have also highlighted the potential benefits of improved glycaemic control in reducing diabetes-related morbidity.

Following its isolation by Banting and Best in 1922, insulin became life-saving treatment for Type 1, or insulin-dependent, diabetic patients. For Type 2, or non-insulin-dependent patients, insulin has often been regarded as a treatment to be considered once patients have well-established poor control, often with severe osmotic symptoms, weight loss, and frequent infection despite maximal doses of oral agents. For elderly subjects, insulin has traditionally been a treatment to be avoided because of concerns about its use in socially isolated, cognitively impaired patients, with poor physical health and who could not identify or manage hypoglycaemia. Although the risks associated with hypoglycaemia are real, they are not confined to those patients on insulin treatment, as the use of sulphonylureas is also associated with significant hypoglycaemic risk. The recognition that elderly diabetic patients can benefit from a structured approach to treatment, with explicit guidelines and outcomes, has been reflected in recent publications (Sinclair, Turnbull and Croxson 1996; Sinclair et al 1997; Hendra and Sinclair 1997).

In addressing the use of insulin for elderly diabetic subjects, there are problems associated with a limited evidence base. As a result, recommendations are an extrapolation from studies in younger adults, taking into account the special needs and problems associated with ageing together with opinion based upon what may be regarded as best practice. For adults of all ages, however, there are limitations of insulin therapy, in that at present it is difficult to achieve normoglycaemia in patients with complete beta-cell failure without resorting to multiple injections, pumps, or accepting a high frequency of hypoglycaemia.

Whereas all Type 1 diabetic patients need insulin from the outset, most Type 2 patients start with diet and then progress to oral medication. For some Type 2 patients, the development of ketosis in the absence of acute illness or starvation and weight loss relatively soon after diagnosis is an indication for insulin; these patients often have beta-cell autoantibodies and are probably best regarded as having Type 1 diabetes. However, some 10% of patients per year with Type 2 diabetes develop unacceptable hyperglycaemia with-

Table 12.1 Indications for insulin treatment

1. Type 1 (insulin-dependent) diabetes mellitus (IDDM)
2. Type 2 (non-insulin-dependent) diabetes mellitus (NIDDM) associated with poor control, weight loss or hyperglycaemic malaise
3. Acute myocardial infarction
4. Acute severe illness
5. Hyperosmolar non-ketotic coma (HONK)
6. Major surgery

Table 12.2 Potential benefits of insulin

Metabolic effects
    inhibits glycogenolysis and hepatic gluconeogenesis
    may improve peripheral insulin sensitivity
    may improve endogenous insulin release
    may enhance responsiveness to oral hypoglycaemic agents
Prevents vascular complications
    reduces the risk of microvascular complications
    reduces mortality in acute myocardial infarction
Ameliorates overt osmotic symptoms and infection
Promotes weight gain
Improves hyperglycaemic malaise and quality of life
Improves cognitive function
Facilitates management of acute illness

out ketosis despite maximal or near-maximal doses of sulphonylureas; these individuals need to be transferred to insulin therapy. Approximately 50% of all Type 2 patients will at some point need to go on to long-term insulin treatment. The term 'secondary sulphonylurea failure' is sometimes used to describe these patients, though this is an inappropriate term since it is the pancreatic beta cell and not the patient's medication that has failed. It is important to explain to patients at the time of diagnosis that beta-cell failure is progressive and that the possible future need for tablets and/or insulin would not reflect any failure on their part to be compliant with dietary advice, medication, or glycaemic monitoring.

This chapter will consider the indications and goals for insulin in elderly patients, the possible benefits and difficulties with this treatment, as well as the rationale for different insulin regimens, insulin analogues and injection devices.

BENEFITS OF INSULIN TREATMENT

Beneficial Metabolic Effects

Whereas the pathogenesis of Type 1 diabetes is related to beta-cell loss and hypoinsulinaemia alone, in Type 2 disease there is a combination of pancreatic beta-cell dysfunction associated with insulin resistance. Following the presentation of Type 2 disease, beta-cell dysfunction progresses at different rates in individual patients, with failure of sulphonylurea treatment to control hyperglycaemia reflecting significant hypoinsulinaemia and the need for insulin therapy. This reduction or absolute lack of endogenous insulin can be assessed by measuring plasma C-peptide levels in the fasting and/or post-prandial state or after intravenous glucagon administration. The presence of autoantibodies to islet cell cytoplasm and glutamic

acid decarboxylase (GAD) in Type 2 diabetes decreases with age at diagnosis, but has been shown in the UKPDS to be predictive of the need for insulin within 6 years (Turner et al 1997).

Exogenous insulin therapy addresses the effects of endogenous insulin deficiency and as a consequence predominantly inhibits glycogenolysis and hepatic gluconeogenesis. It has also been suggested that insulin may improve peripheral insulin sensitivity, resulting in increased glucose uptake in peripheral tissues, and may also directly improve endogenous insulin release by reducing the toxic effect of glucose on beta cells (Yki-Jarvinen 1992). In this context there is some evidence to support the suggestion that a short course of intensive insulin treatment producing short-term near-normoglycaemia can produce improvements in beta-cell function sufficient to induce long periods of responsiveness to oral hypoglycaemic agents (Glaser 1998) —a potentially new indication for the relatively early use of insulin in Type 2 disease.

It follows that insulin therapy would be particularly beneficial for those thin elderly Type 2 patients whose hyperglycaemia is due to hypoinsulinaemia rather than peripheral insulin resistance. In addition, the former patients may be expected to be more sensitive to insulin, require lower maintenance dosages, and have more to gain from this treatment than patients who are already hyperinsulinaemic but who have poor glycaemic control.

Prevention of Vascular Complications

In Type 1 patients of mean age 27 years, the DCCT demonstrated that improved glycaemic control prevented or slowed the development of diabetic retino-pathy and nephropathy, though there was a high in-cidence of hypoglycaemia despite close clinical supervision (DCCT 1993). In this study, the in-tensively treated group achieved a mean glycated haemoglobin (HbA$_{1c}$) level of 7.1%, compared with 9.0% in the conventionally treated group. Extrapolat-ing these results to the relatively small numbers of elderly Type 1 diabetic subjects should be done with caution because of the risks of hypoglycaemia. How-ever, selected elderly Type 1 patients may benefit from tighter control of their disease and cope with increased doses of insulin without excessive hypoglycaemia if adequate monitoring is performed and healthcare professionals provide support.

In the UKPDS, intensive blood glucose control with either sulphonylurea or insulin produced mean HbA$_{1c}$ levels of 7.0% over 10 years, compared with 7.9% in the conventionally treated group. This was associated with a significant 25% reduction in microvascular endpoints. A 10% reduction in any diabetes-related death and a 6% reduction in all-cause mortality did not achieve statistical significance. The overall conclu-sions from this part of the study were that tight gly-caemic control with either insulin or sulphonylureas substantially reduces the risk of microvascular com-plication, but not macrovascular disease, in Type 2 patients (UKPDS 1998).

In this 9-year study, monotherapy with insulin was more effective than sulphonylurea in achieving fasting plasma glucose levels of less than 7.8 mM (42% versus 24%) though similar numbers of 28% and 24% only achieved HbA$_{1c}$ levels below 7% (Turner et al 1999). The average insulin dosage in this study was 30 units/day. This highlights the difficulties of achieving nor-moglycaemia with an insulin regimen which started with a single evening injection of ultralente insulin until a daily dosage of 16 units was reached. Patients then either added pre-meal soluble insulin or switched to a combination of soluble and isophane insulins. However, the previously published Veterans Affairs Cooperative Study had suggested that intensive insulin therapy in Type 2 patients of mean age 60 years and who had poor glycaemic control on oral therapy was effective in maintaining near-normal glycaemic control without excessive weight gain or hypoglycaemia (Abraira et al 1995).

The Diabetes Mellitus Insulin Glucose Infusion in Acute Myocardial Infarction (DIGAMI) study also demonstrated that, in patients of mean age 67 years, standard treatment plus insulin–glucose infusion for 24 hours after myocardial infarction followed by multi-dose insulin treatment resulted in a 11% reduction in mortality, and a reduction in relative risk of 0.72 (Malmberg 1997). These results extend to one year post-infarction and were most pronounced in those patients without previous insulin treatment who were predefined as being at relatively low risk.

Amelioration of Overt Osmotic Symptoms and Infection

Unlike with younger adults, the presence of polyuria and polydipsia in an elderly person can be a poor guide to hyperglycaemia because of the altered renal threshold to glucose excretion with ageing, and also the high prevalence of diuretic medication prescribed for cardiac failure and hypertension in elderly people. However, conversely, elderly people often do not well tolerate the osmotic symptoms of glycosuria because of coexisting poor mobility owing to neurological or degenerative joint disease, which can make getting to the toilet difficult. Similarly, pre-existing difficulties with voiding urine can be exacerbated by poor gly-caemic control, with urinary incontinence a common problem. Recurrent urinary tract infection in women is a common problem, particularly with chronically high glucose values greater than 15 mM.

Promotion of Weight Gain

For Type 2 patients, progressive weight loss on oral treatment should alert the physician to the need for insulin regardless of the patient's current dose of medication. Weight loss is often an insidious problem for those elderly patients with moderate or poor gly-caemic control who have progressive beta-cell failure. Often patients continue with progressive cachexia while taking high but not maximal doses of sulpho-nylureas because of their physician's concerns about hypoglycaemia associated with insulin. Alternatively many thin elderly patients, who would benefit from insulin, are inappropriately taking metformin when they have a low BMI when this agent should be re-served for morbidly overweight subjects.

In the UKPDS, weight gain was significantly greater in the intensively treated group (mean of 2.9 kg) compared with the conventional group. Patients treated with insulin had greater weight gain (mean of 4 kg) compared with those receiving chlorpropamide (2.6 kg) or glibenclamide (1.7 kg) (UKPDS 1998).

Changes in bodyweight may be inversely related to change in HbA$_{1c}$ and directly related to the change in free insulin levels (Yki-Jarvinen et al 1992). Initially weight gain after a long period of poor glycaemic control may be associated with a reduction in basal metabolic rate and rehydration resulting from the amelioration of the osmotic diuresis associated with glycosuria (Makimattola, Nikkila and Yki-Jarvinen 1999). However, about two-thirds of subsequent long-term weight gain is associated with an increase in adipose tissue (Groop et al 1989), with the remaining weight gain due to an increase in lean muscle mass. Since excessive weight gain is undesirable for elderly patients with poor mobility, it is relevant that combination therapy of a single evening dose of intermediate acting insulin may be associated with less weight gain than a single morning injection, twice-daily injections and a multiple injection regimen (mean weight gain 1.2 kg, 2.2 kg, 1.8 kg, and 2.9 kg respectively over three months). In one study, however, multiple insulin injections were associated with an average weight gain of 4.2 kg over 6 months compared to a high-fibre diet (Scott et al 1988).

Improvements in Hyperglycaemic Malaise and Quality of Life

Many elderly diabetic patients with high fasting glucose values and elevated HbA$_{1c}$ levels deny typical osmotic symptoms of thirst, polyuria and polydipsia but have malaise, lassitude and admit to feeling generally unwell. The latter symptoms are sometimes not admitted at the time but are recognized in retrospect after starting insulin. These covert symptoms of the syndrome of 'hyperglycaemic malaise' may persist for many years until progressive weight loss or overt osmotic symptoms develop and the need for insulin is recognized. Classically, patients resist going on to insulin because they claim to be 'well' but then return to clinic wishing that insulin had been started a long time previously.

Correction of hyperglycaemic malaise and improvement in quality of life (QOL), as well as a reduction in the frequency and progression of microvascular complications, are all important goals of insulin treatment. An early study of elderly Type 2 patients with fasting glucose values of >9 mM showed improvements in well-being after 8 months of insulin treatment (Berger 1988). In a randomized study of different insulin regimens (single injection plus oral therapy, twice-daily injection, and multiple injection regimens), significantly more patients reported an improvement in the subjective sense of well-being compared with a control group who stayed on oral treatment (Yki-Jarvinen et al 1992).

In selected poorly controlled elderly Type 2 patients, (mean age 77 years) insulin treatment was associated with improvements in some domains of the Short Form 36 QOL questionnaire (Reza et al 1998). This generic instrument showed improvements in the vitality, social function, and role emotional domains at 3 months compared with a group of control subjects who remained on their oral medication. These improvements were associated with a low incidence of hypoglycaemia, a reduction in hyperglycaemic malaise and improvements in patient satisfaction with treatment, without an increase in carer strain, while achieving a near 4% reduction in HbA$_{1c}$ from 13.6% to 9.8%.

This contrasts with a randomized study of younger patients (age 57–61 years) with moderately controlled disease (HbA$_{1c}$ 8.5–9.1%) who did not show improvements in a 'well-being' QOL questionnaire 24 weeks after switching to insulin (Barnett et al 1996). However, a Dutch study demonstrated that improved glycaemic control with either insulin or increased dosage of oral agents was associated with improvements in quality of life using disease-specific and generic measures (Goddijn et al 1999). In the insulin group this was at the expense of problems with social functioning and pain, though the QOL scores were similar in both groups and there was no direct relationship between HbA$_{1c}$ levels and QOL outcomes.

Improvement in Cognitive Function

There are some cross-sectional and prospective associations between Type 2 diabetes mellitus and cognitive impairment, which may reflect both vascular and non-vascular factors (Stewart and Liolitsa 1999). Studies of the effect of improved glycaemic control with oral agents have also demonstrated some improvements in certain parameters of cognitive function (Gradman et al 1993; Meneilly et al 1993), though there are no studies were insulin was used to lower glucose levels. In extrapolating these studies to the use of insulin, there are concerns that an increased incidence of insulin-induced hypoglycaemia may offset any benefits from improved glycaemic control.

Facilitation of Management of Acute Illness

Insulin-treated patients should be advised not to stop their injections, and that an increase in their insulin dosage may be needed during acute illness. Type 2 patients on oral medication may need to switch to insulin temporarily if hyperglycaemia is not controlled and osmotic symptoms develop. In most cases these patients will require hospital admission, where their disease can be controlled with either intermittent doses of short-acting insulin or a continuous insulin infusion. Some short courses of treatment for other conditions, such as steroids, may also cause temporary loss of diabetic control and require concomitant insulin treatment. Whether due to illness or iatrogenic causes, insulin prescribed in this context should always be stopped as soon as possible and the patient's original medication restarted; unfortunately this is sometimes not the case and there are instances of patients unnecessarily remaining on expensive insulin treatment for life.

POTENTIAL DISADVANTAGES OF INSULIN TREATMENT

Risk of Hypoglycaemia

In newly diagnosed Type 2 patients, the UKPDS demonstrated that those treated intensively with insulin or sulphonylureas had better glycaemic control but more hypoglycaemic episodes and gained more weight than those treated conventionally (UKPDS 1998). The rates for major hypoglycaemic episodes per year were 0.7% with conventional treatment, 1.0% with chlorpropamide, 1.4% with glibenclamide, and 1.8% with insulin. In the DCCT study, intensive treatment of Type 1 patients was also associated with an increased frequency of severe hypoglycaemia compared with conventional therapy (DCCT 1991). These concerns should affect the generalizability of these studies to the elderly population as a whole, though the risk of hypoglycaemia should be assessed on an individual basis.

Table 12.3 Potential disadvantages of insulin treatment

Risk of hypoglycaemia
Excessive weight gain
Risk of atherogenesis
Increased healthcare costs
Increased caregiver support

Concerns about the ability of an elderly person to recognize and deal with hypoglycaemia are a major worry with sulphonylurea as well as insulin treatment. The avoidance of hypoglycaemia, particularly at night, should be a particular goal when starting insulin for elderly patients living alone. Although there will always be an emphasis on self-care, with elderly people it is often the formal and informal caregivers who bear the responsibility for identifying and managing hypoglycaemia. When caregivers are not present, or are themselves elderly or infirm, these issues must be taken into account when establishing the goals of therapy and blood glucose targets.

Several studies have shown serious deficiencies in knowledge of the symptoms of hypoglycaemia in elderly insulin-treated patients (Mutch and Dingwell-Fordyce 1985; Pegg et al 1991; Thomson et al 1991). One study demonstrated an inverse relationship between symptom knowledge and glycaemic control but showed a stepwise loss of hypoglycaemia-related knowledge and treatment with age which was more marked for patients taking sulphonylureas than insulin-treated patients (Mutch and Dingwell-Fordyce 1985). As well as the effects of ageing on learning and recall of information, there may be limitations on the ability to deal with hypoglycaemia owing to poor mobility and manual dexterity, resulting in delay in getting to and opening glucose-containing foodstuffs. Furthermore, the manifestations of hypoglycaemia can be subtle and may result in fluctuating confusion, which may go unrecognized in insulin-treated patients living alone.

Excessive Weight Gain

Patients who are overweight often have peripheral insensitivity to insulin. They may, therefore, develop symptomatic hyperglycaemia and be diagnosed with diabetes at an earlier stage of their decline in beta-cell function than someone who has normal insulin sensitivity. Insulin may exacerbate weight problems for patients who are morbidly overweight and may also increase or aggravate existing insulin resistance. Very often these patients gain more weight than the expected 4 kg when started on insulin because of poor glycaemic control. This is a reflection that the original cause of the patient's hyperglycaemia may have a significant dietary component and is an indication for further strict dietetic advice, concentrating on avoidance of refined carbohydrates and reduced fat intake. Some patients who strongly comply with diet and oral medication in an attempt to avoid conversion to insulin may become less strict with their diet when insulin is introduced. In addition, some patients may overeat because they are concerned about hypoglycaemic episodes. For these reasons combination therapy of a single injection of bedtime isophane insulin and metformin is worthy of consideration rather than twice-daily mixtures of isophane insulin.

Risk of Atherogenesis

In the past, it had been suggested that insulin may itself be atherogenic and contribute directly to the association between macrovascular disease and diabetes (Stout 1990). This led to a debate as to whether the possible benefits of using insulin to improve glycaemic control and reduce microvascular complications were outweighed by the possibility of increasing acute macrovascular endpoints with this treatment. Although there was never any convincing experimental or epidemiological evidence for this hypothesis, it was a concern until the results of the UKPDS demonstrated no difference in macrovascular endpoints between patients treated with oral agents and insulin despite both agents achieving the same degree of improved glycaemic control.

THE PROCESS OF STARTING INSULIN

Although insulin treatment is best started at home on a trial basis, it is important to involve the multidisciplinary diabetes team from the outset since a coordinated package of care will be needed (Da Costa 1997). Although this usually involves hospital-based secondary care services, there is no reason why transferring a patient from oral therapy to insulin cannot be performed exclusively in the primary care setting. The key person is the diabetes specialist nurse who links medical support with the wishes and concerns of the patient and caregivers, while ensuring that insulin injection technique, blood glucose monitoring and insulin dosage adjustment are appropriate.

Before starting, patients should be reviewed by their dietician and should either be able to perform capillary glucose monitoring themselves or have this performed by a third party. For many patients, formal assessment of cognitive function and their ability to perform the activities of daily living should be assessed and recorded. Appropriate tests of cognition include the Abbreviated Mental Test (Jitapunkul, Pillay and Ebrahim 1991) or the Mini-Mental State Examination (Folstein et al 1975). Functional status is most often measured on the Barthel Scale (Collins et al 1988). General practitioners should be aware of all patients starting insulin and it is desirable for district nurses to be involved at the outset for those patients living alone in the community. Education and support from diabetes nurse specialists and/or practice nurses are essential. Although group education sessions together with individualized care planning are the ideal, for many elderly people with poor mobility, cognitive impairment, impaired vision and hearing, one-to-one education sessions are vital. The content of such sessions is important and should emphasize the symptoms and signs of hypoglycaemia as well as the practical aspects of insulin injection and storage, and available devices. It has been suggested that information about the physiology of glucose metabolism and insulin action is less important to an elderly insulin-requiring population (Watson and Parker 1999).

Many elderly patients are understandably anxious about starting insulin. Particular concerns tend to focus on pain from subcutaneous injection and the common misconception that insulin is to be given intravenously. Although starting insulin for Type 2 patients is often suggested as a trial, with the promise of reversion to tablets if there are problems after 3 months, frequently patients feel substantially better within 48–72 hours of their first injection. The reason for this is unclear, though it is possible that it represents a direct effect of insulin on the brain, improved well-being due to the anabolic effects of insulin, the rapid correction of hyperglycaemia, or an alternative and as yet unknown mechanism. Whatever the mechanism, very few patients choose to revert to oral medication once started on insulin.

INSULIN SPECIES AND REGIMENS

Once-daily Insulin

Theoretically a single bedtime injection of intermediate-acting insulin should improve pre-breakfast fasting glucose levels by inhibiting hepatic glucose output overnight. This would then leave endogenous meal-stimulated insulin release to control post-prandial glucose levels. The expectation would be that lowering fasting glucose levels would reduce the toxic effects of hyperglycaemia on beta-cell function and lead to an increase in endogenous insulin release. Although this hypothesis supports the use of a combination of nocturnal insulin and sulphonylurea therapy during the day, the important issue is that once-daily insulin produces adequate glycaemic control only in the presence of endogenous insulin production. It therefore will not work in those patients who have low C-peptide levels. In addition, it may be expected that the efficacy of a single injection of insulin given at bedtime will also be dependent upon the ability of residual beta-cell function to control hepatic glucose output overnight.

Studies of single injections of insulin have shown improved glycaemic control when compared with diet plus oral sulphonylureas. In one study of carefully selected patients, a single morning injection of intermediate insulin did produce acceptable HbA_{1c} levels without an unacceptable risk of nocturnal hypoglycaemia and the need for some patients to have additional short-acting insulin to correct morning hyperglycaemia (Tindall et al 1988). A single bedtime injection of isophane insulin (0.3 U/kg) has also been shown to produce better glycaemic control than a similar dose of insulin in the morning (Seigler, Olsson and Skyler 1992).

Once-daily morning injections of intermediate and/or long-acting insulin are recommended only for selected patients, particularly when the goals of treatment are the relief of hyperglycaemic symptoms and the avoidance of intercurrent infection. Such goals may be appropriate, for example, in the context of terminal illness and severe cognitive impairment. In the past, a common scenario for this strategy has been for patients who live alone and who are dependent only upon a community nurse who visits once daily to give the injections. Sometimes this situation may need to be tolerated in order to keep patients living in the community when they might otherwise require residential care. However, such a strategy is suboptimal as it is associated with a risk of hypoglycaemia owing to the variable absorption of large insulin dosages, and is unlikely to achieve a satisfactory degree of glycaemic control.

Combinations of Insulin and Oral Diabetic Medication

As indicated above, this regimen assumes that there is residual beta-cell function sufficient to control post-prandial hyperglycaemia. By using combinations of bedtime insulin with sulphonylureas, improved metabolic control can be achieved in hyperglycaemic patients. Compared with insulin monotherapy, combined therapy with sulphonylureas requires smaller insulin dosages and results in less weight gain (Johnson, Wolf and Kabadi 1996). A recent study has also indicated that combination therapy of bedtime insulin plus metformin over one year may be associated with less weight gain, a lower frequency of hypoglycaemia, and better glycaemic control than twice-daily insulin, or combinations of glibenclamide plus insulin or metformin (Yki-Jarvinen et al 1999). However, the combination of morning insulin with a sulphonylurea may be associated with more hypoglycaemic episodes, but a similar degree of glycaemic control compared with a combination of bedtime insulin with sulphonylurea (Soneru et al 1993).

Twice-daily Insulin

Elderly patients will need twice-daily or multiple insulin injections when endogenous insulin production is insufficient to control post-prandial glucose levels. In this situation, a once-daily or combination regimen runs into the problem of post-prandial hyperglycaemia, associated with dose-limiting pre-meal hypoglycaemia. These problems are frequently encountered when the insulin dosage in a single injection regimen exceeds 30 U. Should this situation arise, there may also be problems with the irregular absorption of a relatively large volume of insulin. The patient's daily insulin should then be divided into two, with approximately two-thirds being injected before breakfast and the rest before the evening meal.

The total daily insulin requirements for a patient with little residual beta-cell function can vary between 0.3 and 0.5 U/kg/day, though higher dosages may be required for overweight patients with peripheral insulin insensitivity as well as patients receiving insulin via continuous subcutaneous infusion. The majority of patients can be started on twice-daily intermediate-acting isophane insulin, or a combination of pre-mixed short- and intermediate-acting insulins which should be injected 25–40 minutes before the meal. Mixtures of short- and intermediate-acting insulin analogues, as well as the more established different fixed ratios of rapid- and intermediate acting human insulins, are also available. Elderly patients should not be expected to mix insulins themselves since this is associated with inaccuracies in dosage owing to a combination of poor manual dexterity, visual impairment and cognitive impairments (Everett 2000). The twice-daily regimen gives flexibility to adjust dosages in order to achieve good glycaemic control without hypoglycaemic risk

Basal Bolus (Multiple-injection) Regimens

For selected patients, a regimen of basal intermediate insulin before bed together with pre-meal boosts of short-acting insulin is also a safe option. This regimen allows patients greater flexibility with mealtimes compared with twice-daily isophane or mixed insulin, and more closely mimics the non-diabetic state where the beta cells respond to meals with pulses of insulin release. When combined with a rapid-onset insulin analogue such as insulin lispro, which can be injected immediately before or after eating, this regimen may be associated with a lower risk of hypoglycaemia than with conventional short-acting insulins.

Continuous Subcutaneous Insulin Infusions (CSII)

CSII is the most physiological way of delivering insulin with continuous infusion of rapid-acting insulin supplemented by pre-meal boosts. In Type 1 disease, this has been demonstrated to produce near-normoglycaemia, with fewer hypoglycaemic episodes than other regimens and in some people a return of hypoglycaemic awareness. For Type 2 disease, it is usually reserved for patients with microvascular complications who need tight glycaemic control which cannot be achieved with a basal/bolus regimen. Since its introduction in the 1980s, technology has improved and this regimen now has a role for selected and appropriately educated and motivated patients. Although there may be the occasional elderly patient for whom this is appropriate and safe to use (Coscelli et al 1992), in the main there is little place for CSII in the elderly and this route of insulin delivery is not readily available in the United Kingdom.

Glucose–Insulin Infusions

During moderate or major surgery, elderly Type 1 and Type 2 diabetic patients should receive insulin, intravenously even if preoperative diabetes control has been good. However, for Type 2 patients undergoing minor surgery, regular glucose monitoring only may be required if their control has been good. For those with poor control, intravenous insulin is appropriate.

During surgery the two options are either a combined infusion of glucose, potassium and insulin, or separate glucose/potassium and insulin infusions. In this context insulin is necessary to maintain good glycaemic control while preventing proteolysis and lipolysis, while glucose provides energy and prevents hypoglycaemia (Alberti 1991). When glucose is given as 100 mL of 5% dextrose per hour, short-acting insulin doses of 1.5–2.0 U/h are usually sufficient together with 10–20 mMol potassium chloride per litre of glucose. Perioperative glucose monitoring is essential. Because of the risks of separate infusions running at different rates, it is generally recommended that a single infusion of glucose, insulin and potassium be used in this context. Following surgery, patients should revert to their original diabetes treatment.

The advantages and disadvantages of some of the options for insulin treatment in elderly Type 2 diabetic patients are compared in Table 12.4.

INSULIN DELIVERY DEVICES

Elderly patients have several options, including disposable plastic syringes designed for single use, reusable insulin pens, prefilled disposable insulin pens, and insulin pumps. The latter, which can provide insulin from either inside or outside of the body, are generally unnecessary for the Type 2 patient who is switching to insulin because of poor glycaemic control. However, an external pump could be of value for an elderly Type 1 patient with an irregular lifestyle trying to achieve tight glycaemic control.

Insulin pens initially contained only short-acting insulin and were used predominantly by young Type 1 patients adhering to a basal/bolus regimen. Subsequently, premixed insulin cartridges have been introduced and pen design has evolved such that relatively few patients now use separate syringes and bottles of insulin. This is undoubtedly a good thing since many elderly patients do not have the dexterity, vision or cognitive function necessary to reliably draw up and inject the same amount of insulin every day. Dialing up an insulin dose is more reliable, and for many elderly patients easier than drawing up insulin. Although these devices have removed one source of error and variation in insulin delivery, and they do cater for patients with poor eyesight and/or hearing difficulties, they are still difficult to use by someone with

Table 12.4 Options for insulin treatment in elderly Type 2 patients

	Once-daily insulin	Twice-daily insulin	Basal bolus insulin	Insulin plus oral agents
Advantages	Single injection	Can achieve good glycaemic control with insulin mixtures in well-motivated patients	Possible to achieve tight glycaemic control while allowing flexible mealtimes	Less weight gain compared with twice-daily insulin
Disadvantages	Cannot achieve good glycaemic control without high risk of hypoglycaemia	Inflexible lifestyle with fixed meal times	Requires frequent monitoring to avoid hypoglycaemia	Inappropriate for patients who are thin or losing weight
	Assumes residual beta-cell function	Cannot achieve normoglycaemia	Expensive	
Indications	Patients reliant on caregiver for injections when aim is to alleviate hyperglycaemic symptoms only	Regimen of choice	Well-motivated cognitively intact patients who need to achieve near normoglycaemia	Overweight poorly controlled patients who may gain weight with twice-daily injections

arthritis or neurological impairment. Patients do need to be able to recognize and change the insulin cartridge when it is empty, change the needle, and 'troubleshoot' when the device fails. The full range of insulins is now available in pens and this has made insulin delivery easier, more reliable and portable than before. These pens are more socially acceptable and may also lessen the burden of diabetes by giving the patient greater freedom than previously. However, it is essential that the ability of each patient to deal with a pen is assessed by a trained registered nurse (preferably a diabetes specialist nurse) who has expertise and knowledge of the range of devices available.

The new finer and shorter needles are well received by, and allay the fears of, elderly patients starting insulin treatment. However, older patients have the same potential delivery problems as younger adults in terms of the irregular and sometimes unpredictable absorption of insulin from differing subcutaneous sites. The length of the needle is important, with a 6–8 mm needle being preferred for cachectic patients, and a 12 mm needle for patients with a normal to morbidly overweight habitus. In view of the changes in body fat distribution and skin thickness with aging, it is possible that the factors that affect insulin absorption, including the site and technique of injection, may differ. In this regard, it is important to pinch up the skin to ensure a subcutaneous deposition site in thin patients. Furthermore, as in younger adults, abdominal injections of soluble insulin may result in a 29% lower postprandial blood glucose level compared with thigh-site injections (Bantle, Neal and Frankamp 1993).

GLYCAEMIC MONITORING, MIXING INSULIN, AND DOSAGE ADJUSTMENT

Many patients can administer insulin themselves and perform capillary glucose monitoring. As with younger adult patients, there is evidence that educating elderly patients and/or their caregivers to regularly adjust insulin dosages on the basis of capillary glucose monitoring may prevent hypoglycaemia as well as improve glycaemic control if this is desired.

In the past many elderly patients performed urinalysis for glycosuria to monitor their disease. However, this method can often underestimate hyperglycaemia owing to a high renal threshold for glucose in elderly people. In addition, this method of monitoring is valueless if a patient has symptoms that may be due to hypoglycaemia. In view of these concerns, all insulin-treated patients are taught capillary glucose monitoring and asked to record levels at least twice a day after starting insulin while their disease is stabilizing. Subsequently once stable, patients may be asked to record a four-point profile (pre-meals) once or twice a week. In addition, patients are asked to test if they have symptoms indicative of hypoglycaemia or if they develop intercurrent illness.

Some apparently able and cognitively intact patients are unable to master the technique of obtaining reliable capillary glucose results and are, therefore, dependent upon a caregiver or district nurse. This can be an unreliable arrangement particularly when district nursing services have insufficient resources to meet the demand for their skills. Where monitoring is dependent upon district nursing services, it may be possible to obtain fasting and post-prandial levels only once or twice a week.

The majority of elderly insulin-treated patients can perform capillary glucose monitoring. However, this may reflect the process or criteria for selecting patients for this treatment, since glucose monitoring is essential for the early evaluation of progress after starting insulin and the decision to continue with insulin. In other words, an ability to perform capillary glucose monitoring tends to bias a decision on converting to insulin. During stabilization the diabetes nurse specialist or practice nurse makes contact with patients once or twice a week. Subsequently, they are available to give advice by telephone if there are problems, though generally once a patient is stabilized, clinic review is usually indicated once or twice a year.

Since the newer glucose monitoring and insulin injection devices vary in the ease with which they can be used by an elderly person with arthritis, impaired vision and hearing, it is important to be aware of the range of available options when starting treatment. In this regard, the local diabetes centre and diabetes specialist nurses can offer particular advice as well as educate, and initiate and monitor the effects of insulin. Review of injection technique and capillary glucose monitoring also needs to be undertaken annually, particularly if a patient develops arthritis or has a new cerebrovascular event.

SETTING TREATMENT TARGETS

All parties involved, and especially the patient and carer, should identify and agree on glycaemic and other treatment targets. Prompt communication between secondary and primary care providers is essential. The decision to aim for moderate/tight glycaemic control in a relatively fit and 'well preserved' patient may need to be reviewed as he or she ages and becomes at increasing risk of hypoglycaemia. At some stage, relief from osmotic symptoms may become a more appropriate goal of management. For many frail elderly patients, however, identification of glycaemic targets will have to take into account that diabetes is only one of several medical problems impacting on the patient's quality of life. Unfortunately many age-related problems and diseases affecting an elderly person are not as easy to manage or control as is their diabetes. In this latter situation, symptomatic relief only may be the appropriate goal from the outset of the diagnosis

and require a single injection of intermediate- or long-acting insulin.

Usually patients with microvascular complications are given targets in terms of achieving fasting capillary glucose values of 4–7 mM when aiming for tight glycaemic control. However, pre-breakfast readings of 7–9 mM are generally acceptable for someone without complications.

There is some evidence that physicians, diabetes nurse specialists and the patient may differ in their expectations and perception of the needs for insulin as currently prescribed (Casparie and van der Waal 1995; Taylor et al 1998). Clinicians tend to concentrate on biomedical outcomes such as capillary glucose values, glycated haemoglobin percentages, and weight loss, whereas many patients just want to feel better and avoid recurrent infection after starting insulin (Taylor et al 1998).

CONCLUSIONS

Recent research, in particular the UKPDS, has clarified the benefits from, and indications for, insulin for elderly Type 2 diabetic patients. There is a recognition that tight glycaemic control with HbA_{1c} levels of less than 7.0% is an appropriate goal for many patients, and will result in many more elderly diabetic patients starting insulin either as monotherapy or in combination with sulphonylureas or metformin.

There is good evidence that many elderly patients may benefit from insulin, with improvements in well-being and gain in weight, while maintaining blood glucose values above the range likely to pose a significant risk of hypoglycaemia. In starting insulin as a trial, the patient's glycaemic goals need to be agreed upon and monitored by caregivers and/or diabetes specialist/practice nurses with clear joint protocols shared between primary and secondary care. Whereas the initiation of insulin is an indication for referral to secondary care, perhaps to a geriatrician with a special interest in diabetes, follow-up for many patients is best done in the community by general practitioners. It is important that GPs liaise closely with patients and their formal and informal caregivers, with the option of referral to secondary services through established protocols if problems develop.

Future developments for elderly diabetic patients may include an expansion in the use of rapid-acting insulin analogues and possibly new routes of insulin administration. In addition, there may be benefits from combining insulin injections with the new class of glitazone agents which improve peripheral insulin sensitivity.

REFERENCES

Abraira C, Colwell JA, Nuttall FQ, Sawin CT, Nagel NJ, Comstock JP, Emanuele NV, Levin SR, Henderson W, Lee HS (1995) Veterans Cooperative Study on glycemic control and complications in Type II diabetes (VA CSDM). Results of the feasibility trial. Veterans Affairs Cooperative Study in Type II Diabetes. *Diabetes Care*, **18**, 1113–1123.

Alberti KGMM (1991) Diabetes and surgery. *Anaesthesiology*, **74**, 209–211.

Bantle J, Neal L, Frankamp L (1993) Effects of the anatomical region used for insulin injections on glycaemia in Type 1 diabetes subjects. *Diabetes Care*, **16**, 1592–1597.

Barnett AH, Bowen Jones D, Burden AC, Janes JM, Sinclair A, Small M, Tindall H (1996) Multicentre study to assess quality of life and glycaemic control of Type 2 diabetic patients treated with insulin compared with oral hypoglycaemic agents. *Practical Diabetes International*, **13**, 179–183.

Berger W (1988) Insulin therapy in the elderly Type 2 diabetic patient. *Diabetes Research and Clinical Practice*, **4** (Supp l.), 24–28.

Casparie AF, van der Waal MA (1995) Differences in preferences between diabetic patients and diabetologists regarding quality of care: a matter of continuity and efficacy of care. *Diabetic Medicine,* **12**, 828–832.

Collins C, Wade DT, Davies S, Horne V (1988) The Barthel ADL index: a reliability study. *International Disability Studies*, **10**, 61–63.

Coscelli C, Calabrese G, Fedele D, Pisu E, Calderini C, Bistoni S, Lapolla A, Mauri MG, Rossi A, Zapella A (1992) Use of premixed insulin among the elderly. *Diabetes Care*, **15**, 1628–1630.

Da Costa S (1997) A coordinated approach to insulin transfer in the older, Type 2 client. *Journal of Diabetes Nursing*, **1**, 123–126.

Diabetes Control and Complications Trial Research Group (1991) Epidemiology of severe hypoglycaemia in the Diabetes Control and Complications Trial. *American Journal of Medicine*, **90**, 450–459.

Diabetes Control and Complications Trial Research Group (1993) The effect of intensive treatment of diabetes on the development and progression of long-term complications in insulin-dependent diabetes mellitus. *New England Journal of Medicine*, **329**, 977–986.

Everett J (2000) Living and learning with insulin pump therapy. *Diabetes Today*, **3**, 20–21.

Folstein MF, Folstein SE, McHugh PR (1975) 'Mini-mental state': a practical method for grading the cognitive state of patients for the clinician. *Journal of Psychiatry Research*, **12**, 189–198.

Gilden JL, Casia C, Hendryx M, Singh SP (1990) Effects of self-monitoring of blood glucose on quality of life in elderly diabetic patients. *Journal of the American Geriatric Society*, **38**, 511–515.

Glaser B (1998) Insulin treatment of Type 2 diabetes mellitus. *Diabetes Reviews International*, **7**, 5–8.

Goddijn PPM, Bilo HJG, Feskens EJM, Groenier KH, van der Zee KI, Meyboom-de Jong B (1999) Longitudinal study on glycaemic control and quality of life in patients with Type 2 diabetes mellitus referred for intensified control. *Diabetic Medicine*, **16**, 23–30.

Gradman TJ, Laws A, Thompson LW, Reaven GM (1993) Verbal learning and/or memory improves with glycaemic control in older subjects with non-insulin-dependent diabetes mellitus. *Journal of the American Geriatric Society*, **41**, 1305–1312.

Groop L, Widen E, Franssila-Kallunki A, Ekstrand A, Saloranta C, Schalin C, Eriksson J (1989) Different effects of insulin and oral antidiabetic agents on glucose and energy metabolism in Type 2 (non-insulin-dependent) diabetes mellitus. *Diabetologia*, **32**, 599–605.

Hendra TJ, Sinclair AJ (1997) Improving the care of elderly diabetic patients: the final report of the St Vincent Joint Task Force for Diabetes. *Age and Ageing*, **26**, 3–6.

Jitapunkul S, Pillay I, Ebrahim S (1991) The abbreviated mental test: its use and validity. *Age and Ageing*, **20**, 332–336.

Johnson JL, Wolf SL, Kabadi UM. (1996) Efficacy of insulin and sulfonylurea combination therapy in Type II diabetes. *Archives of Internal Medicine*, **156**, 259–264.

Makimattola S, Nikkila K, Yki-Jarvinen H (1999) Causes of weight gain during insulin therapy with and without metfomin in patients with Type 2 diabetes mellitus. *Diabetologia*, **42**, 406–412.

Malmberg K, for the DIGAMI Study Group (1997) Prospective randomised study of intensive insulin treatment on long term survival after acute myocardial infarction in patients with diabetes mellitus. *British Medical Journal*, **314**, 1512–1515.

Meneilly GS, Cheung E, Tessier D, Yakura C, Tuokko H (1993) The effect of improved glycemic control on cognitive functions in the elderly patient with diabetes. *Journal of Gerontology*, **48**, 117–121.

Mutch WJ, Dingwell-Fordyce I (1985) Is it a hypo?. Knowledge of the symptoms of hypoglycaemia in elderly diabetic patients. *Diabetic Medicine*, **2**, 54–56.

Pegg A, Fitzgerald D, Wise D, Singh BM, Wise PH (1991) A community-based study of diabetes-related skills and knowledge in elderly people with insulin-requiring diabetes. *Diabetic Medicine*, **8**, 778–781.

Reza M, Taylor C, Towse K, Ward JD, Hendra TJ (1998) Insulin treatment in elderly non insulin dependent diabetes mellitus (NIDDM): quality of life and impact on carers. *Diabetic Medicine*, **15** (Suppl. 1), S17.

Scott AR, Attenborough Y, Peacock I, Jeffcoate WJ, Tattersall RB (1988) Comparison of high fibre diets, basal insulin supplements, and flexible insulin treatment for non-insulin dependent (Type II) diabetics poorly controlled with sulphonylureas. *British Medical Journal*, **297**, 707–710.

Seigler DE, Olsson GM, Skyler JS (1992) Morning versus bedtime isophane insulin in Type 2 (non-insulin dependent) diabetes mellitus. *Diabetic Medicine*, **9**, 826–833.

Sinclair AJ, Turnbull CJ, Croxson SCM (1996) Document of care for older people with diabetes. *Postgraduate Medical Journal*, **72**, 334–338.

Sinclair AJ, Turnbull CJ, Croxson SCM (1997) Document of diabetes care for residential and nursing homes. *Postgraduate Medical Journal*, **73**, 611–612.

Soneru IL, Agrawal L, Murphy JC, Lawrence AM, Abraira C (1993) Comparison of morning or bedtime insulin with and without glyburide in secondary sulphonylurea failure. *Diabetes Care*, **16**, 896–901.

Stewart K, Liolitsa D (1999) Type 2 diabetes mellitus, cognitive impairment and dementia. *Diabetic Medicine*, **16**, 93–112.

Stout RW (1990) Insulin and atheroma, a 20 yr perspective. *Diabetes Care*, **13**, 631–654

Taylor CD, Towse KW, Reza M, Ward JD, Hendra TJ (1998) Reasons and goals of insulin treatment for elderly patients with poorly controlled Type 2 diabetes: a prospective study. *Diabetic Medicine*, **15** (Suppl. 2), S33.

Thomson FJ, Masson EA, Leeming JT, Boulton AJM (1991) Lack of knowledge of symptoms of hypoglycaemia by elderly diabetic patients. *Age and Ageing*, **20**, 404–406.

Tindall H, Bodansky HJ, Stickland M, Wales JK (1988) A strategy for selection of elderly Type 2 diabetic patients for insulin therapy, and a comparison of two insulin preparations. *Diabetic Medicine,* **5**, 533–536.

Turner R, Stratton I, Horton V, Manley S, Zimmet P, Mackay IR, Shattock M, Bottazzo GF, Holman R (1997) UKPDS 25: autoantibodies to islet-cell cytoplasm and glutamic acid decarboxylase for prediction of insulin requirement in Type 2 diabetes. *Lancet*, **350**,1288–1293.

Turner RC, Cull CA, Frighi V, Holman RC (1999) Glycaemic control with diet, sulphonylurea, metformin, or insulin in patients with Type 2 diabetes mellitus: progressive requirement for multiple therapies (UKPDS 49). *Journal of the American Medical Association*, **281**, 2005–2012.

United Kingdom Prospective Diabetes Study Group (1998) Intensive blood-glucose control with sulphonylureas or insulin compared with conventional treatment and risk of complications in patients with Type 2 diabetes. *Lancet*, **352**, 837–853.

Watson J, Parker L (1999) Providing quality care: evaluation of group education sessions for people changing to insulin treatment. *Diabetes Today*, **2**, 20–21.

Yki-Jarvinen H (1992) Glucose toxicity. *Endocrine Reviews*, **13**, 415–431.

Yki-Jarvinen H, Kauppila M, Kujansuu E, Lahti J, Marjanen T, Niskanen L, Rajala S, Ryysy L, Salo S, Seppala P, Tulokas T, Viikari J, Karjalainen J, Taskinen M-J (1992) Comparison of insulin regimens in patients with non-insulin-dependent diabetes mellitus. *New England Journal of Medicine*, **327**, 1426–1433.

Yki-Jarvinen H, Ryysy L, Nikkila K, Tulokas T, Vanamo R, Heikkila M (1999) Comparison of bedtime insulin regimens in patients with Type 2 diabetes mellitus. *Annals of Internal Medicine*, **130**, 389–396.

13

Managing Surgery in the Elderly Diabetic Patient

Geoffrey Gill, Susan Benbow

University Hospital Aintree and Hairmyres Hospital, East Kilbride

INTRODUCTION

During their lifetime, most patients with diabetes will require some form of surgery, and the likelihood increases as age advances. Nowadays a considerable amount of major surgery is undertaken in the elderly (e.g. coronary artery bypass grafts, peripheral vascular and aneurysm surgery, removal of malignancies etc.), of whom more are proportionately likely to have diabetes than at earlier stages of their lives. Though carefully planned and executed surgery is highly successful in the elderly, such patients with diabetes may tolerate metabolic and infective complications less well than younger subjects. Diabetes per se should never be a reason to decide *not* to operate on an elderly patient; but it *is* a reason for careful planning and management, pre-, peri- and postoperatively. In this chapter we examine the potential problems, the basis of current management systems, and practical methods of treatment.

METABOLIC AND OTHER PROBLEMS INDUCED BY SURGERY

Anxiety, anaesthetic drugs and possibly the underlying disease requiring surgery may all contribute to metabolic destabilization in the diabetic surgical patient. The most important factors, however, are starvation and the pathophysiological metabolic and humoral response to trauma. All but the most minor of operations involve some interruption of normal food intake, and this may not infrequently last for several days. This poses obvious practical difficulties for diabetic patients whose tablets or insulin injections must be accompanied by food. Of more sinister note, however, is that starvation leads to catabolism, and in the presence of

insulin deficiency (i.e. the diabetic state), ketosis becomes likely and eventually inevitable (Allison, Tomlin and Chamberlain 1979; Elliott and Alberti 1983).

Such problems are greatly enhanced by the well-known humoral and metabolic changes associated with trauma, which also greatly enhance catabolism. Surgical trauma disturbs the usual fine balance between anabolism (effectively controlled only by insulin) and catabolism (driven by a variety of hormones—notably cortisol, catecholamines, growth hormone and glucagon). These latter hormones are often collectively known as the 'stress' or 'counter-regulatory' hormones, and they are hypersecreted in traumatic states. Cortisol and adrenaline levels, in particular, rise promptly (within minutes or hours after the initiation of trauma) and often massively (to some extent in proportion to the degree of trauma). In addition, insulin secretion is relatively reduced, and a state of insulin resistance ensues (Allison et al 1979; Elliott and Alberti 1983; Nordenstrom, Sannenfield and Arner 1989). Many of these changes are neurally mediated via afferent nerves from the injured tissue (cortisol for example is secreted secondarily to ACTH release) (Hume and Egdahl 1959). The result of these changes is a massive catabolic drive (see Figure 13.1), with increased gluconeogenesis and glycognolysis leading to glucose release into the circulation. Lipolysis and protein breakdown also occur, though in the non-diabetic patient, even small amounts of insulin ('basal') secretion are sufficient to contain dangerous hyperglycaemia and lipolysis. This of course is not true in the insulin-deficient or diabetic state. The danger of this metabolic scenario to the diabetic patient depends on its degree (as previously mentioned, roughly proportional to the severity of trauma), and to the level of insulin reserves available.

Diabetes in Old Age. Second Edition. Edited by A. J. Sinclair and P. Finucane. © 2001 John Wiley & Sons Ltd.

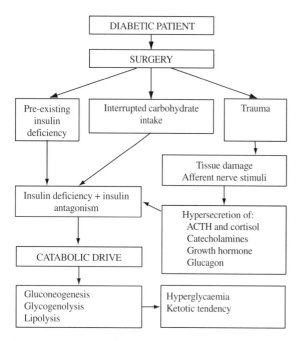

Figure 13.1 Hormonal and metabolic effects of surgery in the diabetic patient

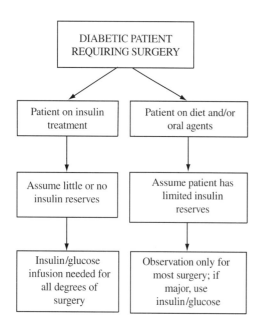

Figure 13.2 Flow chart demonstrating the principles of managing diabetes during surgery

IMPLICATIONS FOR MANAGEMENT

The foregoing basic principles can be translated logically into principles of management for diabetic patients undergoing surgery (Gill and Alberti 1989). The major requirement is to ensure adequate insulinization; and the important variables are the degree of surgical trauma and the individual level of endogenous insulin reserves. Practically, patients can be divided into those on insulin treatment and those on diet and/or oral hypoglycaemic agents (OHAs). The insulin-treated group may or may not be truly insulin-dependent (Type 1 diabetes); but even insulin-treated Type 2 patients can be assumed to have little or no insulin reserves, to have been deemed to need such treatment. These patients need continuous exogenous insulin treatment for all types of surgery.

Those not on insulin must have at least limited insulin reserves, and for minor to moderate degrees of surgical trauma can usually be closely observed only. Major surgery, however, will require continuous insulin as for the first group above. These principles are summarized in Figure 13.2.

POTENTIAL RISKS OF SURGERY IN DIABETIC PATIENTS

There have been surprisingly few studies on post-operative mortality and morbidity comparing diabetic with non-diabetic subjects. Diabetes was certainly considered to be a major risk factor for surgery in past decades. An American study in 1963 reported a 5% mortality postoperatively in a large (487) group of surgical diabetic patients, the major causes of death being ketoacidosis, infection and myocardial infarction (Galloway and Shuman 1963). It is likely, however, that methods of management were highly sub-optimal compared with modern management principles. A more recent study (Hjortrup et al 1985), using modern treatment methods, has shown no difference in mortality between diabetic and non-diabetic subjects (2.2% versus 2.7% respectively). Some specific surgical procedures may have increased risk in diabetic patients, however, notably vascular procedures. Thus, aortic and lower limbs revascularization procedures carry increased mortality in diabetic compared with non-diabetic patients (Melliere et al 1999). However, this is obviously a selected diabetic group with established advanced large vessel disease, and such an outcome difference may not be surprising. Nevertheless, such results are of relevance to surgery in the elderly, as in this study the mean age of the diabetic group was 68 years.

Turning to morbidity, there is little conclusive evidence that diabetes per se causes increased risk. Diabetic patients with pre-existing cardiac or renal problems may have increased morbidity, but not if surgery is relatively uncomplicated and properly managed (MacKenzie and Charlson 1988; Sandler, Maule and Baltus 1986). Risk of postoperative infection also does not appear definitely increased, contrary to normally accepted clinical dogma (Hjortrup et al 1985; Sandler et al 1986). In the Danish study of Hjortrup et al (1985), for example, the wound infection rate was identical amongst diabetic (13/224 or 5.8%) and non-diabetic (12/224 or 5.4%) patients. A recent study of diabetic patients undergoing coronary artery surgery showed an increased risk of post-surgical infections, but this was accounted for by excessive postoperative hyperglycaemia (Golden et al 1999). Overall, critical assessment of the available literature does not support a generally increased risk for diabetic patients undergoing surgery, in terms of both mortality and postoperative complications.

SPECIAL PROBLEMS IN THE ELDERLY

Increased age is known to increase postoperative morbidity, and possibility mortality, in general. This includes diabetic patients, but again there is no convincing evidence in the literature that the effect is significantly greater among such patients. In general, however, diabetic surgical patients are frequently older and 'sicker' than their non-diabetic counterparts (Sandler et al 1986) (e.g. amputees, coronary bypass surgery etc.); but when these factors are taken into account, any increased morbidity amongst diabetics becomes insignificant or much less significant.

When preparing the elderly for surgery, preoperative assessment should be particularly thorough because of comorbidity and polypharmacy. The patient may not be able to give an accurate history because of memory problems or communication difficulties. Ischaemic heart disease may be underestimated as the patient may not give a typical history of chest pain on exertion if exercise is limited by another pathology such as osteoarthritis. Pressure management is important in the elderly throughout the period of immobility, but particularly so if the individual has diabetes, where peripheral vascular disease and peripheral neuropathy increase the risks. Nutritional status can already be

compromised in the elderly hospitalized patient and be further exacerbated by surgery. Prophylaxis against venous thromboembolic disease must also be considered.

Later, we will be discussing potential iatrogenic complications of diabetes management during surgery. Elderly diabetic patients tolerate hypoglycaemia poorly (Jennings, Wilson and Ward 1989), and are less efficient at maintaining water homeostasis than their younger counterparts (Faull, Holmes and Baylis 1993), increasing the risk of fluid and electrolyte imbalance in the postoperative period. Renal impairment can be precipitated or exacerbated by these changes, but hydration can already be compromised by drugs, vomiting, preparation for the operation (e.g. bowel clearance), preoperative starvation or simply inability to obtain or reach fluids.

PRACTICAL MANAGEMENT

Aims of Treatment

Obvious aims of treatment are avoidance of excess mortality and morbidity. As discussed above, with modern management there should nowadays be little or no excess mortality or post-surgical infection risk. Ideally, the period of hospitalization should not be unduly prolonged, though admission a day or two earlier than usual is often required (see later). Postoperative ketoacidosis should no longer occur, but hypoglycaemia is always a risk with intravenous insulin delivery. Avoidance of hypoglycaemia is very important—the surgical patient may be unable to perceive or report hypoglycaemia, and low blood glucose levels may therefore be allowed to become profound and serious before detection and treatment. Elderly diabetic patients in general may present atypically with hypoglycaemia and, for instance, appear to be confused. Additionally, there is no evidence that overzealous attempts at achieving normoglycaemia are of benefit in the surgical situation. Indeed, paradoxically Hjortrup and colleagues (1985) found that patients with particularly 'good' control appeared to be at greater risk of postoperative complications, though other studies have not confirmed this (Golden et al 1999).

Glycaemic aims should therefore be to avoid hypoglycaemia at all costs, but in addition to not allow excessive hyperglycaemia or to risk ketoacidosis. In numerical terms, plasma glucose levels in the region of 6.0–12.0 mM would be a reasonable compromise target.

Preoperative Assessment

Preoperative assessment of the elderly diabetic patient is aimed at checking general fitness for surgery, ensuring that diabetic management is appropriate, and confirming that glycaemic control is reasonable. By 'inappropriate' management is meant potentially hazardous drugs such as the potent and/or long-acting sulphonylureas, glibenclamide and chlorpropamide. Regrettably a number of older diabetic patients remain on such preparations and treatment may need to be updated prior to surgery. There are theoretical reasons for avoiding metformin also if possible (because of lactic acidosis risk), though this is not strictly evidence-based (Gill and Alberti 1992).

Assessment of glycaemic control should be by 'bedside' blood glucose monitoring with reagent strips, but the potential inaccuracies of such measurement needs to be borne in mind (Hutchison and Shenkin 1984), and occasional laboratory plasma glucose levels should be checked, and if possible a preoperative glycosylated haemoglobin (HbA_{1c}). As previously mentioned, 'excellent control' is not necessary, but significant hyperglycaemia (e.g. consistently >10.0 mM) needs action. This may involve moving patients from diet to sulphonylureas, increasing tablet doses if already on oral agents, or perhaps introducing insulin on a temporary basis. If the latter step is required, thrice-daily short-acting insulin (e.g. Actrapid, Humulin S), with or without evening isophane insulin, or twice-daily 30/70 premixes (e.g. Humulin M3, Mixtard 30/70) are usually suitable. Such patients will of course need pre-operative treatment as for 'insulin-requiring' diabetic patients.

Other preoperative assessment in the elderly should include checking for autonomic neuropathy. This can be done by simple ECG tests (e.g. RR ratio standing and lying—the '30/15 ratio'; or during deep breathing) (Ewing et al 1985). However, postural hypotension in the elderly diabetic patient does not always indicate autonomic neuropathy, as it can be secondary to a wide variety of precipitants, especially drugs. This is important because autonomic neuropathy (which is more common in the elderly) may occasionally be associated with sudden perioperative death (Page and Watkins, 1978) and also increased intraoperative morbidity (Burgos et al 1989). Anaesthetists need to be

Table 13.1 Checklist for preoperative diabetic assessment

1. Assess as outpatient and/or admit 2–3 days earlier than usual
2. Full medical assessment; CXR and ECG, electrolytes, serum creatinine
3. Full diabetic assessment; four times daily bedside blood glucose levels, HbA_{1c}, autonomic function etc.
4. Optimize diabetic management; avoid excessively long-acting hypoglycaemic agents
5. Ensure reasonable glycaemic control (see text)
6. Liaise closely with the anaesthetist

aware of such information, so that patients can have close cardiac monitoring.

It can be appreciated that much of the standard preoperative assessment can be done prior to admission, either by liaison with the patient's physician or at a pre-admission anaesthetic clinic. Though this has been advocated for many years (Gill and Alberti 1989), regrettably it rarely occurs, and patients continue to need admission at least a day or two earlier than usual. Moreover, surgery may need to be further delayed if unforeseen problems are discovered following admission.

Finally, Table 13.1 gives a summary checklist of preoperative diabetic assessment. Note the important final step of liaising with the anaesthetist.

Management in Non-insulin-requiring Diabetes

There is general agreement that diabetic patients *not* on insulin treatment, undergoing surgery of less than major severity, can be managed conservatively by observation only (Allison et al 1979; Podolsky 1982; Hirsch et al 1991; Alberti and Marshall 1998; Schade 1988). Surprisingly, there has been very little critical evaluation of this presumed optimal therapy, though the information that is available does support a conservative approach. Thus Thompson and colleagues (1986) measured plasma glucose and metabolite responses to three groups of male patients undergoing transurethral surgery to the bladder or prostate gland. The groups were non-diabetic, Type 2 diabetic patients treated with intravenous glucose and insulin ('GKI infusion') (Alberti, Gill and Elliott 1982), and Type 2 patients treated conservatively. There was no significant difference between the two diabetic groups in terms of peri- and postoperative blood glucose levels. Plasma insulin and metabolite levels were actually closer to the non-diabetic group in the diabetic patients

Table 13.2 Guidelines for surgical care in diabetic patients *not* on insulin treatment[a]

1. Operate in the morning if possible
2. Frequently monitor bedside blood glucose levels (e.g. 2-hourly)
3. If on oral agents, omit on morning of surgery, and restart with first postoperative meal
4. Avoid glucose and lactate-containing fluids intravenously
5. Liaise with anaesthetist

[a]Unless surgery is of major severity, or preoperative control poor—in which case GKI infusion is advisable.

not treated with insulin. The authors concluded that 'GKI' in this situation induced an abnormal metabolic state with no overall glycaemic benefit. This study is of general importance, but is especially so for those caring for elderly diabetic patients requiring surgery. The patients studied had a mean age of about 65 years, and had Type 2 disease—by far the commonest type of diabetes in the elderly.

Guidelines for the conservative management of diabetes in surgery for Type 2 patients are shown in Table 13.2. It must again be emphasized that *major* surgery in such patients (e.g. opening the abdominal or thoracic cavity) should be managed as for insulin-treated patients. Note the importance of avoiding glucose-containing intravenous solutions, which can greatly destabilize glycaemic control. Lactate-containing fluids (e.g. Ringer lactate and Hartmann's) should also not be used as they can have hyperglycaemic effects (Thomas and Alberti 1978). Close plasma glucose monitoring is of course essential, and again liaison with the anaesthetist important (it is often in theatre that the dextrose or Ringer's drip is erected!). Surgery in the morning is advisable for all types of diabetes; there are no special metabolic reasons for this, but from a practical point of view it is much easier (and safer) to manage postoperative control problems in the afternoon rather than the middle of the night.

These simple management principles are successful in almost all Type 2 patients. Very rarely excessive postoperative hyperglycaemia may occur. This should be managed by subcutaneous short-acting insulin with meals; or if the patient cannot tolerate food, a 'GKI' infusion.

Management in Insulin-requiring Diabetes

This section includes true Type 1 diabetes patients, Type 2 patients on insulin treatment (including those on a combination of oral hypoglycaemics and insulin), and patients with Type 2 diabetes requiring temporary perioperative insulin because of poor glycaemic control or planned major surgery. Historically, a confusing number of systems have been advocated at various times; including early bizarre systems such as complete omission of insulin, or insulin with no subsequent glucose (Gill and Alberti 1982; Alberti and Thomas 1979). Not surprisingly, these systems did not work well! Later systems involved subcutaneous insulin with subsequent intravenous glucose infusions. Many such systems were complex, with widely varying types, amounts and proportions of insulin, and equally varied concentrations and rates of glucose infusion. Results with such methods were variable, though in good hands they were comparable with more modern methods (Thomas, Platt and Alberti 1984; Gill 1991).

Subcutaneous methods of insulin delivery have, however, now been generally abandoned because they are awkward and inflexible. Continuous intravenous insulin and glucose delivery was introduced in the late 1970s (Taitelman, Reece and Bessman 1977), and became rapidly popular because of its flexibility and simplicity. There are two major methods of use

The 'separate-line' system. (see Figure 13.3). Here, insulin is infused continuously via a syringe pump, with glucose infused separately. The glucose infusion is usually 10% dextrose, delivered at a rate of 100 mL/h (10 g/h) via an electric drip counter. Insulin is usually delivered via a 50 mL syringe driver: 50 units soluble insulin (e.g. Acrapid, Humulin S) in 50 mL 0.9% saline. Thus, 1 mL/h is equivalent to 1 unit/h. An average starting infusion rate is 3 units/h. The glucose infusion rate is kept constant throughout, and the insulin rate varied according to frequent (e.g. 1–2 hourly) bedside blood glucose measurements, aiming to maintain levels in the range of 6–12 mM.

It can be appreciated that this system is highly flexible and simple. However, it is very 'high tech', and requires expensive equipment which may not always be available. There is also a potential for metabolic 'disaster' if one of the lines comes adrift; thus interruption of glucose will lead to dangerous hypoglycaemia and cessation of insulin will conversely lead to hyperglycaemia and possibly ketosis.

The 'GKI' infusion (see Figure 13.3). A simpler and more 'user-friendly' version of the above method is to combine glucose and insulin in the same infusion bag, and give them together. A small amount of potassium

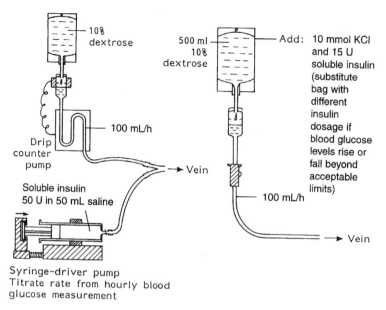

Figure 13.3   The 'separate line' (left) and GKI infusion systems of delivering intravenous insulin and glucose to diabetic patients undergoing surgery. Reproduced by kind permission of Blackwell Scientific Publications Ltd

is added to avoid hypokalaemia—hence the term 'GKI' (glucose–KCl–insulin). Interestingly this method was first advocated in 1963 by Galloway and Shuman, but did not become popular until redescribed by Alberti and Thomas in 1977, and modified by the same group in 1982 (Alberti et al 1982). The present most widely used 'mix' is 500 mL 10% dextrose with 15 units soluble insulin and 10 mMol KCl, delivered at 100 mL/h. This gives 3 units of insulin and 10 g glucose per hour, as does the 'separate-line' technique described above, but without the need for pumps and drip counters. The European Diabetes Policy Group (1999) suggests that 16 units of soluble insulin be used in the 10% dextrose bag, and that the infusion be run at 80 mL/h. No reason is given for the variation but either system will work, as the differences are inconsequential.

Because the insulin and glucose in GKI infusions are delivered together, the potential metabolic problems of rate alterations, line blockages etc. do not exist. The main disadvantage of GKI is that if dose changes are needed, the whole bag has to be discarded and a fresh one made up and erected. In practice this occurs in only 10–20% of cases (Alberti et al 1982).

Comparing the two systems.   As well as being practically effective, glucose–insulin infusion systems have advantageous metabolic effects, reducing the counter-regulatory hormone stress response, and

improving insulin sensitivity (Nygren et al 1998). The actual method of delivering insulin and glucose ('GKI' or 'separate line') is of no metabolic consequence, and it is a matter of practicalities as to which is chosen. Many hospitals use GKI in the general ward situation, and 'separate lines' in high-dependency or intensive care situations. The GKI system certainly works well in practice and is supported by a study of 85 episodes of surgery using GKI, in which mean plasma glucose levels ranged from 8.3 to 10.2 during the operative and first two postoperative days (Husband, Thai and Alberti 1986).

Figure 13.4 shows a summary algorithm for the management of the surgical diabetic patient, including a suggested scheme for altering GKI infusions if necessary according to bedside blood glucose monitoring.

One study has compared the 'GKI' and 'separate line' systems in a random fashion (Simmons et al 1994). Separate lines were generally preferred by nursing staff, and resulted in more blood glucose levels in the target range. Length of hospital stay, duration of insulin infusion and untoward incidents were similar with both systems. Importantly, the report did not give details of the level of nursing care available; a major advantage of GKI is that it is relatively safe on busy low-dependency wards.

Electrolytes should be measured daily in patients on GKI infusion, in case hyponatraemia develops. Finally,

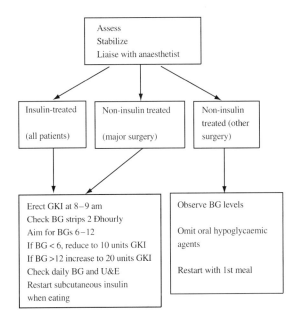

Figure 13.4 Summary chart for managing diabetes in surgery. GKI, glucose–potassium–insulin infusion (standard: 500 mL 10% dextrose + 15 units soluble + 10 mMol KCl; infused at 100 mL/h); BG, blood glucose; U and E, urea and electrolytes)

it should be noted that both systems described here can be used with 5% dextrose if desired, halving the insulin dose delivered appropriately. Similarly, if infused volume needs to be reduced—as may be the case in elderly patients with cardiac problems—20% dextrose at half the volume can be used, or a standard 10% GKI system used at 50 mL/h rather than 100 mL/h (this would be equivalent to a 5% dextrose system).

Management of insulin-requiring diabetic patients being fed pre- or postoperatively via a nasogastric tube or with parenteral nutrition may cause some management difficulties. Insulin infusions are safe if the patient is in a high-dependency or intensive care area, but in general wards subcutaneous insulin can be used. Provided the feed has continuous carbohydrate provision, 12-hourly subcutaneous isophane insulin may be satisfactory.

SPECIAL SURGICAL SITUATIONS

Emergency Surgery

Truly urgent surgery is fortunately relatively rare in diabetic patients, but it does occur, and is perhaps more common in the elderly; examples are peripheral and mesenteric embolization, ruptured aneurysms and trauma. Urgent plasma glucose, urea and electrolyte estimates are of course mandatory, and if the glycaemic and metabolic status is adverse it is best to correct this as far as possible prior to surgery. The urgency of the surgical situation will need to be assessed carefully in each case, and no 'blanket' rules can be made. Similarly, as regards the method of peroperative glycaemic control, this too has to be decided individually. Generally, a GKI system will be advisable in these unplanned situations, but the amounts of insulin needed cannot always be predicted. For example, if the patient requiring urgent surgery has had a sulphonylurea drug or insulin injection with the last 12 hours, the amount of insulin in the GKI infusion may need to be reduced. Each situation needs to be judged individually and very frequent bedside BG monitoring is necessary. In many cases, it may be judged that a 'separate line' system of delivery may be indicated to give extra flexibility.

Open Heart Surgery

Cardiac surgery is now very common, and coronary artery bypass grafting in particular is well established as a symptom-relieving and sometimes life-prolonging operation of low mortality. As such it is now being offered to many relatively elderly patients. Compared with other forms of surgery, coronary artery bypass grafting (CABG) is unusual. It is a long and unusually traumatic operation and patients are also rendered hypothermic and later given large doses of inotropic agents after restoration of cardiac activity. All these factors will promote increased insulin demands. Additionally, however, it was traditional to use a dextrose 'priming solution' to fill the cardiopulmonary pump, often amounting to a glucose load of about 75 g at the start of surgery (Gill, Sherif and Alberti 1981). Not surprisingly, initial results using standard GKI systems in this situation were poor (Gill, Sherif and Alberti 1981; Stephens et al 1988). However, changing to a non-glucose priming solution greatly improved perioperative glycaemic control (Stephens et al 1988; Crock et al 1988). A 'separate line' system for glucose and insulin provision is essential, with frequent BG monitoring. Relatively large insulin doses are needed (Elliott et al 1984), but results are good and algorithms have been produced to aid insulin delivery decisions (Watson et al 1986). Using modern systems such as these, the results of open heart surgery in diabetic patients are comparable with non-diabetic counterparts (Lawrie, Morris and Glaeser 1986; Devinen and McKenzie 1985), thus fulfilling the most important aims of diabetes management during surgery—acceptable glycaemic control by a simple and logical system without excess mortality or morbidity.

CONCLUSION

Though few centres are currently researching practical and theoretical aspects of the operative care of the diabetic patient, the subject continues to be a popular topic for review articles (Hirsch et al 1991; Anonymous 1999). Perhaps this is not surprising. As a clinical problem it is very common, and though current management procedures are well accepted, their detailed application continues to cause confusion.

Safe and effective perioperative diabetic care requires the acceptance of hospital-based agreed protocols of care which must be widely distributed. Transferring these protocols to safe and effective patient treatment depends on a team approach by physician, surgeon and anaesthetist.

REFERENCES

Alberti KGMM, Marshall SM (1988) Diabetes and surgery. In: Alberti KGMM, Krall LP (eds). *The Diabetes Annual*. Amsterdam Elsevier, 248–271.

Alberti KGMM, Thomas DJB (1979) The management of diabetes during surgery. *British Journal of Anaesthesia*, **51**, 603–710.

Alberti KGMM, Gill GV, Eliott MJ (1982) Insulin delivery during surgery in the diabetic patient. *Diabetes Care*, **5**, 65–77.

Allison SP, Tomlin PJ, Chamberlain MJ (1979) Some effects of anaesthesia and surgery on carbohydrate and fat metabolism. *British Journal of Anaesthesia*, **41**, 588–593.

Anonymous (1999) Drugs in the peri-operative period: corticosteroids and therapy for diabetes mellitus. *Drug and Therapeutics Bulletin*, **37**, 68–70.

Burgos LG, Ebert TJ, Asiddao C, Turner LA, Pattison CZ, Wang-Cheng R, Kampine JP (1989) Increased intraoperative cardiovascular morbidity in diabetics with autonomic neuropathy. *Anaesthesiology*, **70**, 591–597.

Crock PA, Ley CJ, Martin IK et al (1988) Humoral and metabolic changes during hypothermic coronary artery bypass surgery in diabetic and non-diabetic subjects. *Diabetic Medicine*, **5**, 47–52.

Devinen R, McKenzie FN (1985) Surgery for coronary artery disease in patients with diabetes mellitus. *Canadian Journal of Surgery*, **28**, 367–370.

Elliott MJ, Alberti KGMM (1983) Carbohydrate metabolism: effects of preoperative starvation and trauma. *Clinical Anaesthesiology*, **1**, 527–550.

Elliott MJ, Gill GV, Home PD et al (1984) A comparison of two regimens for the management of diabetes during open-heart surgery. *Anaesthesiology*, **60**, 364–368.

European Diabetes Policy Group (1999). A desktop guide to Type 1 (insulin-dependent) diabetes mellitus. *Diabetic Medicine*, **16**, 253–266.

Ewing DJ, Martyn CN, Young RJ, Clarke BF (1985) The value of cardiovascular autonomic function: 10 years' experience in diabetes. *Diabetes Care*, **8**, 491–498.

Faull CM, Holmes V, Baylis PH (1993) Water balance in elderly people: is there a deficiency of vasopression? *Age and Ageing*, **22**, 114–120.

Galloway JA, Shuman CR (1963) Diabetes and surgery. *American Journal of Medicine*, **34**, 177–191.

Gill GV (1991) Surgery and diabetes mellitus. In: Pickup J, Williams G (eds). *Textbook of Diabetes*. London: Blackwell, 820–826.

Gill GV, Alberti KGMM (1989) Surgery and diabetes. *Hospital Update*, **15**, 327–336.

Gill GV, Alberti KGMM (1992) The care of the diabetic patient during surgery. In: Alberti KGMM, deFronzo RA, Keen H, Zimmet P (eds) *International Textbook of Diabetes Mellitus*. Chichester: John Wiley, 1173–1183.

Gill GV, Sherif IH, Alberti KGMM (1981) Management of diabetes during open heart surgery. *British Journal of Surgery*, **68**, 171–172.

Golden SH, Kao WHL, Peart-Vigilance C, Broncati FL (1999) Perioperative glycemic control and the risk of infectious complications in a cohort of adults with diabetes. *Diabetes Care*, **22**, 1408–1414.

Hirsch IB, McGill JB, Cryer PE, White PF (1991) Perioperative management of surgical patients with diabetes mellitus. *Anaesthesiology*, **74**, 346–359.

Hjortrup A, Sorenson C, Dynemose E, Hjortso NC, Kehlet H (1985) Influence of diabetes mellitus an operative risk. *British Journal of Surgery*, **72**, 783–785.

Hughes TAT, Borsey DQ (1994) The management of diabetic patients undergoing surgery. *Practical Diabetes*, **11**, 7–10.

Hume DM, Egdahl RH (1959). The importance of the brain in the endocrine response to injury. *Annals of Surgery*, **150**, 697–712.

Husband DJ, Thai AC, Alberti KGMM (1986) Management of diabetes during surgery with glucose–insulin–potassium infusion. *Diabetic Medicine*, **3**, 69–74.

Hutchison ASA, Shenkin A (1984) BM strips: how accurate are they in general wards? *Diabetic Medicine*, **1**, 225–226.

Jennings AM, Wilson RM, Ward JD (1989) Symptomatic hypoglycaemia in NIDDM patients treated with oral hypoglycaemic agents. *Diabetes Care*, **12**, 203–208.

Lawrie GM, Morris GC, Glaeser DH (1986) Influence of diabetes mellitus on the results of coronary bypass surgery: follow-up of 212 diabetic patients 10 to 15 years after surgery. *Journal of the American Medical Association*, **256**, 2967–2971.

MacKenzie CR, Charlson ME (1988) Assessment of perioperative risk in the patient with diabetes mellitus. *Surgical Gynaecology and Obstetrics*, **167**, 293–299.

Mellière D, Berrahal D, Desgranges P et al (1999) Influence of diabetes on revascularisation procedures of the aorta and lower limb arteries: early results. *European Journal of Vascular and Endovascular Surgery*, **17**, 438–441.

Nordenstrom J, Sannenfield J, Arner P (1989) Characterisation of insulin resistance after surgery. *Surgery*, **105**, 28–35.

Nygren JO, Thorell A, Soop M et al (1998) Perioperative insulin and glucose infusion maintains normal insulin sensitivity after surgery. *American Journal of Physiology*, **275**, E140–E148.

Page MM, Watkins PJ (1978) Cardiorespiratory arrest with diabetic autonomic neuropathy. *Lancet*, **i**, 14–16.

Podolsky S (1982) Management of diabetes in the surgical patient. *Medical Clinics of North America*, **66**, 1361–1372.

Sandler RS, Maule WF, Baltus ME (1986) Factors associated with post-operative complications in diabetics after biliary tract surgery. *Gastroenterology*, **91**, 157–162.

Schade DS (1988) Surgery and diabetes. *Medical Clinics of North America*, **72**, 1531–1543.

Simmons D, Morton K, Laughton S, Scott DJ (1994) A comparison of two intravenous insulin regimens among surgical patients with insulin-dependent diabetes mellitus. *Diabetes Educator*, **20**, 422–427.

Stephens JW, Krause AH, Petersen CA et al (1988) The effect of glucose priming solutions in patients undergoing coronary artery bypass grafting. *Annals of Thoracic Surgery*, **45**, 544–547.

Taitelman U, Reece EA, Bessman AN (1977) Insulin in the management of the diabetic surgical patient: continuous intravenous administration versus subcutaneous administration. *Journal of the American Medical Association*, **237**, 658–660.

Thomas DJB, Alberti KGMM (1978) The hyperglycaemic effects of Hartmann's solution in maturity-onset diabetics during surgery. *British Journal of Anaesthesia*, **51**, 693–710.

Thomas DJB, Platt HS, Alberti KGMM (1984) Insulin-dependent diabetes during the peri-operative period. *Anaesthesia*, **39**, 629–637.

Thompson J, Husband DJ, Thai AC, Alberti KGMM (1986) Metabolic changes in the non-insulin dependent diabetic undergoing minor surgery: effect of glucose–insulin–potassium infusion. *British Journal of Surgery*, **73**, 301–304.

Watson BG, Elliott MJ, Pay DA et al (1986) Diabetes mellitus and open heart surgery: a simple practical closed loop insulin infusion system for blood glucose control. *Anaesthesia*, **41**, 250–257.

14

Metabolic Risk Factors and their Treatment

Hosam K. Kamel, John E. Morley

St Louis University School of Medicine, and St. Louis VA Medical Center

INTRODUCTION

Type 2 diabetes is the most prevalent form of diabetes in older adults. This metabolic disorder is characterized by defects in both insulin secretion and insulin action. In recent years, it has become increasingly recognized that Type 2 diabetes is a part of a cluster of cardiovascular risk factors that constitute what is now referred to as the 'metabolic syndrome' (Beck-Nielsen et al 1999). Although most of the individual components of the syndrome were described more than 20 years ago (Zimmet and Albert 1999), it was not until 1988 that Reaven and coworkers focused attention on the cluster and named it 'syndrome X' (Reaven 1988). A World Health Organization expert committee proposed that the syndrome be called the 'metabolic syndrome' and focused its definition mainly on its relationship to cardiovascular disease (CVD) (Alberti and Zimmet 1998). As central visceral obesity was not included in the original description by Reaven, the term 'metabolic syndrome' is preferred to 'syndrome X'. Each of the factors described in the metabolic syndrome represents an important cardiovascular risk factor on its own. These factors contribute cumulatively to macrovascular diabetic complications (Zimmet et al 1999). Furthermore, patients with one of these factors (e.g. diabetes or central obesity) often have one or more of the other cardiovascular risk factors described in the metabolic syndrome (Zimmet 1992).

Atherosclerosis is the most frequent complication of Type 2 diabetes (Zimmet and Alberti 1997). Cardiovascular disease accounts for at least 66% of deaths in individuals with Type 2 diabetes (Panzram 1987). In addition, coronary, cerebrovascular and peripheral vascular disease are 2–5 times more common in persons with diabetes (Zimmet and Alberti 1997). These findings, in addition to the frequent association of Type 2 diabetes with other cardiovascular risk factors, indicate that the management of diabetic individuals should not only focus on tight blood glucose control, but should also involve minimizing other cardiovascular risk factors such as obesity, hypertension, hyperinsulinemia and dyslipidaemia (Zimmet 1995). This chapter discusses the metabolic syndrome and the management of metabolic risk factors in individuals with Type 2 diabetes mellitus.

THE METABOLIC SYNDROME: AN OVERVIEW

A WHO expert committee in 1998 proposed that the metabolic syndrome should be diagnosed in patients who show evidence of glucose intolerance and/or insulin resistance together with two other components of the syndrome (Table 14.1). The expert committee decided to define insulin resistance as insulin sensitivity under hyperinsulinemic euglycemia clamp conditions below the lowest quartile for the population under investigation. This definition of insulin resistance matches the degree of insulin sensitivity in patients with Type 2 diabetes mellitus (Beck-Nielsen et al 1999). Epidemiological studies indicate that the metabolic syndrome is prevalent in industrialized countries. When applying the WHO definition of the metabolic syndrome to the European Group for the study of Insulin Resistance (EGIR) database (Ferranninni et al 1996), the prevalence of the syndrome was estimated at 15.6% among healthy Caucasians in Europe (Beck-Nielson et al 1999). Data from the Danish Twin Register (Kyvik, Green and Beck-Nielsen 1995) indicate a prevalence rate of 12.5% among Danish twins (Beck-Nielsen et al 1999). The actual

Table 14.1 World Health Organization definition of the metabolic syndrome

---

1. *Insulin resistance*: insulin sensitivity below lowest quartile for the population
2. *Glucose intolerance*: 2-hour oral glucose tolerance test plasma glucose levels >7.8 mM
3. *Central obesity*: waist/hip ratio—female >0.85, male >0.95
4. *Hypertension*: blood pressure >160/95 mmHg
5. *Hypertriglyceridemia*: triglycerides >1.7 mM
6. *High-density lipoprotein–cholesterol*: female <1.1 mM, male <0.9 mM

---

prevalence of the metabolic syndrome in these two populations is likely to be greater, however, since these estimates excluded individuals with overt diabetes mellitus. Studies from the US and Australia also indicate high prevalence of the metabolic syndrome, (Zimmet 1992; Hoffner et al 1990).

The occurrence of Type 2 diabetes is probably best represented as the 'top of a pyramid' formed of a cluster of cardiovascular risk factors that together constitute the metabolic syndrome (Figure 14.1) (Zimmet and Collier 1999). Paradoxically, studies have clearly demonstrated that some patients may show the other features of the metabolic syndrome up to 10 years before they develop overt hyperglycaemia (Panzram 1987; Haffner et al 1990). This indicates that the risk of developing CVD in some individuals may actually start well before the manifestations of glucose intolerance become apparent, and that early aggressive management of the metabolic risk factors in such individuals may help prevent the development of Type 2 diabetes and CVD (Zimmet and Collier 1999).

The EGIR database, the largest database currently available on the metabolic syndrome, demonstrates a

statistically significant correlation between the degree of insulin resistance and the other components of the metabolic syndrome; including fasting plasma insulin levels ($r = -0.48$; $p < 0.01$), waist:hip ratio ($r = -0.14$, $p < 0.01$), fasting plasma triglyceride levels ($r = -0.26$; $p < 0.01$), high density lipoprotein (HDL)–cholesterol levels ($r = 0.14$, $p < 0.01$), and diastolic blood pressure ($r = -0.22$, $p < 0.01$). Multiple regression analysis, however, indicated that insulin resistance is a determinant of only fasting plasma insulin levels but not the other factors (Beck-Nielsen et al 1999). It is possible that the effect of insulin resistance on the other components of the syndrome is secondary to the associated hyperinsulinemia. This conclusion is supported by findings from other studies that showed hyperinsulinemia to be a causative factor of both dyslipidaemia and hypertension (Beck-Nielsen and Groop 1994). The EGIR database also provides evidence that only 50% of the variations in insulin resistance could be explained by the other components of the syndrome, which could indicate that other variables (e.g. physical fitness) may play a role in determining the severity of insulin resistance. Poulsen and coworkers (1999) studied the frequency of the metabolic syndrome among twins and showed an overall genetic contribution in the order of 40% to insulin resistance. This finding points towards a more important role for environmental factors in the pathogenesis of the metabolic syndrome (Figure 14.2).

Studies of the offspring (Martin et al 1992) and first-degree relatives (Vaag, Hemriken and Beck-Nielsen 1992) of patients with Type 2 diabetes mellitus indicate that insulin resistance may appear as early as 30 years prior to the onset of hyperglycaemia. We now know that insulin resistance alone rarely gives rise to hyperglycaemia. Insulin secretion usually rises in compensation, thus maintaining a euglycemic state. As long as this compensatory hyperinsulinemia is sufficient to overcome insulin resistance and hepatic glucose overproduction, hyperglycaemia does not develop. With time, however, many individuals develop Type 2 diabetes mellitus. Whether the effect of insulin resistance with time leads to impaired beta-cell function and subsequently its ability to maintain adequate insulin secretion, or whether the presence of insulin resistance adds to the predisposition to Type 2 diabetes in individuals who independently inherit or acquire insulin secretary defects, remains uncertain (DeFronzo and Ferrannini 1991). The sequence of events in the development of Type 2 diabetes is shown in Figure 14.3.

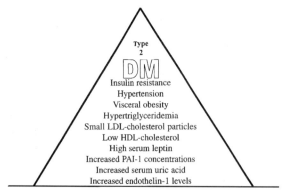

Figure 14.1 Type 2 diabetes at the top of a pyramid of a cluster of cardiovascular risk factors forming the metabolic syndrome. LDL, low-density lipoprotein; HDL, high-density lipoprotein; PAI-1, platelet activator inhibitor-1

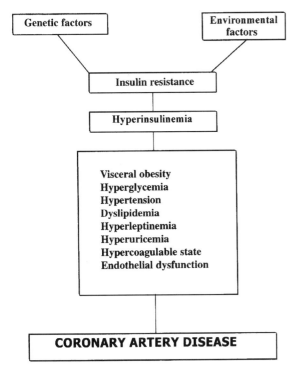

Figure 14.2 Pathogenesis of the metabolic syndrome

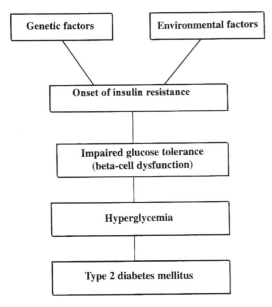

Figure 14.3 Pathogenesis of Type 2 diabetes mellitus

INSULIN RESISTANCE AND HYPERINSULINEMIA

Insulin resistance represents the earliest biochemical characteristic associated with the development of Type 2 diabetes mellitus (Lillioja et al 1993). Thus, screening for insulin resistance may represent the earliest phase at which subjects at risk for diabetes may be identified. At the present time, no simple screening method to measure insulin resistance is available. Fasting hyperinsulinemia in non-diabetic subjects has been shown to be closely related to insulin resistance. Insulin assays currently available, however, are not sufficiently standardized to permit categories of normal and abnormal insulin ranges to be defined for this purpose (Robbins et al 1996). In addition, it is estimated that 25% of the population can be shown to be insulin-resistant (Reaven 1988) yet only 6% of the population develop Type 2 diabetes. This indicates that most insulin-resistant individuals do not develop diabetes. Chronic insulin resistance, in addition to being associated with the development of Type 2 diabetes, has also been linked to increased prevalence of dyslipidaemia, hypertension, a procoagulant state, and CVD (DeFronzo and Ferrannini 1991).

Fifty percent of the variability in insulin action may be attributed to differences in lifestyle; for example obesity, physical inactivity and cigarette smoking all increase the degree of insulin resistance. The other 50% of the variability is likely to be related to genetic differences. In addition, it is now clear that hyperglycaemia itself may produce insulin resistance—a phenomenon known as glucotoxicity (DeFronzo et al 1992). Insulin resistance is common in individuals with Type 2 diabetes mellitus, and this phenomenon is implicated as a major factor in the development of overt hyperglycaemia. In the Insulin Resistance and Atherosclerosis Study (IRAS), Haffner and coworkers (1997) reported that insulin resistance was present in 85% of subjects with diabetes. Insulin resistance may also be found in conditions that are not necessarily associated with glucose intolerance (Table 14.2). (Ferrannini 2000). DeFronzo and Ferrannini (1991) have shown that patients with Type 2 diabetes, obese individuals, and patients with essential hypertension may all have the same degree of insulin resistance relative to individuals with normal insulin sensitivity. Insulin resistance in diabetic individuals, however, is associated with metabolic alterations linked to the metabolic syndrome (Reaven 1988). This association was fully apparent in the EGIR database (Del Prato et

Table 14.2 Conditions commonly associated with insulin resistance

Type 2 diabetes
Thyroid disease (hyper/hypothyroidism)
Cushing's syndrome
Pheochromocytoma
Acromegaly
Essential hypertension
Liver cirrhosis
Rheumatoid arthritis
Acanthosis nigricans
Surgery
Trauma/burns
Pregnancy

al 1999). Even in individuals with a body mass index (BMI) $\leq 27\,kg/m^2$, those with evidence of insulin resistance had higher systolic and diastolic blood pressures and higher plasma triglycerides and cholesterol levels than those with normal insulin sensitivity. This indicates that insulin resistance may be a marker for the future development of diabetes and cardiovascular disease.

Over the past decade, many investigators have tested the hypothesis that lifestyle modification or pharmacological interventions may decrease insulin resistance, prevent diabetes and modify other cardiovascular risk factors. The effects of lifestyle modification on insulin resistance are reviewed in other sections of the chapter. Here we focus on available pharmacological interventions. Two drug classes that have been shown to be promising in this regard were the thiazolidinediones and the biguanides.

Troglitazone was the first of the thiazolidinediones to become available for clinical use. Other drugs in this category include pioglitazone and rosiglotazone, ciglitazone, and englitazone. The thiazolidinediones directly improve insulin sensitivity in muscle and liver through the activation of the nuclear transcription factor, peroxisome proliferator-activated receptor gamma (PPARγ), enhancing insulin-mediated glucose uptake as well as inhibiting hepatic glucose production. Significant clinical data are available only for troglitazone. This drug has been shown to inhibit *in vitro* hyperglycaemia-induced insulin resistance (Kroder et al 1996), to lower the triglyceride content of pancreatic islets in rats (Shimabukuro et al 1997), and to improve the reduced beta-cell response to glucose found in subjects with impaired glucose tolerance

(IGT) (Cavaghan et al 1997). In addition to its advantageous effects on insulin and glucose, troglitazone lowers serum triglycerides and free fatty acids (Iwamoto et al 1996), has antihypertensive and antioxidant properties (Nolan et al 1994) as well as an antiproliferative action on smooth muscle cells (Law et al 1996). These effects may have significant benefits in the prevention of progression of IGT to diabetes as well as on the risk of developing CVD. In a 12-week, multicenter trial of 51 subjects with IGT who were randomized to 400 mg/day troglitazone or placebo, 80% of the troglitazone-treated subjects reverted to normal glucose tolerance versus 48% of the placebo group. In addition, fasting insulin and C-peptide response to glucose and fasting triglyceride levels were reduced in the troglitazone group (Antonucci et al 1997). In another study, 3 months', treatment with troglitazone resulted in improvement of insulin action in subjects with IGT who have not yet developed diabetes (Cavaghan et al 1997). Troglitazone has been withdrawn from the market in the United States and most of Europe because of serious drug-related hepatic toxicity. Pioglitazone and roseglotazone have been introduced recently in the US market. Data from the limited clinical trial with these two drugs indicate effects similar to those of troglitazone on insulin resistance, triglycerides, insulin, and glucose without significant hepatic toxicity (Yamasaki et al 1997; Kawamori et al 1998; Shibata et al 1999).

In a double-blind, placebo-controlled study, the biguanide metformin was found to reduce insulin secretion rate, while increasing insulin sensitivity and metabolic clearance rate without increasing glucose tolerance in 15 overweight subjects with IGT (Scheen, Letiexhe and Lefebvre 1995). The BIGPRO study is a multicenter primary prevention trial being conducted in France with the aim of examining the effects of metformin in 324 subjects with the insulin resistance syndrome, normal glucose tolerance, and upper-body obesity in a randomized, placebo-controlled trial. At one year, metformin-treated individuals had lost weight and had lower fasting glucose and insulin levels (Fontbonne et al 1996). Metformin is included in the Diabetes Prevention Program (1999) a multicenter study initiated in the United States in June 1996 aimed at testing the effects of lifestyle interventions and/or pharmacotherapy on progression to diabetes in 4000 subjects with IGT (Goldberg 1998). Troglitazone was included initially but discontinued because of associated liver toxicity.

HYPERGLYCAEMIA

There is strong evidence linking the occurrence of diabetic complications to the degree of hyperglycaemia. Klein (1995), in a 10-year follow-up of older patients with Type 2 diabetes, demonstrated that each 1% rise of HBA_{1c} is associated with an increased risk of retinopathy by 60% and nephropathy by 65%. The mechanism for this apparent glucotoxicity probably involves multiple metabolic pathways. Some of these pathways are modulated by glucose directly, while others are probably indirect consequences of glycosylation of proteins and changes in oxidative stress, (Mooradian and Thurman 1999).

One of the important accomplishments of the last decade is the completion of two important diabetes clinical trials, namely the Diabetes Control and Complications Trial (DCCT) in the United States and Canada, and the United Kingdom Prospective Diabetes Study (UKPDS). The DCCT (1993) demonstrated conclusively that normalization of blood glucose in individuals with Type 1 diabetes mellitus would reduce the risk of microvascular complications as well as neuropathy. The impact of tight glucose control on the frequency of cardiovascular complications could not be addressed by the DCCT trial. Following the release of the DCCT results, the American Diabetes Association (1993) issued a position statement indicating that the DCCT findings in individuals with Type 1 diabetes mellitus should be readily applicable to individuals with Type 2 diabetes mellitus since the underlying mechanisms responsible for the complications are similar in the two types of disease. This recommendation at the time lacked supportive evidence, however. Even more confounding is the available evidence at the time from the University Groups Diabetes Program study that was not in favor of intensification of blood glucose control (UGDP 1970). Subsequently, two smaller interventional trials in individuals with Type 2 diabetes mellitus yielded conflicting messages. In the Kumamoto study, (Ohkubo et al 1995), tightening of blood glucose control with insulin reduced the risks of microvascular disease to the same extent found in the DCCT. On the other hand, in the pilot study of the Veteran Administration (VA) Cooperative Study (Abraira, Colwell and Nuttall 1995) a disturbing trend of increased cardiovascular mortality was noted in individuals with Type 2 diabetes mellitus randomized to the intensive glucose control arm of the study.

With this background of conflicting messages as to the importance of intensive blood glucose control, the

Table 14.3 Summary of key findings of the UK Prospective Diabetes Study

1. Strict blood glucose control lowers the incidence of microvascular diabetic complications
2. Insulin, sulfonylureas and metformin had similar effectiveness in lowering HbA_{1c} level
3. Type 2 diabetes mellitus is a progressive disease over time
4. Intensification of blood glucose control requires pharmacological intervention in addition to lifestyle changes
5. Insulin or sulfonylurea treatment is not associated with increased or decreased incidence of cardiac events
6. Metformin monotherapy is associated with reduced overall mortality and reduced incidence of cardiovascular events in overweight individuals
7. Addition of acarbose results in additional improvement of blood glucose control irrespective of concomitant therapy
8. Lowering blood pressure <150/85 mmHg reduced diabetes-related microvascular and macrovascular complications
9. Using ACE inhibitors compared to beta-blockers had no distinct advantage on clinical outcomes

UKPDS (1998a–d; Holman et al 1999; see also Mooradian and Chehada 2000) was an important and timely contribution. The key findings from the UKPDS are summarized in Table 14.3. In general these indicate that tight diabetic control is associated with lower microvascular complications. The improvement seen in the frequency of microvascular complications was proportionate to the microvascular benefits observed in the DCCT or the Kumamoto study when HBA_{1c} differences are accounted for. Unlike the effects on microvascular complications, tight glucose control in the UKPDS resulted in only marginal reduction in the incidence of macrovascular complications (16%) that did not achieve statistical significance (UKPDS 1998a). This smaller effect of tight glycemic control on the frequency of cardiovascular complications in individuals with Type 2 diabetes mellitus greatly emphasizes the importance of managing other cardiovascular risk factors (e.g. hypertension, smoking, dyslipidaemia, and central obesity) in such patients. In another prospective study, however, intensive insulin therapy was shown significantly to decrease mortality in diabetic patients who suffered acute myocardial infarction (Malmberg et al 1999).

HYPERTENSION

Hypertension has been established as a powerful risk factor to all of the major cardiovascular diseases, including coronary artery disease, stroke, peripheral arterial disease, renal disease and heart failure. Epidemiological data have shown clearly that hypertension usually occurs in association with other metabolically linked risk factors, and that less than 20% occurs in isolation. Associated risk factors include glucose intolerance, obesity, left ventricular hypertrophy, and dyslipidemia (elevated total, low-density lipoprotein (LDL), and small dense LDL cholesterol levels, raised triglycerides, and reduced HDL cholesterol levels). Clusters of three or more of these additional risk factors occur at four-fold times the rate expected by chance. Based on data from the Framingham Study (Kannel 2000), the risk of coronary artery disease increased stepwise with the extent of risk factor clustering. Among persons with hypertension, about 40% of coronary events in men and 68% in women are attributable to the presence of two or more additional risk factors. Only 14% of coronary events in hypertensive men and 5% of those in hypertensive women occurred in the absence of additional risk factors. Clinical trials have demonstrated conclusively that control of blood pressure will result in decreased total and cardiovascular mortality. The Hypertension Optimization Trial (HOT) (Hansson and Zanchetti 1997) studied the potential impact of aggressive antihypertensive therapy with target diastolic blood pressures being >90, >85 and >80 mmHg. The HOT trial demonstrated that more effective blood pressure lowering was associated with improvement in cardiovascular outcomes.

Hypertension is prevalent in patients with Type 2 diabetes mellitus and its occurrence increases the risk of cardiovascular complications in such individuals (Laakso 1998). In the UKPDS, 1148 individuals with hypertension and Type 2 diabetes mellitus were randomized to tight blood pressure control (blood pressure goal <150/85 mmHg and mean value achieved was 144/82 mmHg) with the use of either an angiotensin-converting enzyme (ACE) inhibitor (captopril), or a beta-blocker (atenolol) as the main treatment, or to a less tight control arm aiming at a blood pressure of less than 180/105 mmHg. Tight blood control in individuals with Type 2 diabetes mellitus and hypertension reduced the risk of diabetes-related deaths by 32%, and diabetes-related complications, notably retinopathy and deterioration of visual acuity, by 47%. The risk of stroke was reduced by 44%. There were no statistically significant differences in the outcomes selectively attributable to ACE inhibitor or beta-blocker therapy (UKPDS 1998d).

CENTRAL VISCERAL OBESITY

Central obesity (obesity localized to central visceral fat depots) is the most prevalent precursor of Type 2 diabetes mellitus (Ohlsson et al 1985). Insulin resistance, which is more prominent in visceral obesity than generalized obesity or that localized to peripheral gluteofemoral depots, is considered to be related to this pattern of obesity (Peiris et al 1986). Free fatty acids have been implicated in the pathogenesis of insulin resistance in muscle through their interface with critical steps in glycolysis. Muscle tissue is the main regulator of systemic insulin sensitivity (Bjorntrop and Rosmond 1999). Compared with subcutaneous fat, visceral fat has increased sensitivity to lipolytic stimuli and has decreased antilipolytic effects to insulin. This means that the potential per unit mass of visceral adipose tissue to mobilize free fatty acid is much larger than that of subcutaneous fat (Bjorntrop 1994).

Acute reductions in caloric intake has been shown to improve insulin sensitivity, and weight reduction further improves insulin action while both decreasing 24-hour insulin secretion and enhancing insulin clearance, thus reducing demand on the beta-cell, particularly in the post-absorptive state (Kelly 1995). In addition, studies have shown that obese individuals with IGT may be prevented from developing diabetes through weight reduction. In a 6-year follow-up study of 109 individuals with IGT and clinically severe obesity who lost more than 50% of their bodyweight after bariatric surgery, only one individual developed diabetes, in comparison to the control group in which 6 out of 27 subjects became diabetic within 5 years (Long, O'Brien and MacDonald 1994). Another study involved 35 non-diabetic elderly men who achieved a 9 kg weight loss after a low-fat, hypocaloric diet maintained over a 9-month period (Colman et al 1995). Of 20 subjects with IGT, glucose intolerance was normalized in nine individuals. The improvement in glucose tolerance was related to the reduction in waist circumference and was associated with reduced insulin level and improvement in insulin action. Studies in animals have shown that high-fat diets may cause insulin resistance (Storlien et al 1991), and several prospective studies of subjects with IGT have demonstrated that fat consumption, especially high saturated fat, significantly predicts conversion to Type 2 diabetes after controlling for obesity (Marshall et al 1994; Feskens et al 1995). In 31 individuals with IGT randomized either to a reduced-fat, polyunsaturated fat-enriched diet, or to a high-fat, monounsaturated fat-enriched diet, fasting glucose levels were slightly lowered by the high monounsaturated-fat diet without significant changes in insulin sensitivity or parameters of insulin secretory response (Sarkkinen et al 1996). There have been no intervention studies in subjects with IGT to evaluate the effect of low saturated-fat diets versus saturated fat-enriched diets on the progression to clinical diabetes.

Several studies have reported the advantage of combining weight-reduction and exercise programs on delaying the progression to diabetes in subjects with IGT. The Oslo Diet and Exercise Study (Torjesen et al 1977) demonstrated that a program combining total fat reduction with moderate increase in physical activity in 219 inactive, normoglycemic men and women with features of the insulin-resistance syndrome reduced fasting glucose levels and body mass index and improved insulin sensitivity and beta-cell function (as well as lipid profile and blood pressure). Insulin sensitivity, estimated using the homeostasis model, improved after one year of a low-fat diet alone as well as in the combined diet and exercise group, but not in the exercise-alone group. The Malmo study (Eriksson and Lindgarde 1991) evaluated the effects of a 5-year program of a low-fat, hypocaloric diet combined with increased physical activity in 41 recently diagnosed Type 2 diabetic subjects and in 181 individuals with IGT, in comparison with 79 subjects with IGT and 114 normoglycemic individuals who did not enroll in the program. In addition to demonstrating significant reductions in body mass index and improvements in fitness (increased maximal oxygen uptake), blood pressure, lipids, and hyperinsulinemia in the intervention group, glucose tolerance was normalized in more than 50% of the subjects with IGT. More than 50% of the diabetic subjects were in remission at the study end. Similar results were obtained in 22 subjects with IGT who completed a 2-year combined diet and exercise program in New Zealand (Borun et al 1994). The Da Qing IGT and Diabetes Study reported from China clearly demonstrated the benefits of lifestyle modification (Pan et al 1994). In this study, the effects of a one-year diet or exercise intervention program were assessed in 577 individuals with IGT. Subjects were randomized to control, diet (low-fat and reduced calories in overweight individuals), exercise, or combined diet and exercise groups. Rates of conversion to diabetes were significantly reduced in both lean and overweight members of the diet (47%), exercise (45%), and diet-plus-exercise (44%) groups when compared with subjects in the control group (66%).

DYSLIPIDAEMIA

Diabetes mellitus and hyperglycaemia are associated with several alterations in lipid metabolism, collectively known as diabetic dyslipidemia (Table 14.4) (Assman and Schulte 1988; Fontbonne et al 1989; Lewis and Steiner 1996) Hypertriglyceridaemia is the key characteristic of diabetic dyslipidaemia. Triglycerides have been shown to be an independent risk factor for coronary artery disease (Hokanson and Austin 1996). This may be attributed to their effect on increasing cholesteryl ester heteroexchange between lipoproteins (Durrington 1994). This may result in low HDL cholesterol and in the formation of small dense LDL particles (Durrington 1997). Small dense LDL particles, although highly atherogenic, do not contribute significantly to total cholesterol serum levels and the only clue to their presence is usually a low HDL cholesterol associated with high triglyceride levels. In a prospective study from Germany (Assman and Schulte 1992), increased triglyceride levels increased the risk of coronary artery disease to a greater extent than did increased LDL cholesterol levels. Triglycerides are also linked to increased plasma fibrinogen levels. Increased plasma fibrinogen has been shown to be a risk factor for coronary artery disease (Hamsten et al 1994), and its levels may be lowered by the use of fibrates with the exception of gemfibrozil (Branchi et al 1993). In the Paris Prospective Study (Fontbonne et al 1989), the strongest predictor for the incidence of CVD during the follow-up period of 11 years in subjects with IGT was the serum triglyceride level. Patients with triglyceride levels higher than 1.5 mM had a relative risk of 3.3 ($p < 0.01$). HDL cholesterol was not measured in this study. A follow-up study among 313 diabetic patients in East Finland (Laakso et al 1993) showed that low HDL cholesterol and high triglyceride levels were the only independent risk factors for the development of coronary artery disease 7 years later. Low HDL (< 0.9 mM) was associated with a relative risk of 3.9 ($p < 0.001$), whereas

Table 14.4 Features of diabetic dyslipidaemia

Increased plasma triglycerides (TG)
Decreased high-density lipoprotein (HDL) – cholesterol
Appearance of small dense low density lipoprotein (LDL) – cholesterol particles
Decreased activity of lipoprotein lipase
Increased serum levels of very-low-density lipoprotein (VLDL) particles
Increased activity of hepatic lipase

the relative risk of high triglycerides (>2.3 mM) was 2.2 ($p = 0.001$).

Nutritional interventions (weight loss and decreased consumption of saturated fat) are recommended as the first step in the management of diabetic dyslipidaemia (Franz et al 1994). However, lifestyle modifications alone often do not result in adequate lowering in serum lipid levels and pharmacological interventions are usually needed. In addition, in older persons therapeutic diets are often linked to the development of protein energy malnutrition.

Two drug groups are often used to manage diabetic dyslipidaemia. These are the statins, which predominantly lower serum cholesterol, and the fibrates, which principally decrease triglycerides. The differential effects of statins and fibrates on cholesterol and triglyceride levels and the impact on cardiovascular outcomes in patients with Type 2 diabetes are being addressed in several clinical trials currently under way. Results from these are expected to be available in the coming few years. The study population of some large lipid clinical trials, however, included patients with diabetes, and results from these studies may help shed some light on some of these issues.

The study population of the Scandinavian Simvastatin Survival Study (4S) (1994), a secondary-prevention randomized controlled trial utilizing the statin simvastatin, included 202 diabetic subjects. Over the 5.4-year follow-up period, total serum cholesterol levels decreased by 29% and cardiac events decreased by 33%. Another secondary-prevention randomized control trial, the Cholesterol and Recurrent Events (CARE), included 586 diabetic subjects (Goldberg et al 1998). This study investigated the effect of another statin, pravastatin, on cardiovascular outcomes. Over the 5-year follow-up period, serum cholesterol decreased by 20% and cardiovascular events by 20%. Unlike the other two trials, the Helsinki Heart Study (Koskinen et al 1992), investigated the effect of a fibrate, gemfibrozil, on the incidence of primary cardiac events in patients with hyperlipidaemia. Over the 5-year follow-up period, the 135 diabetic subjects in this study showed 34% reduction in the incidence of cardiac events, and a 10% reduction in serum cholesterol levels. The greater impact on cardiovascular events in this study in spite of a minimal effect on serum cholesterol levels (3.4% decrease in CVD incidence for 1% decrease in serum cholesterol), compared with the 4S study (1.1%) and the CARE study (1.2%) indicated that an additional benefit appears to accrue from triglyceride lowering (Durrington 1997). Thus when both cholesterol and triglycerides are increased in diabetic

patients, combining the benefits of both statins and fibrates should be considered. The recently introduced statin, atorvastatin, appears to combine the cholesterol-lowering properties of a statin with a greater effect on serum triglycerides compared with other statins (Black 1995). Recently, atorvastatin was found to be more powerful than simvastatin in lowering insulin resistance in 195 elderly diabetics (Paolisoo et al 2000). In this study, the degree of decline in plasma triglyceride concentration was a significant determinant for the effect of stains on insulin resistance.

OTHER METABOLIC RISK FACTORS

Since the introduction of the concept of the metabolic syndrome, several other metabolic abnormalities have been defined to be related to insulin resistance and increased risk of CVD. The plasminogen activator inhibitor-1 (PAI-1) levels have been shown to be elevated in subjects with insulin resistance (Bastard and Pieroni 1999). In one study, PAI-1 levels were directly associated with the amount of visceral fat in obese men but not women. These levels decreased substantially when subjects lost weight (Kocks et al 1999). High PAI-1 levels may cause reduced endogenous fibrinolytic activity and have been linked to increased risk of CVD (Nordt et al 1999). Data from the Framingham offspring study (Meigs et al 2000) demonstrated an association between insulin resistance and abnormalities in several other hemostatic factors. In this study, elevated fasting insulin levels were associated with increased serum concentration of tissue-type plasminogen activator (tPA) antigen, and von Willebrand factor (VWF) antigen in addition to elevated PAI-1 serum levels. In another study (Carmassi et al 1999), intra-arterial infusion of insulin in the forearm resulted in increased local PAI-1 and tPA concentrations. These reported alterations in hemostatic factor levels place subjects with insulin resistance in a hypercoagulable state that may enhance their potential for acute thrombosis and places them at increased risk for CVD. Insulin resistance has been linked also to impaired endothelial function. Piatti and coworkers (2000) demonstrated that both glycosylated hemoglobin (HbA$_{1c}$) and triglyceride serum levels were found to be independently correlated with endothelin-1 (ET-1) serum levels in 200 subjects with the insulin resistance syndrome. Elevated circulating ET-1 concentrations is a well-recognized marker of endothelial dysfunction.

Hyperuriceamia is another factor that has been linked recently to insulin resistance and the metabolic syndrome. In a population of 380 Caucasian subjects, fasting serum uric acid was negatively correlated to the insulin sensitivity index, a measure of insulin resistance (Clausen et al 1998). Data from the First National Health and Nutrition Examination Survey (NHANES I) and the NHANES I Epidemiologic Follow-up Study (NHEF) in the US indicate that an increased serum uric acid level is an independent risk factor of cardiovascular mortality (Fang and Alderman 2000). In addition, a study of 7978 hypertensive patients showed that elevated uric acid levels were associated with increased frequency of cardiovascular events. Blood pressure control did not lower serum uric acid levels (Alderman et al 1999).

Elevated serum leptin levels is another factor that lately has been shown to be associated with insulin resitance (Liuzzi et al 1999). Hyperleptinemia was shown to be a strong predictor of first-ever acute myocardial infarction in obese individuals (Soderberg et al 1999).

CONCLUSION

Over the past decade there have been major strides in our understanding of the pathogenesis of Type 2 diabetes mellitus. It is now clear that Type 2 diabetes is one of several cardiovascular risk factors that collectively constitute what is now best referred to as the 'metabolic syndrome'. A key feature of this is the presence of insulin resistance. Other important features include abnormalities of glucose, uric acid, lipid metabolism as well as the occurrence of hypertension, central obesity, and a hypercoagulable state. These abnormalities tend to cluster in the same individual, and collectively increase his/her risk for the development of CVD. Optimum management of patients with Type 2 diabetes mellitus should target all the cardiovascular risk factors and should only not focus on managing hyperglycaemia. This comprehensive approach is crucial in order to decrease the incidence of CVD, the primary killer of patients with Type 2 diabetes mellitus.

REFERENCES

Abraira C, Colwell JA, Nuttall FQ (1995) Veterans Affairs Cooperative Study of Glycemic Control and Complications in Type II Diabetes. (VACSDM). *Diabetes Care*, **18**, 1113–1123.

Alberti KGMM, Zimmet PZ, for the WHO consultation (1998) Definition, diagnosis and classification of diabetes and its complications: 1. Diagnosis and classification of diabetes mellitus. Provisional report of a WHO consultation. *Diabetic Medicine*, **15**, 539–553.

Alderman MH, Cohen H, Madhavan S, Kivligan S (1999) Serum uric acid and cardiovascular events in successfully treated hypertensive patients. *Hypertension*, **34**, 144–150.

American Diabetes Association (1993) Implications of the Diabetes Control and Complications Trial. *Diabetes*, **42**, 1555–1558.

Antonucci T, Wicomb R, Mclain R et al (1997) Impaired glucose tolerance is normalized by treatment with the thiazolidinedione troglitazone. *Diabetes Care*, **20**, 188–193.

Assman G, Schulte H (1988) The prospective cardiovascular Munster (PROCAM) study: prevalence of hyperlipidemia in persons with hypertension and or diabetes mellitus and the relationship to coronary heart disease. *American Heart Journal*, **116**, 1713–1724.

Assmann G, Schulte H (1992) Relation of HDL-cholesterol and triglycerides to incidence of atherosclerotic coronary artery disease (The PROCAM experience). *American Journal of Cardiology*, **70**, 733–773.

Bastard JP, Pieroni L (1999) Plasma plasminogen activator inhibitor-1, insulin resistance and android obesity. *Biochemistry and Pharmacotherapy*, **53**, 455–461.

Beck-Nielsen H and the European Group for the study of Insulin Resistance (EGIR) (1999) General characteristics of the insulin resistance syndrome. *Drugs*, **1**, 7–10.

Beck-Nielsen H, Groop L (1994) Metabolic and genetic characterization of prediabetic states: sequence of events leading to non-insulin dependent diabetes mellitus. *Journal of Clinical Investigations*, **94**, 1714–1721.

Bjorntrop P (1994) Fatty acids, hyperinsulinemia, and insulin resistance: which comes first? *Current Opinion in Lipidology*, **5**, 166–174.

Bjorntrop P, Rosmond R (1999) Visceral obesity and diabetes. *Drugs*, **58** (Suppl. 1), 13–18.

Black DM (1995) Atorvastatin: a step ahead for HMG-COA reductase inhibitors. In: Woodford FP, Davignon J, Snidman A (eds). *Atherosclerosis X*. Amsterdam: Elsevier Science, 307–310.

Borun DM, Waldron MA, Mann JI et al (1994) Impaired glucose tolerance and NIDDM: does a lifestyle intervention program have an effect? *Diabetes Care*, **17**, 1311–1319.

Branchi A, Rovellini A, Sommariva D et al (1993) Effects of three fibrate derivatives and of two HMG-CoA reductase inhibitors on plasma fibrinogen level in patients with primary hypercholesterolaemia. *Thrombosis and Haemostasis*, **70**, 241–243.

Carmassi F, Morale M, Ferrini L et al (1999) Local insulin infusion stimulates expression of plasminogen activator inhibitor-1 and tissue-type plasminogen activator in normal subjects. *American Journal of Medicine*, **107**, 344–350.

Cavaghan MK, Ehrmann DA, Byme NM et al (1997) Treatment with the antidiabetic agent troglitazone improves P cell responses to glucose in subjects with impaired glucose tolerance. *Journal of Clinical Investigations*, **100**, 530–537.

Clausen JO, Borch-Johnsen K, Ibsen H, Pedersen O (1998) Analysis of the relationship between fasting serum uric acid and the insulin sensitivity index in a population-based sample of 380 young healthy Caucasians. *European Journal of Endocrinology*, **138**, 63–69.

Colman E, Katzel LI, Rogus E et al (1995) Weight loss reduces abdominal fat and improves insulin action in middle-aged and older men with impaired glucose tolerance. *Metabolism: Clinical and Experimental*, **44**, 1502–1509.

DCCT Research Group (1993) The effect of intensive diabetes treatment on the development and progression of long-term complications in insulin-dependent diabetes mellitus: the Diabetes Control and Complications Trial. *New England Journal of Medicine*, **329**, 978–986.

DeFronzo RA, Ferrannini E (1991) Insulin resistance: a multifaceted syndrome responsible for NIDDM, obesity, hypertension, dyslipidemia and atherosclerotic cardiovascular disease. *Diabetes Care*, **14**, 173–194.

DeFronzo RA, Bonnadonna RC, Ferrannini E (1992) Pathogenesis of NIDDM. *Diabetes Care*, **15**, 318–368.

Del Prato S, Maran A, Bonora E et al (1999) The metabolic syndrome in the European population: the experience of the European Group on Insulin Resistance (EGIR). *Diabetes*, **48** (Suppl. 1), A167 (abstract).

Diabetes Prevention Program (1999) Design and methods for a clinical trial in the prevention of Type 2 diabetes. *Diabetes Care*, **22**, 623–634.

Durrington P (1997) Statins and fibrates in the management of diabetes dyslipidaemia. *Diabetic Medicine*, **14**, 513–516.

Durrington PN (1994) *Hyperlipidaemia: Diagnosis and Management*, 2nd edn. London: Butterworth-Heinemann.

Eriksson KF, Lindgarde F (1991) Prevention of Type 2 (non-insulin-dependent) diabetes mellitus by diet and physical exercise: the 6-year Malmo feasibility study. *Diabetologia*, **34**, 891–898.

Fang J, Alderman MH (2000) Serum uric acid and cardiovascular mortality: the NHANES I epidemiologic follow-up study, 1971–1992. *Journal of the American Medical Association*, **283**, 2404–2410.

Ferrannini E (2000) Insulin resistance: the prime mover in Type 2 diabetes? In: Betteridge (ed). *Diabetes: Current Perspective*. London: Martin Dunitz, 93–110.

Ferrannini E, Vichi S, Beck-Nielsen H et al (1996) European Group for the study of Insulin Resistance (EGIR): insulin action and age. *Diabetes*, **45**, 947–953.

Feskens EJM, Stenard J, Viranen SM et al (1995) Dietary factors determining diabetes and impaired glucose tolerance: a 20-year follow-up of the Finnish and Dutch cohorts of the Seven Countries Study. *Diabetes Care*, **18**, 1104–1111.

Fontbonne A, Eschwege E, Cambien F et al (1989) Hpertriglyceridemia as a risk factor of coronary heart disease mortality in subjects with impaired glucose tolerance or diabetes: results from the 11-year follow-up of the Paris Prospective Study. *Diabetologia*, **32**, 300–304.

Fontbonne A, Charles MA, Juhan-Vague I et al (1996) The effect of metformin on the metabolic abnormalities associated with upper-body fat distribution. *Diabetes Care*, **19**, 920–926.

Franz MJ, Horton ESB, Bantle J Sr et al (1994) Nutrition principles for the management of diabetes and related complications. *Diabetes Care*, **17**, 490–518.

Goldberg RB (1998) Prevention of Type 2 diabetes. *Medical Clinics of North America*, **82**, 805–821.

Goldberg RB, Mellies MJ, Sacks FM et al (1998) Cardiovascular events and their reduction with pravastatin in diabetic and glucose-intolerant myocardial infarction survivors with average cholesterol levels: subgroup analyses in the cholesterol and recurrent events (CARE) trial. *Circulation*, **98**, 2513–2519.

Haffner SM, Howard G, Mayer E et al (1997) Insulin sensitivity and acute insulin response in African-Americans, non-Hispanic Whites, and Hispanics with NIDDM: the Insulin Resistance Atherosclerosis Study. *Diabetes*, **46**, 63–69.

Haffner SM, Stem MP, Hazuda HP et al (1990) Cardiovascular risk factors in confirmed prediabetic individuals: does the clock of coronary heart disease start ticking before the onset of clinical diabetes? *Journal of the American Medical Association*, **263**, 2893–2898.

Hamsten A, Eriksson P, Karpe F, Silveira A (1994) Relations of thrombosis and fibrinolysis to atherosclerosis. *Current Opinion in Lipodology*, **5**, 382–389.

Hansson L, Zanchetti A (1997) The Hypertension Optimal Treatment (HOT) Study: 24-month data on blood pressure and tolerability. *Blood Pressure*, **6**, 313–317.

Hokanson JE, Austin MA (1996) Plasma triglyceride level is a risk factor for cardiovascular disease independent of high-density lipoprotein cholesterol level: a meta-analysis of population-based prospective studies. *Journal of Cardiovascular Risk*, **3**, 213–219.

Holman RR, Cull CA, Turner RC et al (1999) A randomized double blind trial of acarbose in Type 2 diabetes shows improved glycemic control over 3 years (UK Prospective Diabetes Study 44). *Diabetes Care*, **22**, 960–964.

Iwamoto Y, Kosaka K, Kuzuya T et al (1996) A new hypoglycemic agent in patients with NIDDM poorly controlled by diet therapy. *Diabetes Care*, **19**, 151–157.

Kannel WB (2000) Risk stratification in hypertension: new insights from the Framingham Study. *American Journal of Hypertension*, **13**, 3S–10S.

Kawamori R, Matsuhisa M, Kinoshita J et al (1998) Proglitazone enhances splanchnic glucose uptake as well as peripheral glucose uptake in non-insulin-dependent diabetes mellitus. AD-4833 Clamp Study Group. *Diabetes Research and Clinical Practice*, **41**, 35–43.

Kelly DE (1995) Effects of weight loss on glucose homeostasis in NIDDM. *Diabetes Review*, **3**, 366–377.

Klein R (1995) Hyperglycemia and microvascular and macrovascular disease in diabetes. *Diabetes Care*, **18**, 258–268.

Kocks M, Leenen R, Seidell J et al (1999) Relationship between visceral fat and PAI-1 in overweight men and women before and after weight loss. *Thrombosis and Haemostasis*, **82**, 1490–1496.

Koskinen P, Manttari M, Manninen V et al (1992). Coronary heart disease incidence in NIDDM patients in the Helsinki Heart Study. *Diabetes Care*, **15**, 820–825.

Kroder G, Bosseninaier B, Kellerer M et al (1996) Tumor necrosis factor-alpha- and hyperglycemia-induced insulin resistance: evidence for different mechanisms and different effects on insulin signaling. *Journal of Clinical Investigations*, **97**, 1471–1477.

Kyvik KO, Green A, Beck-Nielsen H (1995) The new Danish Register: establishment and analysis of twining rate. *Epidemiology*, **24**, 589–596.

Laakso M (1998) Hypertension and macrovascular disease: the killing fields of NIDDM. *Diabetes Research and Clinical Practice*, **39**, S27–33.

Laakso M, Lehto S, Penttila I, Pyorala K (1993) Lipids and lipoproteins predicting coronary heart disease mortality and morbidity in patients with non-insulin-dependent diabetes. *Circulation*, **88**, 1421–1430.

Law RE, Meehan WP, Xi XP et al (1996) Troglitazone inhibits vascular smooth muscle cell growth and intimal hyperplasia. *Journal of Clinical Investigations*, **97**, 1471–1477.

Lewis GF, Steiner G (1996) Hypertriglyceridemia and its metabolic consequences as a risk factor for atherosclerotic cardiovascular disease in non-insulin-dependent diabetes mellitus. *Diabetes: Metabolism Reviews*, **12**, 37–56.

Lillioja S, Mott DM, Spraul M et al (1993) Insulin resistance and insulin secretory dysfunction as precursors of non-insulin dependent diabetes mellitus. *New England Journal of Medicine*, **329**, 1988–1992.

Liuzzi A, Savia G, Tagliaferri M et al (1999) Serum leptin concentration in moderate and severe obesity: relationship with clinical anthropometric and metabolic factors. *International Journal of Obesity*, **23**, 1066–1073.

Long SD, O'Brien K, MacDonald KG et al (1994) Weight loss in severely obese subjects prevents the progression of impaired glucose tolerance to Type II diabetes: a longitudinal intervention study. *Diabetes Care*, **17**, 372–375.

Malmberg K, Norhammar A, Wadel H et al (1999) Glycometabolic state at admission: important risk marker of mortality in conventionally treated patients with diabetes mellitus and acute myocardial infarction. Long-term results from the Diabetes and Insulin-Glucose Infusion in Acute Myocardial Infarction (DIGAMI) Study. *Circulation*, **99**, 2626–2632.

Marshall JA, Shetterly S, Hoag S et al (1994) Dietary fat predicts conversion from impaired glucose tolerance to NIDDM: the San Luis Valley Diabetes Study. *Diabetes Care*, **17**, 5–56.

Martin BC, Warram JH, Krolewski AS et al (1992) Role of glucose and insulin resistance in development of Type 2 diabetes mellitus: results of a 25-year follow-up study. *Lancet*, **340**, 925–929.

Meigs JB, Mittleman MA, Bathan DM et al (2000) Hyperinsulinemia, hyperglycemia, and impaired hemostasis. *Journal of the American Medical Association*, **283**, 221–228.

Mooradian A, Chehade J (2000) Implications of the UK Prospective Diabetes Study. *Drugs and Aging*, **16**, 159–164.

Mooradian AD, Thurman JE (1999) Glucotoxicity. *Clinics in Geriatric Medicine*, **15**, 255–263.

Nolan JJ, Ludvik B, Beersen P et al (1994) Improvement in glucose tolerance and insulin resistance in obese subjects treated with troglitazone. *New England Journal of Medicine*, **331**, 1188–1193.

Nordt TK, Peter K, Ruef J et al (1999) Plasminogen activator inhibitor-1 (PAI-1) and its role in cardiovascular disease. *Thrombosis and Haemostasis*, **82**, 14–18.

Ohkubo Y, Kishikawa H, Araki E et al (1995) Intensive insulin therapy prevents the progression of diabetic microvascular complications in Japanese patients with noninsulin-dependent diabetes mellitus: a randomized prospective 6-year study. *Diabetes Research and Clinical Practice*, **28**, 103–117.

Ohlsson LO, Larsson B, Svardsudd K et al (1985) The influence of body fat distribution on the incidence of diabetes mellitus: 13.5 years of follow-up of participants in the study born 1913. *Diabetes*, **34**, 1055–1058.

Pan XR, Li GW, Hu YH et al (1997) Effects of diet and exercise in preventing NIDDM in people with impaired glucose tolerance. The Da Qing IGT and Diabetes Study. *Diabetes Care*, **20**, 537–544.

Panzram G (1987) Mortality and survival in Type 2 (non-insulin-dependent) diabetes mellitus. *Diabetologia*, **30**, 123–131.

Paolisoo G, Barbagallo M, Petrell G et al (2000) Effects of simvastatin and atorvastatin administration on insulin resistance

and respiratory quotient in aged dyslipidemic noninsulin dependent diabetic patients. *Atherosclerosis*, **150**, 121–127.

Peiris AN, Mueller RA, Smith GA et al (1986) Splanchnic metabolism in obesity: influence of body fat distribution. *Journal of Clinical Investigations*, **78**, 1648–1657.

Piatti PM, Monti LD, Galli L et al (2000) Relationship between endothelin-1 concentration and metabolic alterations typical of the insulin resistance syndrome. *Metabolism: Clinical and Experimental*, **49**, 748–752.

Poulsen P, Kyvik KO, Vaag A et al (1999) Heritability of Type 2 diabetes mellitus and abnormal glucose tolerance: a population based twin study. *Diabetologia*, **42**, 139–145.

Reaven GM (1988) Role of insulin resistance in human disease. *Diabetes*, **37**, 1595–1607.

Robbins DH, Anderson L, Bosher R et al (1996) Report of the American Diabetes Association's Task Force on Standardization of the Insulin Assay. *Diabetes*, **45**, 242–256.

Sarkkinen E, Schwab U, Niskanen L et al (1996) The effects of monounsaturated-fat enriched diet and polyunsaturated-fat enriched diet on lipid and glucose metabolism in subjects with impaired glucose tolerance. *European Journal of Clinical Nutrition*, **50**, 592–598.

Scandinavian Simvastatin Survival Study Group (1994) Randomized trial of cholesterol lowering in 4444 patients with coronary heart disease: the Scandinavian Simvastatin Survival Study (4S). *Lancet*, **344**, 1383–1389.

Scheen AJ, Letiexhe MR, Lefebvre PJ (1995) Short administration of metformin improves insulin sensitivity in android obese subjects with impaired glucose tolerance. *Diabetic Medicine*, **12**, 985–989.

Shibata T, Matsui K, Yonemori F, Wakitani K (1999) Triglyceride-lowering effect of a novel insulin-sensitizing agent, JTT-501. *European Journal of Pharmacology*, **373**, 85–91.

Shimabukuro M, Zhou YT, Lee Y et al (1997) Induction of uncoupling protein-2 MRNA by troglitazone in the pancreatic islets of Zucker diabetic fatty rats. *Biochemical and Biophysical Research Communications*, **237**, 359–361.

Soderberg S, Ahren B, Jansson JH et al (1999) Leptin is associated with increased risk of myocardial infarction. *Journal of International Medicine*, **246**, 409–418.

Storlien LH, Jenkins AB, Chisholm DJ et al (1991) Influence of dietary fat composition on development of insulin resistance in rats: relationship to muscle triglyceride and omega-3 fatty acids in muscle phospholipid. *Diabetes*, **40**, 280–289.

Torjesen PA, Birkeland KI, Anderssen SA et al (1997) Lifestyle changes may reverse development of the insulin resistance syndrome. *Diabetes Care*, **20**, 26–31.

UGDP (University Group Diabetes Program) (1970) A study of the effect of hypoglycemic agents on vascular complications in patients with adult-onset diabetes. *Diabetes*, **19**, (Suppl. 2), 747–830.

UKPDS (UK Prospective Diabetes Study) Group (1998a) Intensive blood-glucose control with sulphonylureas or insulin compared with conventional treatment and risk of complications in patients with Type 2 diabetes. *Lancet*, **352**, 837–853.

UKPDS (UK Prospective Diabetes Study) Group (1998b) Effect of intensive blood-glucose control with metformin on complications in overweight patients with Type 2 diabetes. *Lancet*, **352**, 854–865.

UKPDS (UK Prospective Diabetes Study) Group (1998c) Tight blood pressure control and risk of macrovascular and microvascular complications in Type 2 diabetes. *British Medical Journal*, **317**, 713–720.

UKPDS (UK Prospective Diabetes Study) Group (1998d) Efficacy of atenolol and captopril in reducing risk of macrovascular and microvascular complications in type 2 diabetes. *British Medical Journal*, **317**, 713-720.

Vaag A, Hemriken JE, Beck-Nielsen H (1992) Decreased insulin activation of glycogen synthase in skeletal muscles in nonobese Caucasian first-degree relatives of patients with non-insulin-dependent diabetes mellitus. *Journal of Clinical Investigations*, **89**, 782–788.

Yamasaki Y, Kawamori R, Wasada T et al (1997) Proglitazone (AD-4833) ameliorates insulin resistance in patients with NIDDM. AD-4833 Glucose Clamp Study Group, Japan. *Tohoku Journal of Experimental Medicine*, **183**, 173–183.

Zimmet PZ (1992) Challenges in diabetes epidemiology—from West to the rest. *Diabetes Care*, **15**, 232–252.

Zimmet PZ (1995) The pathogenesis and prevention of diabetes in adults: genes, autoimmunity, and demography. *Diabetes Care*, **18**, 1050–1064.

Zimmet PZ, Alberti KG (1997) The changing face of macro-vascular disease in non-insulin dependent diabetes mellitus in different cultures: an epidemic in progress. *Lancet*, **350** (Suppl.), S1–S4.

Zimmet PZ, Collier G (1999) Clinical efficacy of metformin against insulin resistance parameters. *Drugs*, **58** (Suppl. 1), 21.

Zimmet PZ, Cox VR, Dowse GK et al (1994) Is hyperinsulinemia a central characteristic of a chronic cardiovascular risk factor syndrome? Mixed findings in Asian Indians, Creole and Chinese Mauritians. *Diabetic Medicine*, **11**, 388–396.

15

Drug Therapy: Current and Emerging Agents

Joe M. Chehade, Arshag D. Mooradian
Saint Louis University School of Medicine

INTRODUCTION

The Diabetes Control and Complications Trial (DCCT 1993) and more recently the United Kingdom Prospective Diabetes Study (UKPDS 1998a, b) have proven the benefit of improved glycemic control beyond any reasonable doubt. Furthermore, in elderly people, diabetes control is an important quality-of-life issue. Type 2 diabetes is very common in old age and the rate of development of some diabetic complications, including macroangiopathy, nephropathy and neuropathy, appear to be accelerated in this age group (Morley et al 1987; Rosenthal and Morley 1992).

With advanced disease, achieving glycemic control can be challenging for both the physician and patient. Often a combination of two or more oral antidiabetic agents is needed (UKPDS 1998a, b). Another challenging aspect of treating Type 2 diabetes is targeting post-prandial hyperglycemia (PPHG). PPGH may be a better predictor of diabetes complications than fasting hyperglycemia and it is now possible to target it with some newer agents (Mooradian and Thurman 1999).

In the last decade, the pharmacologic options for treating Type 2 diabetes have grown considerably. Table 15.1 summarizes the characteristics of five classes of agents now available that target hyperglycemia through four different mechanisms (Figure 15.1):

1. Sulfonylureas and meglitinides increase insulin secretion from pancreatic beta-cells.
2. Biguanides decrease hepatic gluconeogenesis and, to a lesser extent, enhance glucose uptake in skeletal muscles.
3. Thiazolidinediones enhance the insulin sensitivity in the liver, muscles and adipose tissue.
4. Alpha-glucosidase inhibitors delay carbohydrate absorption from the gut.

Although additional pharmacological agents are needed in managing other risk factors such as hypertension and dyslipidemia, this review is concerned only with agents that control blood glucose.

SULFONYLUREAS

Sulfonylureas (SFUs) have been used extensively worldwide since the introduction of tolbutamide and carbutamide in 1956. Shortly thereafter, other compounds were developed: acetohexamide, tolazamide and chlorpropamide. These so called 'first generation sulfonylureas' were followed by the development of 'second-generation sulfonylureas' glyburide or glibenclamide, glipizide, gliclazide, gliquidone and glimeperide (Table 15.2).

The primary mechanism of action of SFUs is through the depolarization of pancreatic beta-cells by blocking ATP-dependent potassium channels, causing an influx of calcium and stimulating insulin release (Groop 1992; Gerich 1989). A decrease in plasma glucagon levels was also noticed in some studies (Pfeiffer et al 1983; Frier et al 1981). Although other extrapancreatic effects have also been described, sulfonylureas are ineffective in patients with Type 1 diabetes or who lack islet beta-cells (Ratzmann et al 1984; Keller, Muller and Berger 1986). The reported increased insulin sensitivity in peripheral tissues is thought to be mainly a consequence of the reduction of hyperglycemia and alleviation of glucotoxicity (Kolterman and Olefsky 1984; Mooradian 1987). A reduced hepatic insulin extraction was demonstrated with glipizide (Almér et al 1982; Groop et al 1988) and glibenclamide (Beck-Nielsen et al 1986). However, this effect is probably secondary to increased insulin secretion.

Diabetes in Old Age. Second Edition. Edited by A. J. Sinclair and P. Finucane. © 2001 John Wiley & Sons Ltd.

Table 15.1 Comparative profile of available oral agents for treatment of Type 2 diabetes

	Sulfonylureas	Meglitinides	Biguanide (metformin)	Thiazolidinediones	Alpha-glucosidase inhibitors
Mode of Action	Stimulate insulin release from pancreatic beta cells	Stimulate insulin release from pancreatic beta cells (target PPH)	Decrease hepatic neoglucogenesis Enhance insulin uptake in periphery, mainly muscle[a]	Enhance insulin sensitivity in muscle and liver	Reversible inhibition of the intestinal brush-border glucosidases (target PPH)
Potency as Monotherapy (decrease in HbA$_{1c}$)	1.5–2%	1.5–2%	1.8%	0.7–1.9%	0.5–0.7%
(decrease in FBG from mM baseline)	3.3–3.9 (60–70 mg/dL)	3.3–3.9 (60–70 mg/dL)	3.27 (59 mg/dL)	2.33–3.11 (42–56 mg/dL)	2.77–3.3% (PPH) (50–60 mg/dL)
Effect on lipid profile					
LDL	↓(minimally improved)	NS	↓	(↑6–19%)[b]	NS
HDL	NS	NS	↑(slight increase)	(↑16–19%)	NS
Triglyceride	↓(minimally improved)	NS	↓	(↓↓26%)[c]	NS
Bodyweight	++	++	− /0	+/0	− /0
Tolerability	+++	+++	++	+++	+
Side-effects	Hypoglycemia	Hypoglycemia	GI, Lactic acid	Hepatotoxicity, anemia	Flatulence, GI
Contraindications	Renal failure	Renal failure	Renal impairment Liver disease, IV CHF	Liver failure NYHA class III and CHF Hypoxemic states	Diarrhea No safety for creatinine clearance < 25 mL/min
Cost	+	++	++	++++	++

PPH: Postprandial Hyperglycemia; CHF, Chronic Heart Failure; GI, gastrointestirial symptons; FBG, fasting blood glucose; NS, not significant.
[a]To a lesser extent. [b] NS for pioglitazone. [c] NS for rosiglatazone.

The pharmacologic characteristics of SFUs are summarized in Table 15.1. They are rapidly absorbed, and detectable levels can be found in the serum within an hour of ingestion (Skillman and Feldman 1981). They are 90–99% bound to serum proteins, mainly albumin (Kahn and Schecte 1993) and can be displaced by other drugs. On a milligram per milligram basis, second-generation SFUs have 100 times the potency of first-generation agents (Groop et al 1987; Melander et al 1989) and since their binding to plasma proteins is mainly to non-ionic sites, drug–drug interactions are less likely than with first–generation agents. Even though there are some differences in the pharmacokinetic and pharmacodynamic properties of various SFUs, to date there is no clinical evidence of superiority for any particular agent. SFUs are mainly converted by the liver to inactive, less active, or in the case of acetohexamide, more active metabolites. First-generation drugs and their metabolites are largely excreted by the kidney, while second-generation agents are excreted in both the kidney and bile in varying proportions. Although differences in absorption, metabolism and elimination do not affect long-term efficacy, they are important in terms of the frequency and severity of adverse effects in elderly people. Of special concern is the prolonged half-life of chlorpropamide, along with its water-retaining properties. Of note is that UKPDS showed that the incidence of hypoglycemia with glyburide (glibenclamide) therapy was as high as with chlorpropamide. Gliclazide is now available as a modified release preparation (MR) and when given once daily appears to be as effective as gliclazide given twice daily in controlling blood glucose and had a low incidence of hypoglycemia (0.2 hypoglycemic events/100 patient months) (Drouin 2000). While the long-acting preparation of glipizide (glipizide GITS) can be administered once daily, its longer duration of activity may result in a higher incidence of hypoglycemia.

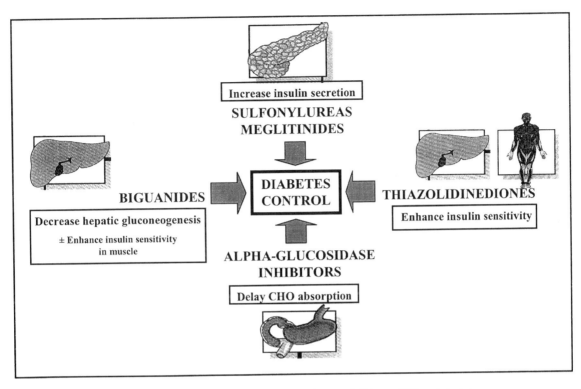

Figure 15.1 Mechanism of action of the currently available oral agents for Type 2 diabetes. CHO, carbohydrate

On average, SFUs lower plasma glucose by 3.3–3.9 mM (60–70 mg/dL) with a concomitant reduction in HbA$_{1c}$ of 1.5–2% (Groop 1992; Scheen 1997; Rosenstock et al 1996;). Some 10–15% of subjects with Type 2 diabetes fail to respond to this class of agents, a situation known as 'primary failure'. Annually, an additional 5–10% of initial responders have 'secondary failure' of response to SFUs (Groop et al 1986, 1989). The most frequent side-effect of SFUs is hypoglycemia (Jennings, Wilson and Ward 1989; Berger 1985; Seltzer 1989). UKPDS data showed that over a 6-year treatment period with SFUs, 45% experienced at least one hypoglycemic episode, and 3% had severe hypoglycemia (UKPDS 1995). It is noteworthy that continuous dextrose infusions for several days may be required to treat sulfonylurea-induced

Table 15.2 Comparative pharmacologic profile sulfonylurea agents

Drug	Dose range (mg)	Duration of Action (h)	Daily dose	Metabolism
First generation				
Acetohexamide	250–1500	8–24	2	60% hepatic; active renal metabolism
Tolbutamide	500–3000	6–12	2–3	Hepatic with renal excretion
Tolazamide	100–1000	12–24	1–2	Hepatic with renal excretion
Chlorpropamide	100–500	24–72	1	30% renal excretion; some hepatic metabolism
Second generation				
Glipizide	2.5–40	16–24	1–2	Hepatic, renal excretion of inactive metabolites
Glipizide XL	5–20	24	1	Hepatic, renal excretion of inactive metabolites
Glyburide	1.25–20	12–24	1–2	Hepatic with renal excretion of active metabolites
Glyburide Micronized	1.25–10	12–24	1	Hepatic with renal excretion of active metabolites
Glimepiride	1–8	12–24	1	Hepatic with renal excretion of active metabolites
Gliquidone	15–60	8–10	1–2	Hepatic with renal excretion of inactive metabolites
Gliclazide	40–320	10–15	1–2	Hepatic with renal excretion of inactive metabolites

hypoglycemia. A retrospective study by the Swedish Board of Health and Welfare from 1975 to 1982 revealed that all serious causes of hypoglycemia secondary to SFUs were associated with advanced age, drug interactions and acute energy deprivation due to gastroenteritis (Asplund, Wiholm and Lithner 1983). Owing to the high prevalence of polypharmacy in elderly people, caution should be taken when SFUs are combined with agents that potentiate their efficacy.

Tolazamide and glyburide have active metabolites that accumulate when creatinine clearance is reduced. Low-dose tolbutamide and glipizide may therefore be preferable for elderly patients with mild renal insufficiency. However, because of its short half-life, tolbutamide may need to be given three times a day, and compliance with such a regimen is often difficult. None of the SFUs, including the more recent glimepiride, should be used in patients whose creatinine clearance is less than 30 mL/min (Pearson et al 1986; Balant et al 1973; Rosenkranz et al 1996).

Other potential disadvantages of SFUs are the associated hyperinsulinemic state and weight gain. Over a 9-year period, subjects assigned to SFUs in the UKPDS gained on average 4 kg compared with 2 kg for those treated with diet alone. In contrast, people in the metformin arm maintained a steady weight (UKPDS 1995, 1998a). This side-effect of SFUs is undesirable in obese subjects. In older subjects where being underweight is common (Mooradian et al 1988), the weight-gain promoting properties of SFU may not be a serious deterrent to their use. The potential advantages of SFUs include their long track record, ease of use, and affordability. However, hypoglycemia remains the main limiting factor in elderly people.

BIGUANIDES

Metformin (dimethylbiguanide) and phenformin (phenethylbiguanide) were introduced for the treatment of Type 2 diabetes in 1957, and buformin was introduced a year later (Bailey 1992). During the 1970s, phenformin and buformin were withdrawn in many countries owing to their association with lactic acidosis (Williams and Palmer 1975). Metformin is now the biguanide of choice and is extensively used worldwide. The bioavailability of metformin after a standard dose of 500 mg is around 50–60%. Food decreases the extent and slightly delays absorption of the drug. In contrast to SFUs, metformin is not sig-

nificantly bound to plasma proteins. Steady-state plasma concentrations are achieved within 24–48 hours (Bristol-Myers Squibb 1995). It does not undergo any hepatic metabolism and is excreted unchanged in the urine (Bailey 1992; Sirtori et al 1978). Because the renal clearance of metformin is 3.5 times greater than the creatinine clearance, tubular secretion appears to be the main route of elimination. In healthy elderly subjects, the total plasma clearance is decreased and thus the half-life of the drug is prolonged. These pharmacokinetic changes with aging are the result of decreased renal function. No pharmacokinetic studies have been conducted in subjects with hepatic insufficiency.

Unlike SFUs, metformin has no insulinotropic effect and does not cause hypoglycemia when used as monotherapy (Bailey and Turner 1996). As such, it is considered as an antihyperglycemic agent rather than a hypoglycemic agent. The antihyperglycemic action of metformin is primarily due to a reduction in hepatic gluconeogenesis, thereby reducing basal glucose output. To a lesser extent, it enhances glucose uptake in the peripheral tissue, mainly muscle (Bailey 1992; Bailey and Turner 1996). The reduction of fatty acid oxidation in metformin-treated subjects may account for some of its antihyperglycemic action (Perriello et al 1994).

A dose–response relationship of the antihyperglycemic effect of metformin was demonstrated in a double-blind, placebo-controlled trial over a 14-week period. At doses between 500 and 2000 mg daily, metformin reduced adjusted mean fasting plasma glucose from baseline by 1.04–4.62 mM (19–84 mg/dL) and adjusted mean HbA_{1c} by 0.6–2.0% (Garber et al 1997). The maximum efficacy is observed at 2000 mg per day (Garber et al 1997).

Metformin has been used extensively both as monotherapy and in combination with SFUs or insulin (UKPDS 1998b; Yki-Jarvinen et al 1999). It is noteworthy that individuals with primary or secondary failure of SFUs are unlikely to respond to metformin alone. However, when metformin is combined with SFUs in individuals who appear to have secondary failure, a substantial blood glucose lowering occurs (DeFronzo and Goodman 1995).

Metformin has a favorable effect on plasma lipid levels and on blood pressure (Stumvoll et al 1995). There is a moderate reduction in triglyceride levels owing to decreased hepatic synthesis of VLDL cholesterol and a slight increase in the HDL level (Wu et al 1990; Grosskopf et al 1997). Perhaps the most attractive feature of this agent is that it is often associated with weight loss and so counteracts the weight gain associated with SFUs or insulin therapy (UKPDS 1998b; Wu et al 1990). However, obesity is not as much of a problem in elderly people as it is in the middle-aged (Mooradian, 1996). In the UKPDS, metformin monotherapy in overweight subjects was the only arm of the study showing a significant reduction in cardiovascular events and overall mortality (UKPDS 1998b). The precise underlying mechanism of this favorable outcome is not known.

The most common and troublesome side-effects of metformin include gastrointestinal discomfort, nausea, diarrhea, anorexia, and rarely a metallic taste (Dandona et al 1983). Starting therapy with 500 mg daily and increasing the dose gradually can attenuate these side-effects. The biguanide-associated malabsorption of vitamin B_{12} (cyanocobalomin) and folate is usually not a major clinical concern (Tomkin 1973; Bergman, Boman and Wilholm 1978). However, this should be borne in mind when prescribing for elderly subjects who have a relatively high incidence of atrophic gastritis and vitamin B_{12} deficiency. Although rare, the most dreaded side-effect is lactic acidosis, the incidence of which is approximately 9 per 100 000 persons per year in metformin users (Stang, Wysowski and Butler Jones 1999), almost 10 times lower than that associated with phenformin. Therefore, any clinical condition associated with or predisposing to lactate generation or decreased ability to clear lactate is a contraindication to the use of metformin. These conditions include hepatic disease, alcoholism, congestive heart failure, peripheral vascular disease, obstructive airway disease and (particularly) renal impairment, all of which are relatively common in elderly people. Metformin is absolutely contraindicated when the serum creatinine level is > 132 mM (1.5 mg/dL) in men or < 124 mM (1.4 mg/dL) in women. Because the risk of lactic acidosis increases with the degree of renal impairment and the patient's age, metformin should not be initiated in patients aged over 80 years. Above the age of 70, careful monitoring of renal function and at least a baseline creatinine clearance is a requirement. Metformin should be withdrawn promptly with the acute onset of dehydration, hypoxemia, sepsis or the use of a contrast media. In this setting, metformin should not be reinstituted unless renal function is demonstrably normal.

Although the efficacy of metformin is comparable to that of SFUs and its use is not limited by hypoglycemia, for the above reasons it is not necessarily the agent of first choice for many older patients with Type 2 diabetes.

ALPHA-GLUCOSIDASE INHIBITORS

More than 50% of Type 2 diabetic patients on oral conventional therapy have persistent post-prandial hyperglycemia (Rabasa-Lhoret and Chiaisson 1998). Alpha-glucosidase inhibitors (AGIs) are a relatively new class of agents that primarily target post-prandial hyperglycemia. Acarbose was the first such agent to be made commercially available. Acarbose and miglitol are now available in many countries and a third agent, voglibose, is available in Japan.

Alpha-glucosidases are hydrolase enzymes within the brush border of the small bowel and are responsible for the cleavage of the non-absorbable oligo- and dissacharides into monosaccharides, which are then rapidly absorbed from the gastrointestinal tract. The improvement of post-prandial hyperglycemia is through a reversible inhibition of the brush border glucosidases, resulting in redistribution of carbohydrate absorption from the upper portion of the gut to a more extended surface area covering the whole length of the small intestine (Hillebrand 1987; Chissold and Edwards 1988). However, this may result in a higher level of fermentable carbohydrate reaching the large bowel where they are metabolized by colonic microflora to short-chain fatty acids and then absorbed (Santeusanio and Compagnucci 1994). There is no substantial caloric loss in the feces. Owing to the high specificity of these agents for α-glucosidases, β-glucosidases, like lactoses, are not inhibited and lactose intolerance is not a clinical problem. Based on its mode of action, several inferences can be made. One is that these agents should be effective in every individual who has post-prandial hyperglycemia and ingests sufficient amounts of carbohydrates. The second inference is that this agent will be effective only when given with meals; being a competitive inhibitor of carbohydrate digestion, it will not be effective when given on an empty stomach. The third inference is that AGIs may cause gastrointestinal flatulence and loose stools in some individuals. Less than 2% of an oral dose of acarbose is absorbed as active drug. Acarbose is metabolized exclusively within the gastrointestinal tract, primarily by the intestinal microflora and to a lesser extent by digestive enzymes. A fraction of these metabolites (34% of the oral dose) is absorbed and subsequently excreted in the urine (Bayer 1998).

Miglitol absorption is saturable at high dose. When an oral dose of 25 mg is given it is almost completely absorbed, whereas a dose of 100 mg is only 50–70% absorbed. Miglitol is not metabolized and is eliminated unchanged by renal excretion. The elimination half-life is 2 hours. In renal failure, plasma concentration increases but a dose adjustment is not recommended because miglitol acts locally. Plasma concentrations of both acarbose and miglitol are increased in renal impairment and no safety data are available when creatinine clearance is less than 25 mL/min (Pharmacia and Upjohn 1998).

Acarbose treatment reduced HbA_{1c} by 0.5–0.7% in monotherapy compared with 0.5–1.2% when combined with a sulfonylurea or biguanide (Chiaisson et al 1994; Coniff 1995; Holman, Cull and Turner 1999). On average, the post-prandial glucose surge was reduced by 2.7–3.3 mM (50–60 mg/dL) but the effect on fasting glucose levels was more modest at 1.1–1.6 mM (20–30 mg/dL) (Chiaisson et al 1994; Coniff et al 1995). In a European comparative dose–response study of miglitol and acarbose, the comparative efficacy based on HbA_{1c} reduction in 603 patients with Type 2 diabetes was similar for acarbose 100 mg t.i.d. and miglitol 50 mg t.i.d. (Rybka, Goke and Sissman 1999).

AGIs are best tolerated when started at low dose (25 mg once-daily with the beginning of the meal), then increasing gradually over a 6–8 week period to a maximum dose of 100 mg t.i.d. with meals. In subjects weighing less than 60 kg, the total daily dose should not exceed 150 mg. In older subjects, a dose–response study showed that the efficacy of acarbose is near maximal at 25 mg when the meal size does not exceed 483 kcal and contains only 61 g of carbohydrates (Mooradian et al 2000). Similarly, in an elderly population with a median age of 70 years, miglitol achieved near maximal metabolic benefits at low dosage of 25 mg t.i.d. (Johnston 1997). Although the efficacy of AGIs may seem less when compared with SFUs, metformin or thiazolidinediones, the Precose Resolution of Optimal Titration to Enhance Current Therapies (PROTECT) study showed that the higher the baseline HbA_{1c}, the greater the drop. When individuals with baseline HbA_{1c} values of >9.1 were compared with those with baseline values of 8.1–9.0%, the drop in HbA_{1c} ranged from 2.1–4.6% to 0.4–0.8%, respectively (Mooradian and Neumann 1997; Baron and Neumann 1997). In this study, there was no difference in efficacy or safety of acarbose when subjects aged over 60 years were compared with younger subjects (Mooradian and Neumann 1997).

Like bigaunides, this class of agents is considered to be antihyperglycemic, since when used as monotherapy they do not result in hypoglycemia. Another potential advantage of AGIs when used as monotherapy is that there is no associated hyperinsulinemia or weight gain. However, if patients are treated with a combination of an AGI and a hypoglycemic agent such as insulin or a sulfonylurea, glucose should be used to treat the hypoglycemic reactions since sucrose or a complex carbohydrate will not be readily effective.

Hypoglycemia is a major concern and limiting factor in treating elderly patients with Type 2 diabetes. Considering the favorable tolerability and safety profile of AGIs, some diabetologists therefore choose these agents as first-line therapy in elderly Type 2 diabetic subjects with fasting blood glucose levels < 11.0 mM (Johnston et al 1998). However, the relatively higher cost of these agents, the need for multiple daily dosing and the gastrointestinal side-effects have limited their widespread use.

THIAZOLIDINEDIONES

Thiazolidinediones (TZDs) are a relatively new class of agents that enhance insulin sensitivity in the liver, adipose tissue and muscle without affecting insulin secretion. Their site of action is believed to be mediated through selective activation of peroxisome proliferator-activated receptor gamma (PPAR Gamma), a nuclear receptor that plays an important role in adipogenesis (Plosker and Faulds 1999; Day 1999). So far, the precise mechanisms that lead to the transcriptional regulation of genes involved in insulin sensitization and lipid metabolism have not been elucidated.

Troglitazone, the first compound in this class to become available, was introduced in 1997 but was subsequently withdrawn in the UK because of hepatic toxicity fears. Two other agents, rosiglitazone and pioglitazone, became available later. TZDs are antihyperglycemic agents and do not cause hypoglycemia when used as monotherapy. However, TZD monotherapy will also fail in patients without enough endogenous or exogenous insulin. TZDs are 99%-bound to plasma proteins, notably albumin. Their plasma elimination half-lives range from 9–34 h for troglitazone to 3–7 h for rosiglitazone and pioglitazone. In the case of rosiglitazone, a twice-daily regimen (4 mg b.i.d.) was more efficacious than a once-daily dosing (8 mg), with a drop in HbA_{1c} from baseline of 0.7% and 0.3%, respectively (SmithKline Beecham 1999). Troglitazone, but not pioglitazone or rosiglitazone, has to be taken with a fatty meal because food increases the extent of absorption by 30–85% and thus enhances the systemic drug bioavailability (Parke–Davis 1997).

All TZDs undergo major hepatic metabolism. Unlike troglitazone, rosiglitazone does not appear to induce P_{450} (CYP)3A4 metabolism. Therefore, it is likely to have less drug–drug interactions. So far, no such data are available for pioglitazone. TZDs are mainly excreted in bile either unchanged or as metabolites and then eliminated by the feces. Therefore, there is no need for dose adjustment in patients with renal impairment. On the other hand, thiazolidinediones are contraindicated in patients with active liver disease or if serum aminotransferase (ALT) is more than twice the normal level at baseline.

The efficacy of TZDs has been shown in multiple clinical trials (Maggs et al 1998; Pioglitazone 001 Study Group 1999; Charbonnel et al 1999). In monotherapy with troglitazone or rosiglitazone, the mean decline in HbA_{1c} from baseline ranged between 0.6 and 1% (Maggs et al 1998; Grunberger et al 1999). A more pronounced drop in HbA_{1c} from baseline (1.0–1.4%) was noticed when combined with insulin (Rubin et al 1999). Monotherapy with pioglitazone resulted in a 1.9% decrease in HbA_{1c} compared with baseline. The reason for this apparent superiority of pioglitazone as monotherapy is not known. Head to head comparisons for TZDs are not available.

On average, 20–50% of the individuals fail to respond to this class of agents (Iwamoto et al 1996; Maggs et al 1998; Mathisen, Geerlof and Houser et al 1999). It appears that obese and hyperinsulinemic individuals are more likely to respond than those who have insufficient insulin. When combined with SFUs, TZDs were as effective as the combination of metformin and sulfonylureas (Schneider, Egan and Houser 1999; Gomis et al 1999). A big disadvantage of the combination of TZDs and SFUs is the associated weight gain that can be as high as 6.5 kg (13 pounds) after one year of therapy. A modest increase in body weight is also observed when TZDs are used as monotherapy (Iwamoto et al 1996).

Both LDL and HDL cholesterol tend to increase with TZD therapy and serum triglyceride level may decrease with troglitazone and pioglitazone but not with rosiglitazone. While rosiglitazone has a pure PPAR Gamma agonist activity, pioglitazone and troglitazone have in addition some PPAR Alpha activity that may account for their effect on lowering serum triglyceride level. Compared with baseline, the reduction in triglyceride level can be as high as 26% with troglitazone and pioglitazone therapy. Although tro-

glitazone may reduce the blood pressure, especially in obese subjects, this effect is minimal and not always consistent.

The major concern of the TZD group is the rare but potentially serious hepatotoxicity. After troglitazone had been released on the US and Japanese markets, more than 150 cases of severe hepatotoxicity were reported, with an estimated incidence of 1:57 000 treated patients. For this reason, troglitazone was withdrawn from the US market. The limited available data suggest that pioglitazone and rosiglitazone may not have an increased incidence of hepatotoxicity. However, until more experience with these new agents is acquired, liver enzymes should be monitored every 2 months.

TZDs are usually well tolerated, and when used in monotherapy there is no associated risk of hypoglycemia. Peripheral edema is occasionally seen, mainly as a result of the plasma volume expansion. Therefore, these agents are not recommended in patients with New York Heart Association (NYHA) class III or IV congestive heart failure (Parke–Davis 1997). A minor decrease in hematocrit and hemoglobin is another observation and this correlates with the dilutional effect of fluid retention.

The once-daily dosing regimen and lack of associated hypoglycemia make TZDs an attractive option in elderly subjects. On the other hand, limited safety data, suboptimal efficacy in underweight subjects and cost limit their usefulness.

MEGLITINIDES

Meglitinides belong to a novel group of insulinotropic agents known as the non-sulfonylurea insulin secretagogues (Malaisse 1995). Repaglinide, a benzoic acid derivative, is one of the meglitinide analogues that recently became available. Like sulfonylureas, the insulinotropic effect is mediated through the ATP-regulated potassium channels but via different binding sites on the beta-cells (Balfour and Faulds 1998; Fuhlendorff 1998). After oral administration, repaglinide is quickly absorbed from the gastrointestinal tract. The maximum plasma concentrations are reached within 0.8 h and the drug is rapidly eliminated with an approximate half-life of one hour (Novo Nordisk 1997). However, the wide variability of the half-life of repaglinide elimination kinetics, ranging between 0.5 h and 8 h is a concern.

Its pharmacokinetic profile makes repaglinide a suitable agent for targeting post-prandial hyperglycemia (Mooradian and Thurman 1999). It is completely metabolized by the liver and some 90% is excreted by the biliary route with only 8% in the urine (Novo Nordisk 1997). When comparing healthy young individuals with people aged 65 years or over, there was no difference in the pharmacokinetic parameters. However, elderly Type 2 diabetic subjects had a significantly higher mean diurnal plasma concentration and a lower clearance than healthy controls (Hatorp et al 1997). Although AUC (area under curve) and C_{max} were significantly increased in subjects with various degrees of renal impairment, a dose adjustment was not necessary. However, the authors recommended a careful and gradual increase in the initial dose (Marbury and Hatorp 1998). After a single dose of repaglinide, patients with moderate to severe liver disease had higher and more prolonged serum concentrations (Hatorp and Haug-Pihale 1998). Although liver disease did not significantly increase the risk of hypoglycemic episodes in the latter study, the safety of repaglinide is still questionable in this subgroup of patients.

One study has compared a fixed dose of 1 mg or 4 mg of repaglinide pre-prandially with placebo over a 6-month period. In previously treated Type 2 diabetics, HbA_{1c} dropped from 8.4% and 8.2% in the 1 mg or 4 mg group respectively, to 8.2% in both groups, while HbA_{1c} rose from 8.4% to 10% in the placebo group (Berger and Strange, 1998). In this study, hypoglycemic episodes occurred in 11%, 27% and 36% in the placebo, 1 mg and 4 mg groups, respectively. The efficacy of repaglinide was compared with glyburide in a multicenter, randomized, double-blind study. Over one year, the reduction in HbA_{1c} was similar in both groups (Marbury and Strange 1998). When added to metformin in suboptimally controlled diabetes ($HbA_{1c} = 8.5\%$), the HbA_{1c} dropped by 1.4% (Moses, Slobodniuk and Donnelly 1997). Combination therapy achieved better control than either drug alone. As with sulfonylurea agents, weight gain and hypoglycemia were the two most frequent adverse effects. However, there is reduced risk of increased hypoglycemic episodes when a meal is omitted and the repaglinide dose is witheld (Tornier et al 1995).

The potential for reduced risk of hypoglycemia is an interesting feature of this new class of agents, especially in older individuals. However, more studies are needed to define the relative value of these agents. Of concern is the wide range of variability in drug elimination kinetics. In addition, a pre-prandial dosing regimen may be an obstacle to achieving long-term compliance in some individuals. Nateglinide is a new meglitinide which is soon to be marketed and has a faster and shorter duration of insulin secretory activity than repaglinide. Thus, nateglinide pharmacokinetics are more favorable in terms of improving post-prandial hyperglycemia (Hirschberg et al 1999; Kalbag et al 1999). Finally, the real advantage of these relatively costly agents over a small dose of short-acting sulfonylurea is still not clear (Mooradian 1998).

INSULIN AND INSULIN ANALOGUES

Insulin therapy in diabetes is discussed in detail in Chapter 13. This section deals mainly with the role of some of the newer insulin preparations. Multiple clinical trials have proven that intensive glycemic control can be achieved with insulin therapy in both Type 1 diabetes (Diabetes Control and Complications Trial Research Group 1993) and Type 2 diabetes (UKPDS 1998 a,b).

Human Insulin Preparations

The most commonly used human insulin preparations are summarized in Table 15.3 (Heinemann and Richter 1993). These preparations differ in their pharmacokinetics. Hypoglycemia is still the most frequently encountered side-effect of insulin therapy and the major limiting factor in intensive glycemic control (Diabetes Control and Complications Trial 1993; UKPDS 1998a). Hypoglycemia is commonly precipitated by erratic meal timing, excessive insulin dosage and unplanned exercise. The failure to give regular insulin in a timely manner (30–45 minutes before a meal) also increases the risk. Besides the increased risk of hypoglycemia, short-acting insulin can disrupt the patient's lifestyle. Ultra-short-acting insulin analogues were developed with the hope of overcoming these limitations. Lispro insulin is identical to human regular insulin with a minor transposition of a lysine and proline in the beta chain. This transposition results in acceleration of the dissociation rate of the insulin hexamers. Lispro insulin acts quickly within 10–20 minutes, peaks on average at 1–2 hours and is essentially cleared from the system within 4–5 hours (Hollerman and Hoekstra 1997; Tornole et al 1994). Thus, Lispro provides greater flexibility in insulin administration and can be given 5–10 minutes before a meal. Another modest advantage of Lispro insulin has been the improvement in the post-prandial hyperglycemia in both Type 1 and Type 2 diabetic subjects and a

Table 15.3 Some of the most commonly used insulin preparations

Preparation	Action profile (h)			Constituents
	Onset	Peak	Duration	
Ultra-rapid acting Lispro (human analogue)	0.2–0.5	0.5–2	3–4	Identical to human regular insulin with transposed lysine and proline in the beta chain
Short-acting				
Regular (human)	0.5–1	2–3	6–8	Solution of unmodified zinc insulin crystals
U-500 (human)	1–3	6–12	12–18	Concentrated unmodified
Intermediate-acting				
NPH (human)	1.5	4–10	16–24	Protamine zinc, phosphate buffer
Lente (human)	1.5–3	7–15	16–24	Amorphous, acetate buffer
Long-acting				
Ultralente (human)	3–4	9–15	22–28	Amorphous and crystalline mix
Mixtures (human)[a]				
70/30	0.5–1	3–12	16–24	NPH 70%, regular 30%
50/50	0.5–1	2–12	16–24	NPH 50%, regular 50%

[a]Mixtures with different proportions of NPH and regular, and more recently a mixture of Lispro insulin and its protamine derivative, are also available but less commonly used.

Souce: Heinemann and Richter (1993)

reduction in the number of hypoglycemic episodes in Type 1 subjects (Hollerman and Hoekstra 1997; Anderson et al 1997). However, this latter advantage over regular insulin has not been consistently demonstrated in Type 2 subjects (Hollerman and Hoekstra 1997). Overall, glycemic control as reflected by HbA_{1c} levels does not differ between Lispro insulin and human regular insulin-treated groups (Anderson et al 1997).

Another short-acting insulin analogue 'Insulin Aspart' (B28 Asp) has a proline at position B28 replaced with a negatively charged aspartic acid (Simpson and Spencer 1999). In addition to its rapid onset of action, insulin Aspart also has a favorable effect on postprandial hyperglycemia in both Type 1 and Type 2. On the other hand, the variability of the metabolic effect of insulin Aspart, even under strict experimental conditions, is 10–20%, which is comparable to that of regular human insulin (Hume et al 1998). Currently, insulin Aspart is still in the late phase of clinical trials. The clinical utility of these short-acting insulin analogues and their advantages over the regular insulin in the elderly population has yet to be established.

Recently, a protamine derivative of Lispro insulin (NPL) became available on some markets. When NPL was premixed with Lispro in a ratio of 75:25%, it was shown to improve post-prandial glycemic control compared with premixed human NPH and regular insulin in 30:70% ratio (Roach, Yuel and Arora 1999). Finally, a new class of long-acting soluble insulin analogues will soon be available (Rosskamp and Park

1999). An example is Glargine (HOE 901) which when injected once a day has a more prolonged action and fewer peak activities, and more reproducible pharmacokinetics than NPH (Lepore et al 1999; Linkeschowa et al 1999). NN304 is another long-acting insulin analogue recently developed. NN304 is a soluble fatty acid acylated insulin that binds to albumin after absorption. The clinical utility of these properties is still to be determined (Heinemann et al 1999).

Amylin Analogues

Amylin was identified in 1987 (Cooper et al 1987), and is a 37-amino-acid hormone secreted in conjunction with insulin by the pancreatic beta-cells in response to a glucose load or other insulin secretagogues (Ogawa et al 1990; Inoue et al 1991). In Type 1 diabetes, the reduction in amylin concentration parallels the decline in insulin secretion (Koda et al 1992). When compared with a population of lean, healthy subjects, basal and stimulated amylin secretion were significantly higher in obese patients with or without impaired glucose tolerance (Ludvik et al 1991). However, this was not the case in patients with Type 2 diabetes. It seems that with longstanding Type 2 diabetes, amylin concentration decreases in conjunction with beta-cell failure (Fineman et al 1996). The effect of amylin on glucose metabolism involves several mechanisms. By mainly slowing the rate of gastric emptying, it limits the proportion of nutrients delivered to the gut, thus preventing the post-prandial hyperglycemic surge (Schmitz et al 1992; Kolterman et al 1995). To a lesser extent, amylin also suppresses postprandial glucagon secretion and helps replenish glycogen stores (Mooradian and Thurman 1999; Gedulin, Rink and Young 1997). However, owing to its short half-life and its tendency to aggregation, amylin is not suitable for clinical use.

The amylin analogue 'pramlintide' is structurally identical to human amylin with the exception of a proline substitution at positions 25, 28, and 29 (Pittner et al 1994; Rink et al 1993; Thompson et al 1997). Early clinical studies have demonstrated a substantial decrease in post-prandial hyperglycemia in healthy individuals as well as in patients with Type 1 or Type 2 diabetes after subcutaneous or intravenous administration (Kolterman et al 1995; Thompson et al 1997, 1998). In a recent randomized clinical trial of 477 patients with Type 1 diabetes treated over one year with pramlintide there was a net 0.3% reduction in HbA_{1c} compared with placebo (Rosenstock et al 1998). A similar study was conducted in 539 Type 2 individuals who were requiring on average 60 units of insulin daily with a baseline HbA_{1c} of 9.15 to 9.27%. In this study, pramlintide treatment resulted in 0.58% reduction in HbA_{1c} at one-year follow-up (Ratner et al 1998). In both studies there was no significant increase in the frequency of hypoglycemic episodes and an associated weight loss ranging from 1.3 to 2.7 kg was also noticed. The main reported side-effect was nausea that usually resolved after a few weeks of therapy (Rosenstock et al 1998; Ratner et al 1998). In a recent news release of the phase III study in Type 2 diabetes comparing Symlin (pramlintide acetate) 120 μg b.i.d. with placebo, after 52 weeks of randomization HbA_{1c} was reduced from baseline by 0.7% in the pramlintide group and 0.1% in the placebo group (Amylin Pharmaceuticals 1999). Although these reports from phase III trials show some encouraging data, the utility and safety of this drug remains to be demonstrated. The frequency and the route of administration of pramlintide raises a major concern about the suitability of such agents in the elderly population.

Glucagon-like Peptide-1

GLP-1 is a very potent insulinotropic peptide hormone secreted by the L-cells of the intestinal mucosa in the lower gut (Holst 1994; Ørskov 1992). The in-

sulinotropic effect is mediated at the level of the L-cells through a stimulation of adenylate cyclase and protein kinase A activity (Drucker et al 1987). Unlike sulfonylurea agents, GLP-1 has no hypoglycemic effect in the absence of glucose (Göke et al 1993). Its secretion increases in response to unabsorbed nutrient within the intestinal lumen. In addition, it also has an inhibitory effect on glucagon secretion and gastric emptying rate (Holst 1994). Although fasting hyperglycemia can be reduced with GLP-1, its primary target is post-prandial hyperglycemia (Cruetzfeldt and Nauck 1996; Gutniak et al 1997). In clinical studies, the two shorter forms of GLP-1, the (7–37) and (7–36) amides have been used. These peptides have a short duration of action and should be given parenterally. A new, mucoadhesive biodegradable buccal tablet was recently developed. However, the main limitation is still the very short half-life of about 17 minutes. Although this agent has an interesting mode of action where it can enhance insulin secretion without the potential risk of hypoglycemia, a new analogue or a better delivery system is needed before it can be made commercially available.

THE CHOICE OF AN ANTIDIABETIC AGENT IN ELDERLY PEOPLE

In general, the management of Type 2 diabetes should be individualized and tailored to the clinical status of the individual, coexistent diseases, bodyweight, goals of therapy, expectations, involvement in care, functional impairment, ease of administration, side-effect profile, cost of therapy, baseline blood sugar and the urgency of blood sugar normalization. Although difficult to generalize when considering all these parameters, some guidelines can be suggested based on blood sugar levels and the known clinical efficacy and tolerability of the various classes of antidiabetic agents.

As in middle-aged individuals, lifestyle modification, including diet-control and exercise, are still the cornerstone of every treatment plan for Type 2 diabetes. However, undernutrition is common in elderly patients with Type 2 diabetes, especially in those who live in nursing homes (Mooradian et al 1990; Mooradian et al 1988). In this sub-group, one should carefully evaluate nutritional status and recommend appropriate caloric consumption. Elderly subjects also have more difficulties with acquisition, preparation and sometimes ingestion of food, and this can affect their nutritional status and increase the risk of hypoglycemic episodes (Reed and Mooradian 1990). A support system that can provide the appropriate meals in a timely manner is helpful. When there is no major physical limitation, physical activity and exercise should be encouraged within reason. On the other hand, a careful medical evaluation and sometimes a limited stress test are needed before starting any exercise program, owing to the high incidence of subclinical coronary artery disease in this population.

Although it should be individualized, the trigger point to starting pharmacological intervention is not generally different from in middle-aged diabetic people (Chehade and Mooradian 2000). The goal for glycemic control in the elderly diabetic is to achieve euglycemia without the undue risk of hypoglycemia. Ideally, the following blood glucose values should be sought: fasting blood glucose (FBG) 4.4–6.6 mM (80–120 mg/dL), one hour post-prandial (PP) glucose <8.8 mM (160 mg/dL) and HbA$_{1c}$ <7%. Additional action is suggested if FBG >7.8 mM (140 mg/dL), PP >10 mM (180 mg/dL) or HbA$_{1c}$ >7%. In order to avoid the deleterious effect of hypoglycemia in the frail elderly diabetic patient, one should not attempt to lower the FBG or bedtime blood glucose below 5.5 mM (100 mg/dL).

Although many physicians have traditionally relied only on the FBG and the HbA$_{1c}$ measurement to guide pharmacological therapy, post-prandial hyperglycemia is becoming an important target of management (Mooradian 1996; Mooradian and Thurman 1999). The rationale behind this approach is that self-monitoring FBG and PP glucose are readily available for the patients and the clinicians and can be used to expedite the titration and changes in drug therapy. In addition, it appears that individuals with isolated PP hyperglycemia are at increased risk of atherosclerotic heart disease. PP hyperglycemia is probably one of the reasons why some individuals with FBG within the target range (4.4–6.6 mM) have already established microvascular and macrovascular complications.

Despite the fact that non-pharmacological interventions alone may be sufficient at early stages of the disease, these measures will fail in most patients as the disease progresses (UKPDS 1998a,b). An initial approach to drug therapy of Type 2 diabetes in elderly people is illustrated in Figure 15.2. When the FBG levels are consistently >16.7 mM (300 mg/dL), it is most likely that the patient has either a profound insulin deficiency or severe insulin resistance or both. Insulin treatment at least initially is the preferred choice for these individuals. Insulin therapy should be

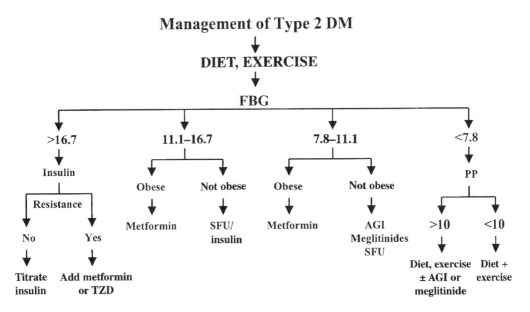

Figure 15.2 Suggested algorithm for the initial choice of therapeutic agents based on fasting blood glucose (FBG) in mM. The initial choice might be only for a brief period of time. Metformin is used only if there are no contraindications. PP, 1-hour post-prandial blood glucose in mM. SFU, sulfonylurea; AGI, alpha-glucosidase inhibitor; TZD, thiazolidinedione

initiated in a hospital setting if the patient is symptomatic with mental status changes or severe dehydration; otherwise it can be started in the physician's office. The dose will be titrated during follow-up visits; and if there is evidence of significant insulin resistance, insulin sensitizers, such as thiazolidinediones or metformin, can be added if there are no contraindications. It is noteworthy, however, that some individuals and especially in obese subjects, who present with FBG over 16.7 mM. may require insulin for only a short period until the glucose toxicity resolves and glycemic goals can then be achieved by switching to oral agents.

When dealing with lean patients with an average FBG between 11.1 and 16.7 mM (200–300 mg/dL) the initial drug of choice can be either a sulfonylurea agent or insulin. For obese subjects (i.e. BMI $>30 \, \text{kg/m}^2$), metformin would be the initial drug of choice, although in many cases a sulfonylurea is started owing to the high prevalence of contraindications to biguanides in the elderly. Pioglitazone and rosiglitazone may be good alternatives to metformin in this sub-group, particularly if further clinical experience confirm their safety. If the FBG is within target, but PP hyperglycemia is still a problem, one should consider adding an AGI.

For obese individuals with FBG between 7.8–11.1 mM (140–200 mg/dL), a trial of an exercise program with a weight-reducing diet for a 2-month period is initially appropriate. After this, if glycemic goals are not within target, metformin should be the initial drug and subsequently a sulfonylurea can be added. Alternatively, one could consider adding a thiazolidinedione or starting insulin. Here also, metformin is often contraindicated and sulfonylurea may be the safest option, at least until the safety of the new thiazolidinediones (pioglitazone or rosiglitazone) is demonstrated.

In lean individuals with a FBG between 7.8–11.1 mM on presentation, a 2-month period of diet and exercise should be initiated, and then an AGI added if one cannot reach the glycemic goals. If with this approach the glycemic goals are still above the target range, then one should add a SFU or a meglitinide and subsequently consider adding insulin or, as an alternative to insulin, adding an insulin sensitizer such as metformin or a thiazolidinedione. With this latter scenario, the cost of a triple therapy is of concern and so are drug interactions. It should probably be reserved for individuals who refuse insulin therapy. When the FBG is less than 7.8 mM (140 mg/dL), one should also check the PP glucose. If the levels are consistently over 10 mM for 1 to 2 week periods, an AGI should be started.

A common problem in clinical practice is that monotherapy with oral agents either fails initially or fails over time. This important clinical observation was confirmed in the UKPDS. In order to achieve an optimal outcome, multiple drug therapy or a combination of oral agents and insulin is often needed. An important question that needs to be explored is whether triple oral therapy when used to avoid insulin use in the elderly has any potential advantages over insulin therapy alone. When using such a regimen, one should consider the high cost of therapy and possible increased adverse events as a result of drug interactions. This latter concern is very legitimate when dealing with a frail population with multiple coexisting medical conditions and where polypharmacy is common. Further studies are needed to evaluate the advantages and disadvantages of triple or quadruple oral therapy in the elderly diabetic and its impact on the quality of life when compared with insulin monotherapy.

Until these data are available, one should try to tailor the management to individual needs. Individuals require different drug regimens and this may change over time as the disease progresses. It should be borne in mind that Type 2 diabetes is a heterogenous disease. Now that we have multiple pharmacological agents with distinct mechanisms of action, it should be more possible than ever to individualize management by matching the appropriate agent to the underlying pathophysiology of Type 2 diabetes.

REFERENCES

Almér L-O, Johannson E, Melander A, Wåhlin-Boll E (1982) Influence of sulphonylureas on the secretion, disposal and effect of insulin. *European Journal of Clinical Pharmacology*, **22**, 27–31.

Amylin Pharmaceuticals (1999) *Positive results for Symlin™ (pramlintide acetate) in Type 2 diabetes study. Data on file Amylin Pharmaceuticals*, San Diego, CA, USA.

Anderson JH, Jr, Brunelle RL, Keohene P, Koivisto VA, Trautmann ME, Vignati L, DiMarchi R (1997) Mealtime treatment with insulin analog improves postprandial hyperglycemia and hypoglycemia in patients with non-insulin-dependent diabetes mellitus. *Archives of Internal Medicine*, **157**, 1249–1255.

Anderson JH, Jr, Brunelle RL, Koivisto VA, Pfutzner A, Trautmann ME, Vignati L, Bimarchi R (1997) Reduction of post-prandial hyperglycemia and frequency of hypoglycemia in IDDM patients on insulin-analog treatment. *Diabetes*, **46**, 265–270.

Asplund K, Wiholm BE, Lithner F (1983) Glibenclamide-associated hypoglycemia: a report of 57 cases. *Diabetologia*, **24**, 412–417.

Bailey CJ (1992) Biguanides and NIDDM. *Diabetes Care*, **15**, 755–772.

Bailey CJ, Turner RC (1996) Metformin. *New England Journal of Medicine*, **334**, 574–579.

Balant L, Zahnd G, Gorgia A, Schwarz R, Fabre J (1973) Pharma-cokinetics of glipizide in man: influence of renal insufficiency. *Diabetologia*, **9**, 331–338.

Balfour JA, Faulds D (1998) Repaglinide. *Drugs and Aging*, **13**, 173–180.

Baron A, Neumann C (1997) PROTECT interim results: A large multicenter study of patients with Type II diabetes. *Clinical Therapy*, **19**, 283–295.

Bayer (1998) *Precose*ᴿ *(acarbose). Prescribing information.* Bayer Corporation, West Haven, CT, USA.

Beck-Nielsen H, Hother Nielsen O, Andersen PH, Pederson O, Schmitz O (1986) In vivo action of glibenclamide. *Diabetologia*, **29**, 515A (abstract).

Berger S, Strange P (1998) Repaglinide, a novel oral hypoglycemic agent in Type 2 diabetes: a randomized, placebo-controlled, double-blind, fixed-dose study. *Diabetes*, **47** (Suppl. 1), 496 (abstract).

Berger W (1985) Incidence of severe side effects during therapy with sulfonylureas and biguanides. *Hormone and Metabolic Research*, **17** (Suppl. 15), 111–115.

Bergman U, Boman G, Wilholm BE (1978) Epidemiology of adverse drug reactions to phenformin and metformin. *British Medical Journal*, **2** (6135), 464–466.

Bristol-Myers Squibb (1995) *Glucophage*ᴿ *(metformin hydrochlor-ide tablets) 500 mg and 850 mg. Prescribing information.* Prin-ceton, NJ: Bristol-Myers Squibb Co.

Charbonnel B, Lönngvist F, Jones NP, Abel MG, Patwardhan R (1999) Rosiglitazone is superior to glyburide in reducing fasting plasma glucose after 1 year of treatment in Type 2 diabetes. *Diabetes*, **48** (Suppl. 1), Poster 494 A114.

Chehade JM, Mooradian (2000) A rational approach to drug therapy of Type 2 diabetes mellitus. *Drugs*, **60**, 95–113.

Chiaisson JL, Josse RG, Hunt JA, Palmason C, Rodger NW, Ross SA, Ryan EA, Tan MH, Wolever JM (1994) The efficacy of acarbose in the treatment of patients with non-insulin dependent diabetes mellitus. *Annals of Internal Medicine*, **121**, 928–935.

Chissold SP, Edwards C (1988) Acarbose: a preliminary review of its pharmacodynamic and pharmacokinetic properties, and ther-apeutic potential. *Drugs* **35**, 214–243.

Coniff RF, Shapiro JA, Seaton TB, Bray GA (1995) Multicenter, placebo-controlled trial comparing acarbose (Bayg 5421) with placebo, tolbutamide, and tolbutamide-plus-acarbose in non-insulin-dependent diabetes mellitus. *American Journal of Medi-cine*, **98**, 443–451.

Cooper GJS, Willis AC, Clark A, Turner RC, Sim RB, Reid KB (1987) Purification and characterization of a peptide from amyloid-rich pancreas of Type 2 diabetic patients. *Proceedings of the National Academy of Sciences USA*, **84**, 8628–8632.

Cruetzfeldt W, Nauck M (1996) Gastric emptying, glucose responses, and insulin secretion after a liquid test meal: effects of exogenous glucagon-like peptide-1 (GLP-1)-(7–36) amide in Type 2 (non-insulin dependent) diabetic patients. *Journal of Clinical Endocrinology and Metabolism*, **81**, 327–332.

Dandona P, Fonseca V, Mier A, Beckett AG (1983) Diarrhea and metformin in a diabetic clinic. *Diabetes Care*, **6**, 472–474.

Day C (1999) Thiazolidinediones: a new class of antidiabetic drugs. *Diabetes Medicine*, **16**, 179–192.

DeFronzo RA, Goodman AM for the Multicenter Metformin Study Group (1995) Efficacy of metformin in patients with non-insulin diabetes mellitus. *New England Journal of Medicine*, **333**, 541–549.

Diabetes Control and Complications Trial Research Group (1993) The effect of intensive treatment of diabetes on the development and progression of long-term complications in insulin-depen-dent diabetes mellitus. *New England Journal of Medicine*, **329**, 977–986.

Drouin P. Diamicron MR Study Group (2000) Diamicron MR once daily is effective and well tolerated in type 2 diabetes. A double-blind, randomised, multinational study. *Journal of Diabetes Complications*, **14**, 185–191.

Drucker DJ, Philippe J, Mozsov S, Chick W, Habener JF (1987) Glucagon-like peptide I stimulates insulin gene expres-sion and increases cyclic AMP levels in a rat islet cell line. *Proceedings the National Academy of Sciences USA*, **84**, 3434–3438.

Fineman MS, Giotta MP, Thompson RG, Kolterman OG, Koda JE (1996) Amylin response following Sustacal ingestion is dimin-ished in Type II diabetic patients treated with insulin. *Diabeto-logia*, **39** (Suppl 1), A149 (abstract).

Frier B, Ashby JP, Nairn IM, Baird JD (1981) Plasma insulin, C-peptide and glucagon concentrations in patients with insulin-dependent diabetes treated with chlorpropamide. *Diabetes and Metabolism*, **7**, 45–49.

Fuhlendorff J (1998) Molecular identification of specific binding site (36 kDa) for repaglinide. *Diabetes* (Suppl. 1), 496 (abstract).

Garber AJ, Duncan TG, Goodman AM, Mills DJ, Rohlf JL (1997) Efficacy of metformin in Type II diabetes: results of a double-blind, placebo-controlled, dose response trial. *American Journal of Medicine*, **102**, 491–497.

Gedulin BR, Rink TJ, Young AA (1997) Dose–response for glucagonostatic effect of amylin in rats. *Metabolism*, **46**, 67–70.

Gerich JE (1989) Oral hypoglycemic agents. *New England Journal of Medicine*, **321**, 1231–1245.

Göke R, Wagner B, Fehmann HC, Göke B (1993) Glucose-dependency of the insulin stimulatory effect of glucagon-like peptide-1 (7–36) amide on the rat pancreas. *Research in Experimental Medicine*, **193**, 97–103.

Gomis R, Jones NP, Vallance SE, Ratwardhan R (1999) Low dose rosiglitazone provides additional glycemic control when combined with sulfonylureas in Type 2 diabetes. *Diabetes*, **48** (Suppl. 1), Poster 266 A63.

Groop L (1992) Sulfonylureas in NIDDM. *Diabetes Care*, **19**, 737–754.

Groop L, Perlkonen R, Koskimies S, Bottazzo GF, Doniach D (1986) Secondary failure to treatment with oral antidiabetic agents in non-insulin dependent diabetes. *Diabetes Care*, **9**, 129–133.

Groop L, Luzi L, Melander A, Groop PH, Ratheiser K, Simonson DC, Defronzo RA (1987) Different effects of glyburide and glipizide on insulin secretion and hepatic glucose production in normal and NIDDM subjects. *Diabetes*, **36**, 1320–1328.

Groop L, Groop PH, Stenman S, Saloranta C, Tötterman KJ,Fyhr-quist F, Melander A (1988) Do sulfonylureas influence hepatic insulin clearance? *Diabetes Care*, **11**, 689–690.

Groop L, Shalin C, Fonssila-Kallunki A, Widen E, Ekstrand A, Eriksson J (1989) Characteristics of non-insulin dependent diabetic patients with secondary failure to oral antidiabetic therapy. *American Journal of Medicine*, **87**, 183–190.

Grosskopf I, Ringel Y, Charach G, Mahurshak N, Mor R, Iaina A, Weintraub M (1997) Metformin enhances clearance of chylo-microns and chylomicron remnants in nondiabetic mildly over-weight glucose-intolerant subjects. *Diabetes Care*, **20**, 1598–1602.

Grunberger G, Weston W, Patwardha R, Rappaport EB (1999) Rosiglitazone once or twice daily improves glycemic control in patients with Type 2 diabetes. *Diabetes*, **48** (Suppl 1), Poster 439 A102.

Gutniak M, Larsson H, Sanders S, Juneskans O, Holst JJ, Ahrén B (1997) GLP-1 tablet in Type 2 diabetes in fasting and postprandial conditions. *Diabetes Care*, **20**, 1874–1879.

Hatorp V, Haug-Pihale G (1998) A comparison of the pharmacokinetics of repaglinide in healthy subjects with that in subjects with chronic liver disease. *Diabetes* (Suppl 1), 496 (abstract).

Hatorp V, Perentesis G, Nielsen K, Wu F (1997) Pharmacokinetics of repaglinide: a comparison between young and elderly healthy subjects and elderly NIDDM patients. *Journal of Clinical Pharmacology*, **37**, 874 (abstract).

Heinemann L, Richter B (1993) Clinical pharamacology of human insulin. *Diabetes Care*, **16** (Suppl. 3), 90–100.

Heinemann L, Sinha K, Weyer C, Loftager M, Hirschbergert S, Heise (1999) Time-action profile of the soluble, fatty acid acylated, long-acting insulin analogue NN304. *Diabetic Medicine*, **16**, 332–338.

Hillebrand I (1987) Pharmacological modification of digestion and absorption. *Diabetic Medicine*, **4**, 147–150.

Hirschberg Y, McLeod J, Gareffa S, Spratt D (1999) Pharmacodynamics and dose response of nateglinide in Type 2 diabetes. *Diabetes*, **48** (Suppl. 1), A100 (abstract).

Hollerman F, Hoekstra JB (1997) Insulin Lispro. *New England Journal of Medicine*, **337**, 176–183.

Holman RR, Cull CA, Turner RC (1999) A randomized double-blind trial of acarbose in Type 2 diabetes shows improved glycemic control over 3 years. (UK Prospective Diabetes Study 44). *Diabetes Care*, **22**, 960–964.

Holst JJ (1994) Glucagon-like peptide-1 (GLP-1): a newly discovered GI hormone. *Gastroenterology*, **107**, 1848–1855.

Hume PD, Lindholm A, Hylleberg B, Round P (1998) Improved glycemic control with insulin aspart: a multicenter, randomized, double-blind crossover trial in Type 1 diabetic patients. UK Insulin Aspart Study Group. *Diabetes Care*, **21**, 1904–1909.

Inoue K, Hisatomi A, Umeda F, Nawata H (1991) Release of amylin from perfused rat pancreas in response to glucose, arginine, gamma-hydroxybutyrate, and gliclazide. *Diabetes*, **40**, 1005–1009.

Iwamoto Y, Kosaka K, Kuzuya T, Akanuma Y, Shigeta Y, Kaneko T (1996) Effects of troglitazone: a new hypoglycemic agent in patients with NIDDM poorly controlled by diet therapy. *Diabetes Care*, **19**, 151–156.

Jennings AM, Wilson RM, Ward JD (1989) Symptomatic hypoglycemia in NIDDM patients treated with oral hypoglycemic agents. *Diabetes Care*, **12**, 203–208.

Johnston PS, Lebovitz HE, Coniff R (1997) Advantages of monotherapy with alpha-glucosidase inhibitors in elderly NIDDM patients. *Diabetes*, **46** (Suppl. 1), 158A (abstract).

Johnston PS, Lebovitz HE, Coniff RF, Simonson DC, Raskin P, Munera CL (1998) Advantages of alpha glucosidase inhibition as monotherapy in elderly Type 2 diabetic patients. *Journal of Clinical Endocrinology and Metabolism*, **83**, 1515–1522.

Kahn CR, Schecte Y (1993) Oral hypoglycemic agents. In: Gilman AG, Rall TW, Nies AS, Taylor P (eds), *The Pharmacologic Basis of Therapeutics*. New York: McGraw-Hill, 1485.

Kalbag J, Hirschberg Y, McLeod JF, Gareffa S, Lasseter K (1999) Comparison of mealtime glucose regulation of nateglinide and repaglinide in healthy subjects. *Diabetes*, **48** (Suppl 1), A206 (abstract).

Keller U, Muller R, Berger W (1986) Sulfonylurea therapy fails to diminish insulin resistance in Type 1 diabetic subjects. *Hormone and Metabolic Research*, **18**, 599–603.

Koda JE, Fineman M, Rink TJ, Daily GE, Muchmore DB, Linarelli LG (1992) Amylin concentrations and glucose control. *Lancet*, **339**, 1179–1180.

Kolterman OG, Gottlieb A, Moyses C, Colburn W (1995) Reduction of post-prandial hyperglycaemia in subjects with IDDM by intravenous infusion of AC137, a human amylin analogue. *Diabetes Care*, **18**, 1179–1192.

Kolterman OG, Olefsky JM (1984) The impact of sulfonylurea treatment upon the mechanisms responsible for the insulin resistance in Type II diabetes. *Diabetes Care*, **7** (Suppl. 1), 81–88.

Lepore M, Kurzhals R, Pampanelli S, Fanelli CG, Bolli GB (1999) Pharmacokinetics and dynamics of s.c. injection of the long-acting insulin glargin (HOE 1) in T1DM. *Diabetes*, **48** (Suppl. 1), A97 (abstract).

Linkeschowa R, Heise T, Rave K, Hompesch B, Sedlack M, Heinemann L (1999) Time-action profile of the long acting insulin analogue HOE 901. *Diabetes*, **48** (Suppl. 1), A97 (abstract).

Ludvik B, Lell B, Hartter E, Schnack C, Prager R (1991) Decrease of stimulated amylin release precedes impairment of insulin secretion in Type II diabetes. *Diabetes*, **40**, 1615–1619.

Maggs DG, Buchanan TA, Burant CF, Cline G, Gumbiner B, Hsueh WA, Inzucchi S, Kelley D, Nolan J, Olefsky JM, Polonsky KS, Silver D, Valiquett TR, Shulman GI (1998) Metabolic effects of troglitazone monotherapy in Type 2 diabetes mellitus: a randomized double blind placebo controlled trial. *Annals of Internal Medicine*, **128**, 176–185.

Malaisse WJ (1995) Stimulation of insulin release by non-sulfonylurea hypoglycemic agents: the meglitinide family. *Hormone and Metabolic Research*, **27**, 263–266.

Marbury T, Hatorp V (1998) Pharmacokinetics of repaglinide after single and multiple doses in patients with renal impairment compared with normal healthy volunteers. *Diabetes*, **47** (Suppl. 1), 496.

Marbury T, Strange (1998) Multicenter, randomized comparison of the therapeutic effects of long-term use of repaglinide with glyburide in Type 2 diabetes. *Diabetes* **47** (Suppl. 1), 496 (abstract).

Mathisen A, Geerlof J, Houser V (1999) Pioglitazone 026 Study Group. The effect of pioglitazone on glucose control and lipid profile in patients with Type 2 diabetes. *Diabetes*, **49** (Suppl. 1), A441 (abstract).

Melander A, Bitzén PO, Faber O, Groop L (1989) Sulphonylurea antidiabetic drugs: an update of their clinical pharmacology and rational therapeutic use. *Drugs*, **37**, 58–72.

Mooradian AD (1987) The effect of sulfonylureas on the in vivo tissue uptake of glucose in normal rats. *Diabetologia*, **30**, 120–121.

Mooradian AD (1996) Drug therapy of non-insulin-dependent diabetes mellitus in the elderly. *Drugs*, **6**, 931–941.

Mooradian AD (1998) Repaglinide: a viewpoint. *Drugs and Aging*, **13**(2), 181.

Mooradian AD, Neumann C (1997) Precose resolution of optimal titration to enhance current therapies (PROTECT) study: experience in the elderly. *Annual Meeting of the American Geriatric Society*, 153.

Mooradian AD, Thurman J (1999) Drug therapy of postprandial hyperglycemia. *Drugs*, **97**, 19–29.

Mooradian AD, Osterweil D, Petrasek D, Morley JE (1988) Diabetes mellitus in elderly nursing home patients: a survey of clinical characteristics and management. *Journal of the American Geriatrics Society*, **36**, 391–396.

Mooradian AD, Kalis J, Nugent CA (1990) The nutritional status of ambulatory elderly Type II diabetic patients. *Age*, **13**, 87–89.

Mooradian AD, Albert SG, Wittry S, Chehade JM, Kim J, Bellrichard BA (2000) Dose-response profile of acarbose in older subjects with Type 2 diabetes. *American Journal of Medical Sciences* (in press).

Morley JE, Mooradian AD, Rosenthal MJ, Kaiser FE (1987) Diabetes mellitus in elderly patients: is it different? *American Journal of Medicine*, **83**, 533–544.

Moses R, Slobodniuk R, Donnelly T (1997) Additional treatment with repaglinide provides significant improvement in glycemic control in NIDDM patients poorly controled on metformin. *Diabetes*, **46** (Suppl 1), 93 (abstract).

Novo Nordisk (1997) *Prandin*[R] *(repaglinide). Prescribing information.* Novo Nordisk Pharmaceuticals, Princeton, NJ, USA.

Ogawa A, Harris V, McCorkle SK, Unger RH, Luskey KL (1990) Amylin secretion from the rat pancreas and its selective loss after streptozotocin treatment. *Journal of Clinical Investigations*, **85**, 973–976.

Ørskov C (1992) Glucagon-like peptide-1, a new homrone of the enteroinsular axis. *Diabetologia*, **35**, 701–711.

Parke–Davis (1997). *Rezulin (troglitazone) tablets. Prescribing information.* Morris Plains, New Jersey, USA.

Pearson JG, Antal EJ, Raehl CL, Gorsch HK, Craig WA, Albert KS, Welling PG (1986) Pharmacokinetic disposition of 14^C-glyburide in patients with varying renal function. *Clinical Pharmacology and Therapeutics*, **39**, 318–324.

Perriello G, Misericordia P, Volpi E, Santucci C, Ferrannini E, Ventura MM, Santeusanio F, Brunetti P, Bolli GB (1994) Metformin in NIDDM: evidence for suppression of lipid oxidation and hepatic glucose production. *Diabetes*, **43**, 920–928.

Pfeiffer MA, Beard JC, Halter JB, Judzewitsch R, Best JD, Porte D Jr (1983) Suppression of glucagon secretion during a tolbutamide infusion in normal and noninsulin-dependent diabetic subjects. *Journal of Clinical Endocrinology Metabolism*, **56**, 586–591.

Pharmacia and Upjohn 1998. *Glyset*[R] *(miglitol). Prescribing information.* Pharmacia and Upjohn Company, Kalamazoo, MI, USA.

Pioglitazone 001 Study Group (1999) Pioglitazone: its effect in the treatment of patients with Type 2 diabetes. *Diabetes*, **48** (Suppl. 1), 469 (abstract).

Pittner RA, Albrandt K, Beaumont K, Gaeta LS, Koda JE, Moore CX, Rittenhouse J, Rink TJ (1994) Molecular physiology of amylin. *Journal of Cell Biochemistry*, **55S**, 19–28.

Plosker LG, Faulds D (1999) Troglitazone: a review of its use in the management of Type 2 diabetes mellitus. *Drugs*, **57**, 409–438.

Rabasa-Lhoret R, Chiaisson JL (1998) Potential of α-glucosidase inhibitors in elderly patients with diabetes mellitus and impaired glucose tolerance. *Drugs and Aging*, **13**, 131–143.

Ratner R, Levetan C, Schoenfeld S, Organ K, Kolterman O (1998) Pramlintide therapy in the treatment of insulin-requiring Type 2 diabetes: results of a 1-year placebo-controlled trial. *Diabetes*, **47** (Suppl. 1), A88 (abstract).

Ratzmann KP, Shulz B, Heinke P, Besch W (1984) Tolbutamide does not alter insulin requirement in Type 1 (insulin-dependent) diabetes. *Diabetologia*, **27**, 8–12.

Reed RL, Mooradian AD (1990) Nutritional status and dietary management of elderly diabetic patients. *Clinics in Geriatric Medicine*, **6**, 883–901.

Rink TJ, Beaumont K, Koda J, Young A (1993) Structure and biology of amylin. *Trends in Pharmacological Science*, **14**, 113–118.

Roach P, Yuel L, Arora V (1999) The Humalog mix 25, a novel protamine-based insulin Lispro formulation. *Diabetes Care*, **22**, 1258–1261.

Rosenkranz B, Profozic V, Metelko Z, Mrzljak V, Lange C, Malerczyk V (1996) Pharmacokinetics and safety of glimepiride at clinically effect doses in diabetic patients with renal impairment. *Diabetologia*, **39**, 1617–1624.

Rosenstock J, Samols E, Muchmore DB, Schneider J (1996) The Glimepiride Study Group. Glimepiride, a new once-daily sulfonylurea: a double-blind, placebo-controlled study of NIDDM patients. *Diabetes Care*, **19**, 1194–1199.

Rosenstock J, Whitehouse F, Schoenfeld S, Dean E, Blonde L, Kolterman O (1998) Effect of pramlintide on metabolic control and safety profile in people with Type 1 diabetes. *Diabetes*, **47** (Suppl. 1), A88 (abstract).

Rosenthal MJ, Morley JE (1992) Diabetes and its complications in older people. In: Morley JE and Korenman SG (eds), *Endocrinology and Metabolism in the Elderly*. Boston: Blackwell Scientific Publications, 373–387.

Rosskamp RH, Park G (1999) Long-acting insulin analogs. *Diabetes Care*, **22** (Suppl. 2), B109–B113.

Rubin C, Egan J, Schneider R for the Pioglitazone 014 Study Group (1999). Combination therapy with pioglitazone and insulin in patients with Type 2 diabetes. *Diabetes*, **48** (Suppl. 1), 473 (abstract).

Rybka J, Goke B, Sissmann J (1999) European comparative study of 2 alpha-glucosidase inhibitors, Miglitol and acarbose. *Diabetes*, **48** (Suppl. 1), 433A (abstract).

Santeusanio F, Compagnucci P (1994) A risk-benefit appraisal of acarbose in the managment of non-insulin-dependent diabetes mellitus. *Drug Safety*, **11**, 432–444.

Scheen AJ (1997) Drug treatment on non-insulin-dependent diabetes mellitus in the 1990s: achievements and future developments. *Drugs*, **54**, 355–368.

Schmitz O, Nyholm B, Orskov L, Gravholt C, Moller N (1992) Effects of amylin and the amylin agonist pramlintide on glucose metabolism. *Diabetic Medicine*, **14** (Suppl. 2), S19–S23.

Schnieder R, Egan J, Houser V for the Pioglitazone 101 Study Group (1999) Combination therapy with pioglitzzone and sulfonylurea in patients with Type 2 diabetes. *Diabetes*, **48** (Suppl. 1), 458 (abstract).

Seltzer HS (1989) Drug-induced hypoglycemia: a review of 1418 cases. *Endocrinology and Metabolism Clinics of North America*, **18**, 163–183.

Simpson KL, Spencer CM (1999) Insulin Aspart. *Drugs*, **57**, 759–765.

Sirtori CR, Franceschini G, Galli-Kienle M, Cighetti G, Galli G (1978) Disposition of metformin (N,N-diemethylbiguanide) in man. *Clinical Pharmacology and Therapeutics*, **24**, 683–693

Skillman TG and Feldman (1981) The pharmacology of sulfonylureas. *American Journal of Medicine*, **70**, 361–372.

SmithKline Beecham (1999). *Avandia (Rosiglitazone) tablets. Prescribing information.* Philadelphia, Pennsylvania, USA.

Stang M, Wysowski DK, Butler Jones D (1999) Incidence of lactic acidosis in metformin users. *Diabetes Care*, **22**, 925–927.

Stumvoll M, Nurijhan N, Perriello G, Dailey G, Gerich JE (1995) Metabolic effects of metformin in non-insulin-dependent diabetes mellitus. *New England Journal of Medicine*, **333**, 550–554.

Thompson RG, Gottlieb A, Organ K, Koda J, Kisicki G, Kolterman OG (1997) Pramlintide: a human amylin analogue reduced postprandial plasma glucose, insulin, and C-peptide concentrations in patients with Type 2 diabetes. *Diabetic Medicine*, **14**, 547–555.

Thompson RG, Pearson L, Shoenfeld S, Kolterman OG for the Pramlintide in Type 2 Diabetes Group (1998) Pramlintide, a synthetic analog of human amylin, improves the metabolic profile of patients with Type 2 diabetes using insulin. *Diabetes Care*, **21**, 987–993.

Tomkin G (1973) Malabsorption of vitamin B_{12} in diabetic patients treated with phenformin: a comparison with metformin. *British Medical Journal*, **3**, 673–675.

Torlone E, Fanelli C, Rambotti AM, Kassi G, Modarethi F, Di Vincenzo A, Epifano L, Ciofetta M, Pampanelli S, Brunetti P (1994) Pharmacokinetics, pharmacodynamics and glucose counterregulation following subcutaneous injection of the monomeric insulin analogue [Lys(B28), Pro(B29)] in IDDM. *Diabetologia*, **37**, 713–720.

Tornier B, Marbury TC, Dambso P, Windfield K (1995) A new oral hypoglycemic agent, repaglinide, minimizes risk of hypoglycemia in well controlled Type 2 diabetic patients. *Diabetes*, **44** (Suppl. 1), 70A (abstract).

UK Prospective Diabetes Study Group (1995) Overview of 6 years' therapy of Type II diabetes: a progressive disease. *Diabetes*, **44**, 1249–1258.

UK Prospective Diabetes Study Group (1998a) Intensive blood-glucose control with sulfonylureas or insulin compared with conventional treatment and risk of complications in patients with Type 2 diabetes (UKPDS 33). *Lancet*, **352**, 837–853.

UK Prospective Diabetes Study Group (1998b) Effect of intensive blood-glucose control with metformin on complications in overweight patients with Type 2 diabetes (UKPDS 34). *Lancet*, **352**, 854–865.

Williams RH, Palmer JP (1975) Farewell to phenformin for treating diabetes mellitus. *Annals of Internal Medicine*, **83**, 567–568.

Wu MS, Johnston P, Sheu WHH, Hollenbeck CB, Jeng CY, Goldfine ID, Chen YD, Reaven GM (1990) Effects of metformin in NIDDM patients. *Diabetes Care*, **13**, 1–8.

Yki-Jarvinen H, Ryysy L, Nikkilä K, Tulokas T, Vanamo R, Heikkila M (1999) Comparison of bedtime insulin regimens in patients with Type 2 diabetes mellitus: a randomized controlled trial. *Annals of Internal Medicine*, **130**, 389–396.

16

Rehabilitation

Paul Finucane, Maria Crotty
Flinders University, Adelaide

INTRODUCTION

Earlier chapters of this book have documented the catastrophic events that can complicate the course of diabetes mellitus. For anybody, the onset of a stroke, a myocardial infarct, an ischaemic limb requiring amputation, or significant loss of vision is potentially devastating. The process of rehabilitation aims to minimize the consequences of such catastrophes. For people young or old, diabetic or otherwise, the principles of rehabilitation are broadly similar. However, special considerations arise when the patient happens to be elderly and diabetic, as problems tend to be complex and more difficult to address.

An understanding of the terms 'impairment', 'disability' and 'handicap' greatly facilitates an appreciation of the process of rehabilitation. Impairment refers to a defect in an organ, a pathological process. Disability refers to the loss of function resulting from the impairment, and handicap to the social disadvantage resulting from the disability. Take, for example, a woman with a thrombotic stroke resulting in hemiplegia. The impairment is the cerebral infarct, indirect evidence of which is found by neurological examination and more direct evidence by computerized tomography or magnetic resonance imaging scanning. Resulting disability may take the form of inability to perform activities of daily living because of a motor deficit, hemianopia and sensory inattention. Consequently, she or he may be handicapped, and unable to continue with former pastimes.

Every impairment has the potential to trigger the onset of disability and handicap. While many definitions of rehabilitation have been advanced, it can simply be regarded as a process that minimizes the disability and handicap resulting from impairment. To understand this process, it is essential to have an understanding of the determinants of disability and handicap.

FACTORS INFLUENCING THE DEVELOPMENT OF DISABILITY AND HANDICAP

It is remarkable how people with similar underlying impairments differ in the extent of their resulting disability and handicap. For example, some people are fully independent and have resumed a normal life-style within a few weeks of having an ischaemic leg amputated, while others are left permanently incapacitated, following months in hospital. Some of the major determinants of disability and handicap (summarized in Table 16.1) need to be recognized. In an individual patient, all these factors interact, and they should not therefore be considered as discrete.

The Impairment

It is a truism that the greater the severity of an impairment, the greater the likelihood of disability and handicap. The site of the impairment may also be important. For instance a small cerebral infarct involving the internal capsule may cause profound disability, while a much larger lesion involving a 'silent' region of the brain may go unnoticed. Some impairments may resolve spontaneously, be halted or be reversed by therapeutic intervention, while others inexorably progress. The chronicity of the impairment may also be important. For some people, long-standing impairment promotes familiarity and the development of adaptive skills, which limit disability. Thus the diabetic person with angina learns to avoid exercise likely to precipitate chest pain and/or use nitrate pro-

Diabetes in Old Age. Second Edition. Edited by A. J. Sinclair and P. Finucane. © 2001 John Wiley & Sons Ltd.

Table 16.1   Factors influencing the extent of disability and handicap

The impairment
Severity
Site
Reversibility
Chronicity

Intrinsic patient factors
Physical status
    Coincidental pathology
    Premorbid health
    Physiological reserve
Mental and psychological status
    Mood
    Ability to adjust
    Motivation

Extrinsic patient factors
Healthcare
Social supports
    Spouse, family, friends, pets
    Housing
Financial status

phylaxis. In other situations, people become gradually worn down by continuing impairment, consequently fail to develop or lose adaptive skills, and so become disabled and handicapped.

Intrinsic Patient Factors

People with long-standing diabetes, irrespective of their chronological age, may well have a number of active impairments at any one time. Thus, retinopathy and nephropathy commonly coexist, and macrovascular disease may involve the coronary, cerebral and peripheral vasculature simultaneously. Furthermore, elderly patients, diabetic or otherwise, often have coincidental diseases that are not necessarily linked aetiologically. For example, a person with chronic chest disease may also have an arthropathy and prostatic hyperplasia.

The elderly diabetic patient tends to have the worst of both worlds, with multiple impairments both related and unrelated to diabetes. Thus, visual impairment may be as much a consequence of macular degeneration as diabetic retinopathy and autonomic neuropathy as much a consequence of Parkinson's disease as diabetes. The presence of multiple impairments is of particular importance in a rehabilitation setting where it can prevent the achievement of goals. Take, for ex-

ample, the patient recovering from a lower limb amputation, whose angina and/or chronic chest disease limit exercise tolerance, or whose mobility is limited by osteoarthritis and/or peripheral neuropathy involving the remaining leg.

The physical status of the patient prior to the onset of the impairment therefore has a major impact on the extent of subsequent disability and handicap. Other things being equal, the person who was fit and active prior to the onset of the impairment has a better prognosis than another with pre-existing disease. Unfortunately, the lifestyles of many old people do not promote cardiorespiratory or neuromuscular fitness. In a Canadian study, for example, less than half of people with Type 2 diabetes participated in any form of exercise program, either formal or informal (Searle and Ready 1991).

A decline in cardiorespiratory and neuromuscular function with aging means that an older person with impairment is more likely to develop disability and handicap than is a younger person with similar impairment (Seymour 1989). In the past, this lack of 'physiological reserve' to meet the challenge of a new impairment has tended to receive undue emphasis, leading to nihilistic and agist attitudes in the area of rehabilitation as elsewhere. In practice, advanced chronological age per se is no barrier to successful rehabilitation.

As will be discussed later (see 'Psychological aspects of rehabilitation'), psychological factors have an enormous impact on the extent of disability and handicap resulting from impairment. Thus the person who rapidly comes to terms with an impairment, perceives it as a challenge rather than as a negative event and is well motivated, is likely to fare better than another with a different attitude.

Extrinsic Patient Factors

Access to high-quality healthcare can do much to prevent impairment in the elderly diabetic patient. Even if impairment develops, medical intervention can retard the progression to disability and handicap. For example, vascular reconstructive surgery can reverse limb ischaemia and laser photocoagulation can retard the development of visual loss in diabetic retinopathy. As will be explained, even when disability and handicap have resulted, a multidisciplinary rehabilitation team can work to restore function and social competence.

Reduced social supports are a particular problem for the elderly diabetic patient. In the UK, for example, over 50 per cent of women and 25 per cent of men aged over 65 years have no living spouse (Hine 1989). As a result, one-third of this age group and an even greater proportion of older groups live alone. The vast majority of such people live full and independent lives, even if they happen to be diabetic. However, for those who struggle to cope with illness, the physical and emotional support that a partner, family members or friends can provide is a major asset in preventing disability and handicap. The important role that pets play in the lives of some people should also be recognized.

Financial resources or their lack can further determine the extent to which impairment results in disability and handicap. Access to personal care and to appropriate housing and technology can be expensive and in all societies is influenced to some extent by ones ability to pay. Here again, elderly people are disadvantaged. In Australia, for example, 78 per cent of older people are reliant on an age pension the equivalent of 25 per cent of the average adult working wage, and 85 per cent of pensioners are eligible for means-tested supplementary benefits (Australian Institute of Health, 1990).

CONDITIONS COMMONLY NECESSITATING REHABILITATION

The chronic complications of diabetes (Table 16.2) have been described in earlier chapters. All of these

Table 16.2 Common impairments and resulting disabilities in people with Type 2 diabetes

Impairment	Disability
Neuropathy	
Peripheral	Impaired mobility
	Impaired manual dexterity
Autonomic	Impaired mobility
	Incontinence
	Impotence
Retinopathy	Visual impairment, blindness
Nephropathy	Reduced exercise tolerance
Coronary artery disease	Reduced exercise tolerance
Cerebrovascular disease	Communication problems
	Impaired cognition
	Visual problems
	Impaired mobility
	Incontinence
Peripheral vascular disease	Impaired mobility

impairments can result in significant disability and handicap. At a glance, it can be seen that some impairments can result in a number of disabilities, and that some disabilities can be due to a number of different impairments. Before discussing specific rehabilitation issues, some general points about rehabilitation should first be understood.

REHABILITATION: SOME GENERAL POINTS

The Process

The principles of rehabilitation are broadly similar, irrespective of the problem with which one is dealing. An understanding of impairment, disability and handicap as previously discussed, helps to explain the process, and the need for a multidisciplinary team approach. A properly resourced rehabilitation team will have input from medical and nursing staff, physiotherapists, occupational therapists, speech pathologists, clinical psychologists and social workers. Diabetic patients in particular benefit from access to dietitians, orthotists and podiatrists.

All rehabilitation programs must be planned. The first step is to accurately assess the patient's current level of impairment, disability and handicap. Diagnostic skills and the appropriate use of investigative technology are required to define the impairment. A plethora of assessment scales are available to assess disability; the Barthel scale (Mahoney and Barthel 1965) is most widely used and, despite its limitations, has stood the test of time. While several 'quality of life' scales have been devised, the extent of handicap has proved difficult to quantify owing to its subjective nature. It is also important to formally assess cognitive function, even in patients who appear alert and orientated. At the very least this will establish a baseline, which may later prove useful. The 30-point Mini Mental Status Examination (Folstein, Folstein and McHugh 1975) has become popular, perhaps because it best combines sensitivity with ease of administration.

Following assessment, the next step is to identify goals and a time frame within which to achieve them. All team members must be involved in these initial steps, and it is essential that consensus be achieved, otherwise cohesion gives way to chaos. The patient is an important (though often forgotten) member of the team. It is crucial that he or she be involved in establishing goals, as any goal that is not shared by the patient is unlikely to be achieved. For goals to be realistic, the patient's level of function prior to the new impairment must be taken into account. As a general rule, it is unrealistic to aim for greater than the pre-morbid level of function, though there may be exceptions to this.

Having established goals, the combined talents of the team are brought to bear in meeting them. A detailed description of the skills used by individual team members when dealing with various impairments and disabilities is beyond the scope of this chapter and is well dealt with elsewhere (Andrews 1987). Medical staff are mainly responsible for the identification and management of impairment. In a rehabilitation setting, they must focus on the current impairment, coincidental impairments, underlying risk factors and potential complications. Thus in a diabetic patient who has had a limb amputation, they may be called upon to supervise the wound, treat phantom limb pain, monitor diabetic control, and manage coexisting angina and hypertension.

Allied health staff are best equipped to manage disability. Occupational therapists primarily assess problems encountered with activities of daily living and help the patient to devise strategies to overcome them. Physiotherapists plan and implement physical therapies that target specific problems, and enhance cardiorespiratory and neuromuscular function. Speech pathologists have particular expertise in the area of communication difficulties and swallowing disorders. For some patients, the main disability may be psychological rather than physical, and input from a clinical psychologist can be invaluable in addressing this. Social workers have particular expertise in helping patients to deal with handicap, the social disadvantage resulting from disability. They can harness the support needed to maintain a disabled person in the community, as well as provide information, advice and practical help with financial and legal matters.

While multidisciplinary team members have discrete areas of expertise, it is essential that each also has a global perspective which spans impairment, disability and handicap. Each must understand what the other is doing. For example, the speech pathologist must have knowledge of neuroanatomy and the medical practitioner must understand the need for home modifications and 'meals on wheels' provision. Nurses are arguably the most holistic of the health professions, as their role encompasses impairment, disability and handicap. In a hospital rehabilitation setting, they en-

sure continuity of patient care while other team members tend to be available only during 'office hours'. In this regard, they are the true linchpins of the rehabilitation process.

For such a disparate group to function with cohesion, there must be effective communication. When team members are co-located in a specific area (e.g. a rehabilitation unit), exchange of information occurs regularly and informally. In addition, most teams have regular formal meetings to review the process of individual patients and revise the rehabilitation goals. A leader or chairperson is required to ensure that all perspectives are aired and that consensus is reached. Team meeting should also be used for discharge planning and to organize follow-up following discharge from the unit.

When to Rehabilitate

To be most effective, rehabilitation should start as soon as possible, so as to prevent further impairment and minimize the risk of disability. This implies that the initial impairment can be compounded if managed inappropriately. Take, for example, the patient with a flaccid hemiplegia and therefore at risk of shoulder subluxation. Inappropriate handling, as might occur when helping the patient to move in bed or to transfer to a chair, can result in serious and persistent shoulder damage (Reding and McDowell 1987). Such a problem is less likely to develop in a rehabilitation setting where staff are sensitized and trained in its prevention.

Selection of appropriate patients for rehabilitation is important and can sometimes be difficult. On the one hand it is unfair to subject a patient who will not benefit to a demanding rehabilitation program and in the process to raise false expectations. This is also wasteful of resources. On the other hand, those who may benefit, even to a limited extent, should not be denied access to rehabilitation. In certain situations, it is appropriate to set modest goals, such as helping a hemiplegic patient to regain sitting balance or an amputee patient to become wheelchair independent. The quality of the person's life can be greatly improved if such goals are achieved.

Patients are most likely to benefit from a rehabilitation program if they are able to actively participate and if they are well motivated. For those who do not benefit, there is usually an identifiable reason, such as an overwhelming physical impairment, cognitive impairment, depression or a personality disorder. A small minority of patients will simply lack the motivation to combat their impairment. As explained later, strategies exist to help such people.

Where to Rehabilitate

The nature and extent of the impairment largely determine this. With some conditions, such as an uncomplicated myocardial infarction, only a few days of in-hospital treatment is required and an out-patient rehabilitation program is most appropriate. Other impairments, such as major strokes and limb amputations, generally require hospital-based rehabilitation, at least in the early stages. In large centres of population, rehabilitation of elderly diabetic patients is often carried out in units specializing in specific impairments. This has the advantage of allowing high levels of expertise to be developed together with complementary facilities such as workshops for artificial limbs and appliances. Having people with similar impairments in a single unit provides opportunities for patient education, the training of health professionals and for research. Specialized units have a role in setting standards of excellence and in the design, implementation and evaluation of new therapeutic tools and techniques. However, the principles of rehabilitation can be applied in any setting, provided that staff with the necessary knowledge, skills and attitudes are available.

There is increasing evidence to support rehabilitation in the home (Shepperd and Iliffe 1998). Randomized trials have suggested that outcomes achieved by offering home rehabilitation to patients with strokes are comparable with those obtained in hospital. These programs do not appear to increase burden on carers (Gunnell et al 2000) and are less expensive (Anderson et al 2000). With the proliferation of geriatric day hospitals in the 1960s, much rehabilitation is now undertaken in an outpatient setting, often after an initial period of more intensive in-patient treatment. Alternative community-based or domiciliary-based rehabilitation programs are increasingly being developed and may have some advantages over traditional day hospital programs (Young and Forster, 1992).

Psychological Aspects of Rehabilitation

The onset of impairment is usually associated with some emotional disturbance, particularly if the event is catastrophic (e.g. a major stroke or loss of a limb).

There may be a feeling of loss with regard to ones physical and/or mental faculties, to relationships with others or to inanimate objects such as ones home or other possessions. Normally, a grief reaction occurs, with phases of denial, anger and depression leading to a level of acceptance sufficient to allow a relatively normal life to be resumed. However, adjustment to impairment is sometimes abnormal. For example, 20% of people have severe and often persistent depression following acute myocardial infarction (Leng 1994). Several studies have documented high levels of psychosocial dysfunction in people following a stroke (Ahlsio et al 1984; Schmidt et al 1986) even despite participation in a rehabilitation program (Young and Forster 1992).

The manner in which people adapt to impairment greatly influences the development of disability and handicap. Some people seem to be inherently more adaptable than others in responding positively to an adverse situation. Such 'highly motivated' people are keen to participate in a rehabilitation program, and work hard to achieve their goals. At the other end of the spectrum are those who appear to succumb to impairment, disengage, surrender power and autonomy and adopt a 'sick role'.

There are psychological theories to explain such different responses. Kemp (1988) has proposed an excellent model, which explains motivation as a dynamic process, determined by four elements: the person's wants; beliefs; the rewards for achievement; and the costs to the patient. Thus if a person really wants something, believes it to be attainable and if attainment is likely to bring reward, they will strive to achieve it, provided the cost (in terms of pain and effort) is acceptable. On the other hand, a lack of achievement can occur if the goal is not strongly wanted, if the person believes that it cannot be attained, if there is little or no reward for attaining the goal, or if the perceived cost of achievement is too high. By using this framework, the rehabilitationist can help individual patients in a number of ways.

First, a patient can be helped to identify wants or, in other words, to establish goals. In a rehabilitation setting, failure to achieve goals is often attributable to their being set by rehabilitationists without reference to the patient. The role of therapists is to ensure that the goals which patients set themselves are realistic. If goals are unrealistic, the patient should be encouraged to modify them. Second, the patient's beliefs should be explored and important misconceptions should be corrected. Third, having established what goals are important to the patient, the rehabilitationist should ensure that he or she is appropriately rewarded when goals are achieved. Interim goals as well as final goals should be set and rewarded. For example, a patient who has regained a certain level of independence might have some weekend leave from hospital, the time spent at home increasing as new goals are met. When progress is gradual, patients will need to be reminded of their achievements. It is often useful to have concrete evidence of progress, as when a hemiplegic patient compares their current status with a video of themselves taken shortly after the onset of impairment. Finally, the patient's perception of the cost of rehabilitation needs to be explored, and any misconceptions should be addressed.

It follows that an understanding of individual patients is a prerequisite for successful rehabilitation. This can be achieved only by listening, not just to the people concerned, but to others who know them intimately. Health professionals should consistently demonstrate a positive approach to patients as well as to their progress at rehabilitation. Respecting patients as people fosters a sense of self-worth and, among other things, further enhances motivation. While providing positive feedback is important, honesty and sincerity should never be compromised, and false expectations should not be generated.

By acting as a 'self-help group' or 'therapeutic community', patients participating in a rehabilitation program can provide each other with support and encouragement. The rehabilitation team should endeavour to create an atmosphere conducive to this and should structure the ward and organize ward activities so as to promote camaraderie. On the other hand, relationships between patients are occasionally destructive and staff may need to intervene if the rehabilitation program is to be salvaged. For example, sleeping and dining arrangements may need to be reviewed so that some people are kept apart.

It is worthwhile remembering that for many patients with diabetes, concerns about the future may be just as significant as concerns about the present. The onset of one disability may trigger justifiable apprehension about further loss in the future. Thus, the onset of angina pectoris may raise fears of a fatal myocardial infarct and calf claudication may raise fears of limb amputation. Indeed anxieties about future morbidity and premature mortality can be an important source of 'dis-ease' in people with 'uncomplicated' diabetes. Again, listening to the patient is the key to identifying and addressing the problem. Unless concerns for the future surface spontaneously, they should be sought by direct questioning.

All members of the multidisciplinary rehabilitation team should at least have a basic understanding of the psychology of loss and motivation and have some practical skills to overcome those problems that commonly surface. More complex problems may require input from a clinical psychologist and having access to such expertise is most valuable. Psychologists also have an educative role in helping other team members to understand their own feelings and behaviour. They can also help to resolve conflict, whether arising within or between patients, within or between team members or between patients and team members.

SPECIFIC REHABILITATION PROBLEMS

For reasons stated earlier, rehabilitation problems seldom exist in isolation in the elderly diabetic patient. Thus, the person whose immediate concern is a lower limb amputation may also have a residual hemiparesis from a previous stroke, together with angina and visual impairment. Efforts to regain mobility can be influenced as much by the remote as the recent problems. It is therefore somewhat artificial to discuss specific problems as if they existed in isolation. In the clinical setting it is essential to have an holistic approach, particularly as attempts to relieve one problem may exacerbate another. Thus, attempts to mobilise a patient who has had a limb amputation may provoke an acute myocardial infarct, while drug therapy for angina may exacerbate peripheral vascular disease, heart failure or renal failure. These considerations should be kept in mind when considering specific rehabilitation problems.

The Patient With Stroke

For the person with diabetes, a stroke is undoubtedly the impairment with the greatest potential to cause disability and handicap. About 20% of those having their first stroke are dead within a month, and one-third of survivors have severe residual disability (Sacco et al 1982). Motor and sensory deficits, gait disorders, cognitive deficits, visual field defects, communication disorders, dysphagia and incontinence are all potentially devastating and all too common sequelae. Some patients will have a number of these disabilities. A detailed description of the rehabilitation process following stroke is beyond the scope of this text. Readers are referred to the admirably concise and informative papers on the topic by Reding and McDowell (1987) and Black-Schaffer, Kirsteins and Harvey (1999).

A few points are worthy of emphasis, however. For the individual, it is often difficult to predict outcome in the immediate aftermath of a stroke and in the process to decide on the utility or futility of a rehabilitation program. Epidemiological evidence indicates that previous health status, the extent and severity of the stroke, and the level of consciousness, cognition and continence following the stroke are the best pointers (Flicker 1989). However, most who survive the acute stage improve to some extent. Serial assessments suggest that the great bulk of recovery occurs in the first 6 months after stroke and most patients reach their best 'activities of daily living' (ADL) function within 13 weeks of stroke onset (Jorgensen et al 1995). Having a range of rehabilitation options to choose from is the ideal, with those most likely to improve being admitted to the more intensive programs. For some people, rehabilitation goals must be modest. They are nonetheless valid, as helping people to recover their ability to swallow, to transfer from bed to chair more easily or to become wheelchair-independent can greatly enhance the quality of life. The role of the various members of the multidisciplinary rehabilitation team is described elsewhere (Reding and McDowell 1987). As with all rehabilitation situations, the role that the patient's family has to play should not be forgotten.

At present there is much interest in early treatments of stroke. For example, thrombolysis offers the hope of reducing the size of an ischaemic stroke and resultant disability, albeit with an increased risk of intracerebral bleeding (Wardlaw, Yamaguchi and Del Zoppo 1998). However, at this stage the window of opportunity for treatment is three hours following the onset of symptoms, and only a small proportion of patients present at this early stage and are managed by services with the potential to deliver treatments within this timeframe. Until larger trials convincingly demonstrate the benefits and identify the most appropriate patient groups, timing and delivery strategies, most patients will need to rely on rehabilitation to reduce their disability following stroke. When provided by a specialist team, stroke rehabilitation reduces mortality and morbidity for stroke victims (Stroke Unit Trialists' Collaboration 1997). However, little is known about which components are effective and the process is often therefore referred to as a 'black box'. Factors assumed to be important are: early mobilization, increased awareness and treatment of medical complications, aggressive treatment of risk factors (e.g. hypertension and atrial fibrillation) and therapy. Increasing interest is now being shown in identifying those therapies which work, when they should be used and how frequently (Kwakkel et al 1999). Therapy directed at specific tasks appears more likely to produce better outcomes. For example, early treadmill training with partial body support may produce better walking (Hesse et al 1995) and the more practice the better the result (Kwakkel et al 1999). However, the relationship between the damaged brain tissue and therapies is poorly understood and the impact of various therapy approaches on neural recovery is only starting to be explored (Pomeroy and Tallis 2000).

The Patient with Myocardial Infarction

Not only are diabetic patients more susceptible to myocardial infarction, they are also at greater risk from its consequences in both the short term and long term. For example, one-quarter of diabetic patients admitted to hospital with acute infarction do not survive to discharge (Malmberg and Ryden 1988). Compared with non-diabetics, the overall mortality of diabetics after infarction is four times higher among men and seven times higher among women (Lundberg et al 1997). Poor pre-infarction cardiac status and greater damage resulting from the infarct, together with the diabetic state itself, all seem to contribute to the relatively poor prognosis. Fatal reinfarction is a particular concern, being over twice as common in diabetic than in non-diabetic people (Malmberg and Ryden 1988).

Rehabilitation programs that aim to improve the long-term prognosis for people after myocardial infarction have been described and evaluated. They tend to be exercise-based, though some also aim to optimize social and psychological recovery and reduce or eliminate risk factors for coronary artery disease. Meta-analyses suggest a survival advantage of 20% (O'Connor et al 1989), and hospital-directed home exercise programs provide similar functional results as group exercise programs (Miller et al 1984), although depressed mood may be less common in those enrolled in group programs (Taylor et al 1986). The benefits were apparent one year after randomization and persisted for at least three years. Almost all studies have excluded elderly subjects and provide no data on the sub-group of subjects with diabetes. There is therefore no evidence of the efficacy of post-infarction rehabilitation programs for elderly diabetic patients. However, because of the relatively poor prognosis of myocardial infarction, this group has potentially the most to gain. At the very least, exercise programs enhance self-esteem, feelings of autonomy and self-confidence (Fentem 1994).

Before embarking on any exercise-based rehabilitation program, it is important to establish that exercise is safe and to quantify the level of cardiorespiratory reserve. An exercise stress test under the supervision of a trained health professional clarifies these issues. Assessing functional reserve allows exercise programs to be tailored to the individual and allows progress to be measured. It is also important to identify factors that limit the ability to exercise, as some of these, for example foot deformities or unsuitable footwear, can be rectified. Aerobic exercise (in which muscular effort is sustained by oxygen) and not anaerobic exercise should be engaged in. In practice, exertion that leads to muscular aches and pains on the following day should be avoided. New guidelines from the Australian National Institute of Health (1996) recommend the accumulation of 30 minutes of moderate intensity physical activity over the course of most, preferably all days of the week. If the patient experiences angina during or following exercise, this regimen must be revised.

An alternative approach is a low-intensity group approach such as that which is often used in Australian cardiac rehabilitation programs. This does not require initial exercise testing for risk stratification or monitoring. Patients are taught to monitor their own exercise levels based on perceived exertion. They are advised to exert themselves to the level at which they breathe more deeply but still talk comfortably while exercising. Low-intensity group programs achieve similar improvements in quality of life and physical fitness as high-intensity exercise programs (Worcester et al 1993).

Assuming that medications (e.g. beta-blockers) which control heart rate are not being prescribed, individual patients should aim to maintain heart rate within a predetermined range when exercising. To this end, the pulse rate should be monitored regularly, and the degree of exercise modified accordingly. An adequate warm-up and cool-down period should begin and end every exercise session. Running, swimming, cycling, tennis and gym workouts are examples of suitable exercise. Exercise that the person finds enjoyable is best. Those struggling to psychologically adjust to a recent myocardial infarction may find it helpful to meet with others who are similarly affected.

Though a graded aerobic exercise program is usually prescribed following a myocardial infarction, there is increasing interest in the role of resistance exercise programs particularly in the elderly cardiac patient. Resistance exercise programs (typically a single set of 8–15 repetitions of 8–10 exercises, performed two to three times each week) have been emphasized in older adults to reduce age-associated reductions in muscle strength and subsequent disability. Evidence suggests that decreases in blood pressure and heart rate can be achieved with such programs (Kelley and Kelley 2000) but controversy surrounds their use after acute myocardial infarction. While many programs include some strength training (Hare et al 1995), recent American Heart Advisory guidelines found that there is insufficient research evidence to support the routine prescription of resistance training for people with moderate to high cardiac risk (Pollock et al 2000).

The Amputee Patient

As peripheral vascular disease is now the main cause of lower limb amputations in Western countries, the majority of amputee patients are elderly and many are diabetic. In the UK, 80% of people undergoing lower limb amputation are aged over 60 years (Chadwick and Wolfe 1992). In the United States, 45% of all patients undergoing lower limb amputation in the late 1970s were diabetic (Most and Sinnock 1983). Furthermore, these authors reported that the incidence of lower limb amputation was some 15 times higher in diabetic than in non-diabetic people. Wide variation has been reported in the incidence of limb amputations, with European rates being consistently lower than those in the US (LEA Study Group 1995). For example, in 1991 the age-adjusted incidence of diabetes-related lower limb amputations was significantly higher in California than in the Netherlands (49.9 compared with 36.1 per 10 000 diabetics), suggesting that access to healthcare and healthcare funding models impact on the incidence of amputations (Van Houtum and Lavery 1996).

The process of rehabilitating the elderly diabetic amputee goes through a number of overlapping stages (Andrews 1996). Getting the stump to heal is the first step, and an adequate blood supply is crucial. Surgeons aim to preserve as much of a limb as possible without compromising the viability of the stump. Whether the initial procedure should be trans-tibial (or below-knee amputation—BKA) or trans-femoral (above-knee amputation—AKA) is a crucial and often difficult decision. On the one hand, there is a particular advantage in preserving the knee joint, as following a BKA people regain and retain mobility far more effectively than those with an AKA. On the other hand, if the stump fails to heal following a BKA, an AKA will be required. The need for a second more radical operation after a prolonged and futile effort to heal the stump delays the rehabilitation process and often demoralizes the patient.

Postoperatively early therapy is directed at stabilizing residual limb volume by decreasing oedema, and this is achieved with rigid or soft dressings such as 'shrinkers' (i.e. fitted elasticated stump socks) and elastic figure-8 bandaging (Andrews 1996). Emphasis is placed on avoiding contractures and maintaining joint mobility. Prolonged periods sitting in a chair without corrective exercises will lead to knee and hip flexion contractures, which will present obstacles to prosthetic fitting and gait training. Patients are encouraged to lie prone for 20–30 minutes a day to promote full extension. During this period training in how to transfer, cardiovascular training and general strengthening is undertaken to prepare for gait retraining when the prosthesis is fitted.

Once the suture line has healed, the patient can be mobilized on a temporary device such as a pylon or on a pneumatic post-amputation mobility (PPAM) aid. When the stump wound is soundly healed, a permanent prosthesis is fashioned. Initially, the stump will be oedematous, with the swelling gradually resolving over a number of weeks. The socket, which interfaces between the stump and prosthesis, will therefore need to be modified or recast as the swelling reduces. The prosthesis needs to be customized for the individual patient. Modern prostheses have a modular design consisting of a socket, a shank, knee (if transfemoral) and an ankle and foot mechanism (Figure 16.1).

The cosmetic appearance is also important, though many people cover their prosthesis with trousers. Strong and lightweight materials are increasingly available, and 'endoskeletal' limbs have a central pillar of carbon fibre or lightweight metal to support the bodyweight. This is surrounded by a soft foam cover which is pleasant to touch and silent when accidentally struck. An artificial foot may be rigid or have an ankle that allows movement in one or more planes. The stages involved in training an amputee to walk are beyond the scope of this chapter. However, they involve stump care (including bandaging the stump), transfer training (bed to chair, chair to toilet), balance training, hopping with crutches or frame (a useful skill

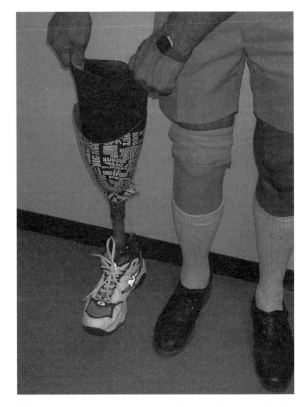

Figure 16.1 A lower limb endoskeletal patella tendon bearing (PTB) prosthesis. That being held by the patient shows the prosthesis without a cover whereas that being worn by the patient shows a covered prosthesis. (Photograph courtesy of Dr Adrian Winsor)

when the patient gets up at night or the prosthesis is being repaired), and gait training (including over slopes, steps and rough ground).

Peripheral vascular disease in the diabetic patient is usually a bilateral condition, so that following amputation, the remaining leg may be critically ischaemic. Over 50% of diabetic patients will have lost their remaining leg within 4 years of their first amputation (Ebskov and Josephsen 1980). This highlights the need to monitor the remaining leg carefully and to educate the patient about optimal diabetic control and footcare. Arteriography and vascular reconstruction should also be considered (LoGerfo and Coffman 1984). Mortality rates among diabetic amputees are also high; survival rates of only 50% at 3 years following amputation have been quoted (Bild et al 1989). The patient's general medical condition must be considered; coincidental cerebrovascular and coronary artery disease should be suspected and be appropriately managed if found.

Pain is sometimes a problem, particularly in the early phase of amputee rehabilitation. Stump pain can be due to infection, ischaemia, a bony spur or a neu-roma. Appropriate management requires an accurate diagnosis. Phantom limb pain is common and some-times debilitating (Jensen et al 1985). Physical treat-ments such as desensitising massage and the use of transcutaneous electrical nerve stimulation (TENS) are usually taught. Carbamazepine is often effective and the pain tends to resolve with time (Baron, Wasner and Lindner 1998).

The Patient With Diabetic Retinopathy

Diabetic retinopathy is a significant cause of visual impairment in elderly people. In the Framingham Study, 3% of all people aged 65–74 y had diabetic retinopathy, with 7% of 75–85 y olds being affected (Kini et al 1978). The duration of diabetes is the cri-tical risk factor in the development of retinopathy; those with Type 2 diabetes have a similar risk as those with Type 1 diabetes mellitus (Nathan et al 1986).

Strategies to prevent or retard the development of diabetic retinopathy are described in Chapter 9. Even if visual impairment does result, much can be done to minimize resulting disability and handicap. Ophthal-mology departments usually have affiliated units spe-cializing in the provision of low vision aids and other appliances. An array of products are also available to help the visually impaired with blood sugar monitoring and insulin administration (Petzinger 1992). In many countries, those registered as visually impaired or legally blind are eligible for special services and ben-efits, which help to reduce the impact of visual im-pairment. Functional vision, however, may be impaired without meeting these criteria. After an assessment, strategies to maximize remaining vision will be iden-tified. Generally speaking the rehabilitation approach is to enhance residual vision using devices which ei-ther magnify objects (glasses, magnifiers) or modify environmental factors such as glare, lighting and contrast. When there is insufficient vision, other compensatory strategies may be possible. If a person is unable to reliably identify a change in surface while walking, a long white cane may be useful.

Other Complications in the Diabetic Patient

Diabetic patients with end-stage renal disease (ESRD) and who are dependent on renal dialysis are obliged to be physically inactive for long periods of time and tend to lose cardiorespiratory and neuromuscular fitness.

Tiredness resulting from uraemia and chronic anaemia limits exercise capacity and leads to further loss of fitness. Renal osteodystrophy is an early complication of renal failure and the loss of bone mass is ex-acerbated by lack of exercise. Exercise programs can reduce disability and handicap in patients with ESRD (Painter 1988), and therefore qualify as valid re-habilitation activities.

Sensory neuropathy sometimes limits the exercise options available to the elderly diabetic patient and loss of fitness can result. For those who do exercise, trauma to the foot can result in blistering and ulceration of the skin, muscular sprains and fractures. Muscles and tendons are at risk from overstretching. Neuropathic weight-bearing joints are easily damaged and a Char-cot joint can result. For these reasons, exercises such as swimming and cycling which minimize weight-bear-ing are best. Sensory loss also makes some patients dependent on vision when performing motor skills, and visual aids may need to be incorporated into the exercise program.

Between 20% and 40% of all diabetic patients have some degree of autonomic dysfunction (Ewing and Clarke 1982). Exercising can be hazardous for the person with diabetic autonomic neuropathy as essen-tial cardiovascular responses and endocrine responses may be blunted or absent (Hilsted, Calbo and Chris-tensen 1980; Hilsted et al 1982). Not only is the ca-pacity for exercise reduced, there is also a risk of silent myocardial ischaemia and infarction, together with sudden cardiac death. It is therefore essential that simple tests of autonomic function (Ewing and Clarke 1982) be performed on all diabetic patients before they embark on an exercise-based rehabilitation program, and that those with abnormalities undergo a formal exercise test. For those with autonomic dysfunction, intensive exercise and activities that require rapid changes in posture must be avoided. For such people, exercising in water or while sitting or lying helps to maintain blood pressure and is particularly suitable (Graham and Lasko-McCarthey 1990).

AIDS AND ADAPTATIONS

Technology has much to offer in minimizing disability and handicap. A large variety of aids (often called assistive devices) can assist with such activities of daily living as dressing, toiletting and housework as well as with recreational pursuits. Those in common use have been described by Mulley (1989); they range

Table 16.3 Aids and orthoses sometimes prescribed for patients with diabetes

Indication	Modification	Goal
Forefoot calluses	Mild rocker sole, high-top footwear	Reduce pressure of metatarsal heads
Transmetatarsal amputation	Rocker sole, molded inside with filler; increased density of material used in sole to increase rigidity	Aids toe off; prevents toe break (forefoot stump is stressed during toe break)
Foot drop (CVA or peripheral neuropathy)	Ankle foot orthosis	Substitute for weak ankle dorsiflexors and provides some mediolateral stability
Foot ulcer	Total contact walking cast or orthotic variant	Relieve pressure
Unable to distinguish ground surfaces	Long white cane	Improve mobility

from the simple and inexpensive to the sophisticated and costly. Mobility can be enhanced by a variety of walking aids, wheelchairs and motorized vehicles. Communication difficulties can be reduced with a range of devices, both simple and complex. Some elderly diabetic people also benefit from low-vision, continence and memory aids. The environment in which the person functions can also be adapted so as to reduce disability and handicap. Requirements can range from the provision of a simple handrail which helps with toilet use to major structural changes to ones home.

It is crucial that aids and adaptations be tailored to meet the needs of the individual. An assessment of need is therefore the preliminary step; the premorbid level of functioning, degree of current disability and aspirations for the future must all be considered. The most important perspective is that of the patient, though it is important to differentiate between the patients perceived needs and actual needs. If the patients perception of need conflicts with that of the health professional, agreement should be reached through negotiation. It should be kept in mind that the inappropriate use of aids or the use of inappropriate aids promotes rather than relieves disability and handicap. For this reason, advice on the suitability of aids and adaptations is best left to occupational therapists or others with particular expertise in this area. Physiotherapists can give advice on the selection of mobility aids, speech pathologists with communication aids and audiologists with hearing aids.

Footwear is particularly important for the patient with diabetes, and if prescribed carefully can prevent further complications. For example, atrophy of intrinsic foot muscles is common in diabetic patients with peripheral neuropathy, creating an 'intrinsic minus foot'. This makes flexion of the MTP joints and straightening of the toes difficult and leads to hammer toes and a heightened plantar arch. This in turn reduces the foot's walking surface, such that much of the support comes from protruding MTP joints and the heel. Appropriate prescription of high-top shoes to avoid pressure on PIP joints of the hammer toes and orthoses to expand the weight-bearing areas of the soles are likely to avoid the development of calluses and pressure areas. Table 16.3 summarizes information on some commonly prescribed aids and orthoses for people with diabetes.

For the diabetic patient with retinopathy or other causes of visual impairment, a number of assistive devices can enhance vision. Most large centres of population have access to a 'low vision clinic' or other centre where specialized advice and equipment is available. Such centres usually work hand in hand with ophthalmology services, with patients regularly being referred from one service to the other. Where stroke has left the patient with a visual field defect, the use of prisms fitted to spectacles can enlarge the field of binocular vision (Roper-Hall 1976).

METABOLIC CONTROL IN THE DISABLED DIABETIC PERSON

While this chapter has focused on disability and handicap resulting from diabetic complications, it should be appreciated that the onset of disability and handicap can have implications for diabetic control. Thus the person with hemiplegia or visual impairment may have difficulty with self-monitoring of glycaemia and with self-administration of insulin. Reduced mobility may lead to weight gain and/or loss of good metabolic control. As part of the rehabilitation program, the ability of the person to manage their diabetes should be assessed and, when necessary, remedial action taken.

EDUCATION AND REHABILITATION

Rehabilitation is essentially an educational activity, in which the patient acquires the knowledge, skills and attitudes (the key components of any educational package) to minimize the disability and handicap resulting from impairment. As far as possible, patient education should be integrated into the rehabilitation program and should be acknowledged as an essential component, which requires time and other resources. It is important that all rehabilitation team members acknowledge their role as educators, preferably to the extent of acquiring formal education skills. If educational resources directed at the diabetic population (e.g. a diabetes educator or education team) are available, their input into a rehabilitation program can be invaluable.

Education can have a number of objectives relevant to rehabilitation. It promotes good metabolic control and behaviours that prevent further impairment and minimize disability and handicap. Furthermore, participation in education programs can foster autonomy, improve self-esteem and coping skills and reduce anxiety and depression (Rubin, Peyrot and Sandek 1989). In other words, education can reduce the psychological handicap resulting from diabetes. Support groups or self-help groups can also have a major impact on psychological rehabilitation, though it is valuable to have input from a health professional, preferably one with some training in psychotherapy (Toth and James 1992).

Of the three components of an educational package, attitudinal learning is more difficult to attain than is knowledge or skills acquisition. For example, the difficulty in getting people to modify their diet, level of exercise and other lifestyle factors is well recognized, even in people with knowledge about what constitutes a healthy lifestyle (Searle and Ready 1991). Health professionals who fail to understand the value of rehabilitation also require education, to counteract nihilistic attitudes. It is important that such people come to understand that neither old age nor diabetes is a barrier to successful rehabilitation. As stated eloquently by Roald Dahl (1975): 'It is possible for anyone, given a lot of guts and a bit of luck, to overcome gigantic misfortunes and terrible illness.'

REFERENCES

Ahlsio B, Britton M, Murray V, Theorell T (1984) Disablement and quality of life after stroke. *Stroke*, **15**, 886–890.

Anderson C, Rubenach S, Mhurchu CN, Clark M, Spencer C, Winsor A (2000) Home or hospital for stroke rehabilitation? Results of a randomized controlled trial: I. Health outcomes at six months. *Stroke*, **31**, 1024–1031.

Andrews K (1987) *Rehabilitation of the Older Adult*. London: Edward Arnold.

Andrews KL (1996) Rehabilitation in limb deficiency: 3. The geriatric amputee. *Archives of Physical Medicine and Rehabilitation*, **77**, S14–S17.

Australian Institute of Health (1990) *Australia's Health 1990*. Canberra: Australian Government Publishing Service.

Baron R, Wasner G, Lindner V (1998) Optimal treatment of phantom limb pain in the elderly. *Drugs and Ageing*, **12**, 361–376.

Bild DE, Selby JV, Sinnock P, Browner WS, Braveman P, Showstack JA (1989) Lower extremity amputation in people with diabetes. *Diabetes Care*, **12**, 24–31.

Black-Schaffer RM, Kirsteins AE, Harvey RL (1999) Stroke rehabilitation: 1. Comorbidities and complications. *Archives of Physical Medicine and Rehabilitition*, **80**, S8–16.

Chadwick SJD, Wolfe JHN (1992) Rehabilitation of the amputee. *British Medical Journal*, **304**, 373–376.

Dahl R (1975) In: Griffith VE (ed) *A Stroke in the Family*. London: Wildwood House.

Ebskov B, Josephsen P (1980) Incidence of reamputation and death after gangrene of the lower extremity. *Prosthetics and Orthotics International*, **4**, 77–80.

Ewing DJ, Clarke BE (1982) Diagnosis and management of diabetic autonomic neuropathy. *British Medical Journal*, **285**, 916–918.

Fentem PH (1994) Benefits of exercise in health and disease. *British Medical Journal*, **308**, 1291–1295.

Flicker L (1989) Rehabilitation for stroke survivors—a review. *Australian and New Zealand Journal of Medicine*, **19**, 400–406.

Folstein M, Folstein S, McHugh P (1975) Mini-mental state: a practical method for grading the cognitive state of patients for clinicians. *Journal of Psychiatric Research*, **12**, 189–198.

Graham C, Lasko-McCarthey P (1990) Exercise options for persons with diabetic complications. *Diabetes Educator*, **16**, 212–220.

Gunnell D, Coast J, Richards SH, Peters TJ, Pounsford JC, Darlow M (2000) How great a burden does early discharge to hospital-at-home impose on carers? A randomized controlled trial. *Age and Ageing*, **29**, 137–142.

Hare DL, Fitzgerald H, Darcy F, Race E, Goble AJ (1995) Cardiac rehabilitation based on group light exercise and discussion: an Australian hospital model. *Journal of Cardiopulmonary Rehabilitation*, **15**, 186–192.

Hesse S, Bertelt C, Jahnke MT, Schaffrin A, Baake P, Malezic M, Mauritz KH (1995) Treadmill training with partial body weight support compared with physiotherapy in nonambulatory hemiparetic partients. *Stroke*, **26**, 976–981.

Hilsted J, Calbo H, Christensen NJ (1980) Impaired responses of catecholamines, growth hormone, and cortisol to graded exercise in diabetic autonomic neuropathy. *Diabetes*, **29**, 257–262.

Hilsted J, Galbo H, Christensen NJ, Parving HH, Benn J (1982) Haemodynamic changes during graded exercise in patients with diabetic autonomic neuropathy. *Diabetologia*, **22**, 318–323.

Hine D (1989) Demography and epidemiology of old age. In: Pathy MSJ, Finucane P (eds), *Geriatric Medicine, Problems and Practice*. New York: Springer-Verlag, 15–30.

Jensen TS, Krebs B, Nielsen J, Rasmussen P (1985) Immediate and long term phantom limb pain in amputees: incidence, clinical characteristics and relationship to preamputation limb pain. *Pain*, **21**, 267–278.

Jongbloed J (1986) Prediction of function after stroke: a critical review. *Stroke*, **17**, 765–776.

Jorgensen HS, Nakayama H, Raaschou HO, Vive-Larsen J, Stoier M and Oslen TS (1995) Outcome and time course of recovery in stroke: II. Time course of recovery. The Copenhagen Stroke Study. *Archives of Physical Medicine and Rehabilitation*, **76**, 406–412.

Kelley GA, Kelley KS (2000) Progressive resistance exercise and resting blood pressure. *Hypertension*, **35**, 838–843.

Kemp BJ (1988) Motivation, rehabilitation, and aging: a conceptual model. *Topics in Geriatric Rehabilitation*, **3**, 41–51.

Kini MM, Leibowitz HM, Colton T, Nickerson RJ, Ganley J, Dawber TR (1978) Prevalence of senile cataract, diabetic retinopathy, senile macular degeneration, and open-angle glaucoma in the Framingham eye study. *American Journal of Ophthalmology*, **85**, 28–34.

Kwakkel G, Wagenaar RC, Twisk JWR, Lankhorst GJ, Koetsier JC (1999) Intensity of leg and arm training after primary middle cerebral artery stroke: a randomised trial. *Lancet*, **354**, 191–196.

LEA Study Group (1995) Comparing the incidence of lower extremity amputations across the world: the global lower extremity amputation study. *Diabetic Medicine*, **12**, 14–18.

Leng CC (1994) Depression following myocardial infarction. *Lancet*, **343**, 2–3.

LoGerfo FW, Coffman JD (1984) Vascular and microvascular disease of the foot in diabetes. *New England Journal of Medicine*, **311**, 1615–1619.

Lundberg V, Stegmayr B, Asplund K, Eliason M, Huhtasaari (1997) Diabetes as a risk factor for myocardial infarction: population and gender perspective. *Journal of International Medicine*, **241**, 485–492.

Mahoney FI, Barthel DW (1965) Functional evaluation: Barthel Index. *MD State Medical Journal*, **14**, 61–65.

Malmberg K, Ryden L (1988) Myocardial infarction in patients with diabetes mellitus. *European Heart Journal*, **9**, 259–264.

Miller N, Haskell W, Berra K, DeBusk R (1984) Home versus group exercise training for increasing functional capacity after myuocardial infarction. *Circulation*, **70**, 645–649.

Most RS, Sinnock P (1983) The epidemiology of lower extremity amputation in diabetic individuals. *Diabetes Care*, **6**, 87–91.

Mulley GP (1989) *Everyday Aids and Appliances*. London: British Medical Journal.

Nathan DM, Singer DE, Godine JE, Harrington CH, Perlmuter LC (1986) Retinopathy in older Type II diabetics. *Diabetes*, **35**, 797–801.

National Institutes of Health Consensus Development Panel on Physical Activity and Cardiovascular Health. (1996) Physical activity and cardiovascular health. *Journal of the American Medical Association*, **276** 241–246.

O'Connor GT, Buring JE, Yusuf S, Goldhaber SZ, Olmstead EM, Paffenbarger RS, Hennekens CH (1989) An overview of randomized trials of rehabilitation with exercise after myocardial infarction. *Circulation*, **80** 234–244.

Painter P (1988) Exercise in end-stage renal disease. *Exercise & Sport Sciences Reviews* **16**, 305–340.

Petzinger RA (1992) Diabetes aids and products for people with visual and physical impairment. *Diabetes Educator*, **18**, 121–138.

Pollock ML Franklin BA, Balady GJ, Chaitman BL, Fleg JL, Fletcher B, Limacher M, Pina IL, Stein RA, Williams M, Bazarre T (2000) Resistance exercise in individuals with and without cardiovascular disease: benefits, rationale, safety and prescription. *Circulation*, **101**, 828–833.

Pomeroy VM, Tallis RC (2000) Need to focus research in stroke rehabilitation. *Lancet*, **355**, 836–837.

Reding MJ, McDowell F (1987) Stroke rehabilitation. *Neurological Clinics*, **5**, 601–630.

Roper-Hall G (1976) The effects of visual fields defects on binocular single vision. *American Journal of Orthopedics*, **26**, 74–82.

Rubin RR, Peyrot M, Saudek CD (1989) Effect of diabetes education on self-care, metabolic control, and emotional well-being. *Diabetes Care*, **12**, 673–679.

Sacco RL, Wolf PA, Kannel WB, McNamara PM (1982) Survival and reocurrence following stroke. The Framingham Study. *Stroke*, **13**, 290–294.

Schmidt SM, Herman LM, Keonig P, Leuze M, Monahan MK, Stubbers RW (1986) Status of stroke patients: a community assessment. *Archives of Physical Medicine and Rehabilitation*, **67**, 99–102.

Searle MS, Ready AE (1991) Survey of exercise and dietary knowledge and behaviour in persons with Type II diabetes. *Canadian Journal of Public Health*, **82**, 344–348.

Seymour DC (1989) The physiology of ageing. In: Pathy MSJ, Finucane P (eds) *Geriatric Medicine, Problems and Practice*. New York: Springer-Verlag, 3–13.

Shepperd S, Iliffe S (1998) The effectiveness of hospital at home care compared with in-patient hospital care: a systematic review. *Journal of Public Health Medicine*, **20**, 344–350.

Stroke Unit Trialists' Collaboration (1997) A collaborative systematic review of the randomised trials of organised (stroke unit) care after stroke. *British Medical Journal*, **314**, 1151–1159.

Taylor CB, Houston-Miller N, Ahn DK, Haskell W, DeBusk RF (1986) The effects of exercise training programs on psychosocial improvement in uncomplicated post myocardial infarction patients. *Journal of Psychosomatic Research*, **30**, 581–587.

Toth EL, James I (1992) Description of a diabetes support group: lessons for diabetes caregivers. *Diabetic Medicine* **9**, 773–778.

Van Houtum WH, Lavery LA (1996) Outcomes associated with diabetes-related amputations in the Netherlands and in the state of California, USA. *Journal of Internal Medicine*, **240**, 227–231.

Wardlaw JM, Yamaguchi T, Del Zoppo G (1998) Thrombolytic therapy versus control in acute ischemic stroke (Cochrane review). In: *The Cochrane Library*, issue 3. Oxford: Update Software.

Warlow CP (1998) Epidemiology of stroke. *Lancet*, **352** (Suppl. III), 1–4.

Worcester MC, Hare DL, Oliver GR, Reid MA, Goble AJ (1993) Early programmes of high and low intensity exercise and quality of life after acute myocardial infarction. *British Medical Journal*, **307**, 1244–1247.

Young JB, Forster A (1992) The Bradford community stroke trial: results at six months. *British Medical Journal*, **304**, 1085–1089.

17

Approaching Primary Care

Klaas Reenders
University of Groningen

INTRODUCTION

The management of elderly people with diabetes is a challenge for all persons involved in diabetes care: patients, health and social care professionals and government agencies. In 1989, representatives of governmental health departments, patients' organisations and diabetes experts agreed on a set of measures to reduce the disabling complications of diabetes in the future. This agreement, the St Vincent Declaration, has stimulated a process not only of redefining of the national guidelines for the quality of care but also of renewing the strategies for diabetes care for the growing number of diabetic patients at both national and regional levels (Keen and Hall 1996).

In 1998, encouraging news emerged with the publication of the UKPDS data (Kinmonth, Griffin and Wareham 1999). Intensive treatment of hyperglycemia and hypertension was associated with increased opportunities for a healthier and longer life. Primary care, mostly provided by general practitioners (GPs) and nurses, plays a key role in reaching the goals of the St Vincent Declaration. The contribution of primary care in the management of patients with diabetes has increased gradually in most countries since the mid-1970s (Griffin 1998). Diabetes care shifted from specialist care in the hospital to general practice (Thorn and Russell 1973; Wilkes and Lawton 1980). The treatment of patients with Type 2 diabetes without serious complications on oral hypoglycemic tablets and diet shifted from hospital to general practice. Newly diagnosed diabetic patients remain under the control of GPs only, whose knowledge of and experience in the management of diabetes has increased (Goyder et al 1998). Overall, the percentage of patients under the control of GPs has increased to 50% (Khunti et al 1999) and this percentage is higher for older adults with diabetes.

The management of diabetes in the elderly differs from the approach in younger diabetics. The presence of coexisting diseases, the shorter longevity, the threat and consequences of hypoglycemia and the psychosocial circumstances (living alone, loss of cognitive function) require a different type of care and approach. Each patient should be treated as an individual, the approach should be flexible, and the therapeutic regimen tailored to the individual requirements of the patient. In many cases the main goal is not to cure but the maintenance of pleasurable and independent living (Hill 1994; Sinclair and Barnett 1993).

This chapter poses the principal question: which type of care is the best for elderly people with diabetes? Should it be primary care by GPs (or a primary care team), or shared care given in close co-operation between GPs and the hospital diabetes team in the same hospital or region? In addition, many other questions need to be asked. Which factors determine the quality of care in a country or region? What can we learn from history, the published experiences in different countries in the last decade? Also, if we decide on a primary care approach, how can we organize this care? What is the structure, process and outcome of diabetes care in general practice? We also need to ask about two other special problems: how to manage emergencies in the care of elderly people with diabetes (intercurrent illnesses and hypoglycemia) and how to organize the care for patients who cannot visit a doctor because they are housebound and/or staying in a nursing or residential home (Sinclair et al 1997a,b).

Diabetes in Old Age. Second Edition. Edited by A. J. Sinclair and P. Finucane. © 2001 John Wiley & Sons Ltd.

CHOOSING THE TYPE OF CARE

Self-care is important for maintaining quality of life in individuals who deal with their symptoms without seeking formal medical advice (Jones 2000). Self-care is also an essential component of the management of chronic illness. The diabetes team should teach the patient to practise self-care. However, self-care alone is not sufficient for an elderly person with diabetes. It is important for the person to visit the diabetes team to monitor the cardiovascular risk factors and to detect early complications of diabetes (Hill 1994).

Primary Care

Primary care is defined as first-contact, continuous, comprehensive and coordinated care provided to populations undifferentiated by gender, disease or organ system (Starfield 1994). Secondary care is consultative, usually short-term in nature, for the purpose of assisting primary care physicians with their diagnostic and therapeutic dilemmas. This is provided by informal consultations of secondary care physicians or by short-term referral of patients. Tertiary care is for patients with disorders requiring additional specialist referral and involves the provision of long-term care. It is important that the three levels of care be integrated for the patient to receive clear and consistent advice.

The role of primary care in a country depends on the presence of the characteristics of a primary healthcare system (Starfield 1991) (Table 17.1).

In most countries of Europe the primary-care physican is a GP, but in the United States this term also refers to internists and pediatricians working in primary care. The funding for primary care in the UK is provided by the National Health Service (NHS), in the Netherlands and Denmark by the health insurance companies, and in the United States by managed care systems for those in employment and by Medicare for the elderly. The mode of payment by the patient is fee-for-service or capitation/salary, and in Belgium, small co-payments ('remgeld') are applied to discourage

Table 17.1 Factors involved in primary healthcare

Distribution of general practices and hospitals
Type of physician who provides primary care
Funding
Mode of payment of the physician
Percentage of active physicians who are specialists

---

excessive utilization of primary care. In Table 17.1, two main features are central to primary care by general practitioners: a defined list of all patients registered in the practice and the gatekeeping role of the GP to secondary care. The GP controls the access to expensive and invasive secondary services. In the Scandinavian countries, the UK and the Netherlands (Starfield 1991) primary care plays a strong role in the healthcare system. Patients have free access to their GP, not only for self-limiting ailments but also for monitoring of their chronic disease (Olesen, Dickinson and Hjortdahl 2000).

In most circumstances, patients in those countries have a personal primary care physician who is responsible for record-keeping and for continuity of care (Koperski 2000). A personal relationship with the same doctor and practice is especially important for elderly people with a chronic disease such as diabetes. Development and implementation of guidelines in primary care is more difficult in countries with a weak primary healthcare system. To fulfil the goals of the St Vincent Declaration there is a task force for primary care (Keen 1996). In Denmark, the Netherlands and the UK, GPs with a special interest in diabetes have organized expert groups to stimulate diabetes primary care. In these latter countries during the last 25 years, diabetes care has shifted from secondary hospital to general practice. Some enthusiastic GPs have already published their experiences of this process (van Weel and Tielemans 1981; Wilks 1973).

Moving the care of diabetic patients from hospital to general practice without valid agreements between all interested parties can create difficulties for the GP. The doctor may have a lack of time, knowledge and experience to manage those patients, although this depends on several factors. In Sheffield (MacKinnon et al 1989), for example, 1000 diabetic patients were discharged from a diabetic clinic in three years. Only one specialist nurse was available to visit the general practices, and yet half of those practices succeeded in improving the care for diabetics in a short period. Important factors were: enthusiasm for diabetes care of the GP, access to a dietitian, organizing diabetes miniclinics (Thorn and Russell 1973; Williams et al 1990), a prompting system (Hurwitz, Goodman and Yudkin 1993), a monthly diabetic day (Koperski 1992), a service for annual review (Higgs et al 1992), a community care service (Hill 1976), and the use of a diagnostic centre (Sonnaville et al 1997).

Wilks (1973) in Bristol wrote an individual study based on his own experience with diabetes care, and concluded: 'diabetes is an ideal disease for general practice to diagnose, observe and treat with interest'. Only one of the 24 diabetic patients in his practice was not under his direct control. Van Weel and Tielemans (1981) treated 75% of the diabetics in their practice in 1979 and concluded that there were shortcomings in the surveillance for complications, although monitoring became easier and more reliable with the introduction of Glucostrips in general practice, and treatment options increased with the introduction of metformin.

Development of guidelines and postgraduate education gave GPs the tools for better management of diabetes. However, each practice in a country is an individual entity, and services vary between practices in the same region (Table 17.2).

Table 17.2 Factors influencing the provision of diabetes care in general practice

Number of GPs: single-handed or group practice (more than two GPs)
Practice team: receptionist, clerk, medical-assistant, (practice) nurse-practitioner, GP.
Facilities: instruments for monitoring diabetes, premises
Access to services: dietitian, chiropodist, ophthalmic optician
Miniclinic versus integrated diabetes care

A primary care team is a group of diverse professionals who communicate with each other regularly about the care of a defined group of patients and participate in that care (Wagner 2000). The potential of the team is the ability to increase the number and quality of services available. Teamwork in a practice is most effective in small (2–5 people) groups focused on a single task (Pearson and Jones 1994). Everyone's role should be clearly defined and explicitly delegated. The different members are trained for their individual roles (Table 17.3).

Table 17.3 Characteristics of a team

Share a common purpose
Clear function of each member
Pooling knowledge, skills and resources
Share responsibility for the outcome

The receptionist/clerk in the UK, and the medical assistant in the Netherlands, are in the front line. They monitor telephone calls and visits, update and maintain the recall registers, compile the appointments list and send invitations.

Not all doctors employ nurses, but in a large group-practice it would be impossible to give satisfactory patient education and surveillance without a nurse. In the Netherlands, the government commissions one nurse for every three GPs. Their task is to improve the care of patients with diabetes or asthma. Most doctors have neither the training nor the time to engage in counselling and the giving of self-management support. The advantage of a nurse trained in behavioural counselling is illustrated in different studies (Wagner 2000; Waine 1992).

The role of the practice nurse especially in managing older patients with diabetes includes: (1) education of the patient and/or his caregivers; (2) advice on diet, smoking, exercise, taking tablets or insulin, self-care of the feet, recognizing and managing hypo- and hyperglycemia, and infection diseases; (3) visiting housebound patients; (4) extra attention for patients at higher risk for diabetic feet problems and visual problems; and (5) communication with nurses and care managers in residential and nursing homes. Leadership in the team is taken by people most committed to the task.

Shared Care

Shared diabetes care is the joint participation of GPs and specialists in the planned delivery of care for patients (Greenhalgh 1994). A scheme of shared care is as follows. Every three months patients are seen by the primary carers, and for their annual review they are seen in hospital. But 'sharing' of patients between GP and specialist can lead to confusion about responsibility for the different aspects of care, so clear boundaries should be established (Sinclair 1998).

Effective shared care requires structured coordination of medical activities in which clinicians agree on guidelines or protocols and trust each other's actions and interventions. Optimal communication is a vital point by means of a common diabetes record and a shared dataset for evaluation and audit.

Shared care is also a system in which the professionals in a district or region make arrangements to divide the care for groups of diabetics. The hospital provides care for Type 1 (insulin-dependent), insulin-treated or complicated Type 2 patients and pregnant woman. The other Type 2 patients are reviewed only in primary care. In a recent study with data from 38 288 diabetic patients in primary care in the UK, 51% were managed by general practice only, 19% by hospital care only and 30% (11–50%) by shared care (Khunti et al 1999). The collating of audit data in a district should form the basis for audit of the quality of care and highlight local deficiencies. Information about levels of performance of process and outcome measures between general practices may have a role in improving care. It is important to evaluate which patients are not included in the audit.

Butler et al (1997) in an audit showed an under-representation of the elderly aged over 75 years who are housebound or in residential care. In a screening program for microvascular complications (Higgs et al 1992), 22 of the 46 patients aged over 80 years were non-attenders; and in Koperskis study (1992) on screening for complications on the so-called 'diabetic day', 12 of the 26 excluded patients were housebound. In Denmark and Germany, shared care includes the referral of newly diagnosed patients to the diabetic clinic for education and start of treatment (Lauritzen 1995; Berger, Jorgens and Flatten 1996). Since 1993, diabetes care in general practice in the UK has been encouraged by specific payments, including for diabetes education and multipractice audits. The new contract in the UK doubled the number of patients reviewed annually in Leicester between 1990 and 1995 (Goyder et al 1998), but the proportion of patients under hospital control only did not fall.

Shared care also involves referral to hospital specialists, not just to the diabetologist and ophthalmologist but also to the geriatrician (Sinclair 1998). The geriatrician can provide an important source of support and advice to the GP in terms of:

- assessment of coexisting disease which impacts on diabetes management
- management of increasing dependency and disability
- recognition and management of cognitive impairment.

Criteria and circumstances for referral of patients to other specialists are shown in Table 17.4.

Table 17.4 Criteria for referral

Secondary failure on oral (insulin) therapy
Diabetic ulcer formation
Absence of footpulses (suggesting peripheral vascular disease)
Severe hypoglycemia or hyperglycemia
Ophthalmological risk
Renal insufficiency (creatinine >200 mM or clearance <30 mL/min
Cardiovascular disease

Table 17.5 Advantages of hospital and general practice in delivering diabetes care

Hospital	General practice
Wider expertise available	Personal doctor
Trained diabetic nurse	Practice staff
Easy referral to:	Easy access also in emergency
dietitian/chiropodist	Short distance: saves time/money
ophthalmologist	Home visits if necessary
Education service	Continuity of care
Insulin therapy	

Finally, the advantages of diabetes care in general practice or hospital are summarized in Table 17.5. Bearing these factors in mind, it is possible to structure the care for diabetics and to improve the quality of this care especially for the elderly. An audit of care for diabetic patients in the author's group practice at the end of 1995 demonstrated that diabetes care was suboptimal, and to improve this care was a major challenge.

IMPROVING THE ORGANIZATION OF CARE IN GENERAL PRACTICE

Designing a Protocol

A doctor with a special interest in diabetes should take the initiative to structure the care. First of all it is important to convince the other GPs in the practice to agree on the plan for an improved structure. The components of the protocol are listed in Table 17.6, and it is necessary to decide who is to be responsible for the different steps and actions. Each year the practice protocol can be adapted according to the audited outcome.

Table 17.6 Steps in restructuring diabetes care

1. Design a protocol which all staff members agree to
2. Make a register of all patients diagnosed with diabetes
3. Undertake a survey and record of every diabetic patient
4. Organize an appointment and recall system
5. Organize a monitoring system (three months and annually)
6. Organize referrals to paramedics and specialists
7. Initiate patient education: who, what and when
8. Set up a regular evaluation/audit of care

Identifying Patients with Diabetes

It is essential to produce a register of all patients in the practice known to have diabetes. The following methods can be used:

- Ask each member of the staff to register every diabetic patient.
- Record the prescriptions for oral hypoglycaemic agents and insulin with the help of the local pharmacist.
- Reread the letters from specialists.

It may be possible in six months to register nearly all the diabetic patients. Remember especially those only on diet, or elderly people housebound or staying in a residential or nursing home. It is important to realize that half of all diabetics are unknown (Mooy, Grootenhuis and de Vries 1995). The reason is that hyperglycaemia is often asymptomatic in older people (Burrows et al 1987). The higher renal threshold for glucose hampers the secretion of glucose into urine. Glycosuria is mostly absent and as a consequence the symptoms of polyuria and thirst may be absent also. Some of these individuals present with serious complications of diabetes and cardiovascular risk factors.

Selective screening of patients at high risk for diabetes is an alternative: blood glucose in patients with obesity, cardiovascular risk factors or diseases, diabetes in the family etc. Be aware of patients with nonspecific symptoms: itching, candida infection, neuropathy, visual problems and recurrent infections.

A Survey of Every Patient with Diabetes

If the diagnosis of diabetes is confirmed in accordance with the local guidelines, a review of the patient is necessary (Table 17.7). An educational program and treatment with diet should be started. Only in patients with the classic symptoms of hyperglycemia and blood glucose levels $> 20\,\text{mM}$ should insulin therapy be considered at this point. Sometimes, external factors are responsible for hyperglycemia: infection, psychological stress and increased a glucose intake. It is wise to wait for a while on the results of educational and dietary measures before starting tablets or insulin.

It is essential to record all data according to the protocol. A record card for every person with diabetes is important; it can be copied for the patient or for the specialist on referral. The advantage of a computerized record card is the ease of transformation to a central database. This facilitates a yearly audit in the practice and audit group (Khunti 1999; Chesover, Tudor-Miles and Hilton 1991). A good example is the DiabCare card (Figure 17.1).

By means of this survey it is possible also to detect the non-attenders: people not under supervision during the previous year. In some studies of good organized practices this percentage is approximately 5% (van Dam et al 1998), but Higgs et al (1992) reported a figure 12% and Burrows et al (1987) one of 20%. A certain number of patients on diet alone, and especially older people, are not under supervision: 30–50%. There are many reasons for non-attendance: being housebound or a great distance from the practice, fear of the doctor etc. The GP can detect the non-attenders and employ a reminder method either by telephone or letter. In one report, most non-attenders visited the GP in the following year (Burrows et al 1987). Consequent follow-up for these patients is very important. Many of the defaulters of an outpatient clinic had more morbidity from their diabetes than the patients under supervision (Hammersley et al 1985).

Appointments and Recall

Follow-up at regular intervals (3–6 months) to measure weight and blood glucose, and a yearly review for signs of complications (eyes, feet, cardiovascular diseases and risk factors evaluation) are the core of structured care. Older diabetics with poor memory and communication problems forget their appointments and become non-attenders. Education about the importance of regular supervision is necessary. An appointment card with the date of a new visit, and a staffmember (receptionist or medical assistant) responsible for the recall system, are a means to prevent non-attendance. In the author's practice with follow-up visits every 3

Table 17.7 Review at diagnosis

Existing diseases?
On medication?
Complications:
    fundus examination
    examination of the feet
    cardiovascular diseases and risk factors
Blood: HbA_{1c}, serum creatinine, lipids
Review goals of care
Education
Monitoring

DIABCARE
Basis Informatie Formulier
Implementatie van de St. Vincentdeclaratie

Nederlands Centrum:_____

Basis Gegevens Patiënt

| initialen | geboorte gegevens | maand | jaar |

N°.: | voorn. achtern. | geslacht m v

IDMM ○ NIDDM ○ andere ○ diabetes sinds: | OAD sinds 1 9 | insuline sinds: 1 9

Reden voor consult/ ZH opname
consult ○ routine consult ○ stabilisatie ○ complicaties ○ andere ○
of: ZH opname ○ nieuwe diagnose ○ zwangerschap ○ acuut probleem ○

Zwanger-schappen
beëindigd in de laatste 12 maanden j n normaal | abortussen | ernst. aangeb. afw. | perinatale doden |

Risicofactoren huidige situatie
roker j n indien ja: sig./dag | alcohol j n indien ja: g./wk. |

Zelfcontrole
zelfcontrole j n bloedglucose/wk. | urineglucose/wk. |

Educatie/ Diabetes-vereniging
gezonde voeding j n voetverzorging j n complicaties j n zelfcontrole j n
hypoglycemie j n therapie aanpassing j n lid van diabetesvereniging j n

Meetwaarden laatste bepaling in de afgelopen 12 maanden

gewicht	kg.	bloeddruk	mmHg.	cholesterol
lengte	cm.	BG		creatinine	HDL-chol.
	HbA1	%	microalbum.	trigliceriden
	HbA1c	%	proteinurie	nuchter j n

ST. VINCENT DOELEN
blindheid j n zo ja: ontstaan in de laatste 12 mnd. j n terminaal nierfalen j n zo ja: ontstaan in de laatste 12 mnd. j n
MI/CABG/angioplastie j n zo ja: gebeurd in de laatste 12 mnd. j n amputat. boven de enkel j n zo ja: gebeurd in de laatste 12 mnd. j n
CVA j n zo ja: gebeurd in de laatste 12 mnd. j n amputat. onder de enkel j n zo ja: gebeurd in de laatste 12 mnd. j n

Symptomen in de laatste 12 maanden
orthostat. hypotensie j n angina pectoris j n perifere neuropathie j n claudicatio intermit. j n

Onderzoeken

OGEN onderzocht in de laatste 12 mnd. j n | **VOETEN** onderzocht in de laatste 12 mnd. j n

lasercoagulatie in de laatste 12 m. j n j n | normale vibratiegevoeligheid j n j n
cataract j n j n | normale naaldprik gevoeligheid j n j n
retina gezien j n j n | voetpulsaties aanwezig j n j n
indien ja: maculopathie j n j n
retinopathie j n j n
indien rp.: niet proliferatieve rp. j n j n | genezen ulcus j n j n
preproliferatieve rp. j n j n | open ulcus/gangreen j n j n
proliferatieve rp. j n j n | bypass/angioplastie j n j n
vergevorderde diab. oogziekte j n j n
visus: L: | R: |

Kwaliteit v. leven/ Acute problemen
hypoglycemie | (n°/jaar) hyperglycemie | (n°/jaar) ziektedagen | (d./jaar) ZH opnamedagen | (d./jaar)

Diabetes therapie

| | | tot nu toe | vanaf nu | | | tot nu toe | vanaf nu |
alleen dieet | j n | j n
biguaniden sinds 1 9 | j n | j n | insuline injecties/dag aantal | | |
sulphonylurea sinds 1 9 | j n | j n | insulinepomp j n j n
glucosidase remm. sinds 1 9 | j n | j n | overige diabetes therapie j n j n

Overige therapie
hypertensie j n j n | hartfalen j n j n | isch. hartlijden j n j n | dyslipidemie j n j n | nefropathie j n j n | neuropathie j n j n | overige j n j n

arts: (niet verplicht) | handteke-ning arts: | datum:

© DIABCARE Munich 2/96

Figure 17.1 DiabCare basic information sheet

months, the percentage of non-attendant patients in every trimester is 10–15%. One of the medical assistants has the task of reminding the non-attenders. Some practices recall patients for their annual review in the month of their birthday. It is possible to recall the non-attenders with a computer system (Hurwitz et al 1993).

Good structured care has as a consequence more follow-up visits. Doctors particularly interested in diabetes detect more cases. In some studies the number of identified diabetic patients in general practice doubled although the number attending hospital clinics remained the same (Goyder et al 1998; Williams et al 1990). When doctors in a general practice do not have the motivation or the opportunity to organize follow-up (mostly due to lack of time, room or staff), it is possible to delegate this task to a specialized diabetes nurse or a community screening service.

In some regions in the Netherlands (Sonnaville et al 1997), Australia (McGill et al 1993) and the UK (Higgs et al 1992), GPs can refer their patients to a service program for screening of diabetic complications. The service includes education if necessary and recall. The service sends the results of its review, with advice from the specialist, to the GP; the GP informs the patient. Not all patients of the participating practices are reviewed. In one study (Higgs et al 1992), 88% of all patients participated, but of the patients aged over 80 years, only 50% did so. The percentage of practices with a recall system is growing in the UK under the new contract. It is now the task of GPs to manage chronic diseases. In a study in 1988 (Chesover et al 1991), 19% of the practices had a recall system; in 1993 in East Dorset the figure was 71% (Dunn and Pickering 1998).

Annual review

Many elderly patients with diabetes live long enough to develop complications. To prevent or delay these disabling complications it is important to organize an annual survey. The goal is to increase the number of complication-free years for elderly patients. In recent studies the percentage of patients with regular eye and foot examinations increase from 40% to 75% in practices with good structured care (Khunti et al 1999; Koperski 2000; Butler et al 1997; Lauritzen 1995). Table 17.8 lists the essential elements of the review.

Table 17.8 Essential elements of an annual review of elderly diabetic patients

HbA_{1c}
Creatinine
BMI
Blood pressure: lying and standing
Lipids
Smoking
Foot examination
Retinal examination and visual acuity
Pharmacotherapy
Coexistent diseases

Footcare. Good footcare combines clinical examination of the risk factors and education of the patient. Age increases the risk of developing a diabetic foot and decreases the ability for self-care. In general practice, performing a good clinical examination and providing information takes only 15 minutes for each patient. Before the visit the patient should receive a written instruction form about the foot examination by the GP and about self-care. The clinical examination includes:

- symptoms: claudication or paresthesia of the feet
- neuropathy: ankle jerks/sensation using nylon monofilament
- circulation: foot and femoral pulses and skin colour/temperature
- joint: deformity/immobility of the joint
- skin/nails: callosity, ulcer formation, infections
- self-care: cutting nails.

After the examination the GP is informed about a foot at risk and about the level of self-care by the patient.

Self-care is a problem in elderly patients. Nearly half are not able to perform self-care (Thomson and Masson 1992). They cannot reach their feet because of joint immobility, they cannot see their feet because of reduced visual acuity, and they cannot practise footcare because of other coexisting diseases such as Parkinson's or previous stroke. In these situations it is important to inform and advise the spouse or carer about the results of the examination. Instruction and education by a nurse or referral to a chiropodist to engage in foot self-care can prevent an amputation. The primary prevention of ulceration and amputation is one of the goals of the St Vincent Declaration.

Eye complications. The prevalence of sight-threatening retinopathy in elderly patients is nearly 10%

(Hirvela and Laatikainen 1997; Cahill et al 1997). In the elderly the advice is for a two-yearly retinal examination (Retinopathy Working Party 1991). It is the task of the GP to organize this examination for the patients under his or her care. Eye examination should be included in the annual survey. Screening should ideally be done by an ophthalmologist, but most countries do not have these specialists in sufficient numbers. Some GPs are able to perform this fundal examination, although intensive training is necessary (Reenders et al 1992). In the UK, GPs can refer their patients to ophthalmic opticians or for retinal photography. In three-quarters of elderly diabetics this is a good alternative (Hirvela and Laatikainen 1997). However, in one quarter of the cases the photograph is not of good quality.

Cardiovascular disease. Life-expectancy, and co-existing diseases including the presence of cardiovascular diseases and risk factors, determine the consequences of screening for the patient. Risk factor management can often result in changes of lifestyle (stopping smoking, taking more exercise, new eating habits). Medication can lower hypertension or dyslipidemia. If older people have a good relationship with 'their' GP, it is preferable that the GP counsels the patient about lifestyle and medication.

Polypharmacy poses great risks for patients with reduced memory or without a caregiver. The practice nurse is the person designated to visit those patients and to advise on compliance. Also the pharmacist can advise in such cases. It is obvious that in the obese smoking patient, with high glucose levels and hypertension, the main effort for primary care is changing the individual's lifestyle. When the patient's resistance to change is great, it is sometimes wise to accept their decision.

MANAGEMENT OF DIABETES

Patient Education

The first step is the education of a newly diagnosed patient. Education should include:

- What is diabetes mellitus?
- Advice on smoking, exercise, alcohol intake.
- Dietary advice from a dietician.
- Management plan: regular monitoring, goals for weight and glucose.
- Information to the principal caregiver.
- Information about the organization of patients.

- How to self-diagnose and manage hypo- and hyperglycemia.

In the author's practice and region, every newly diagnosed patient and his partner are invited for two 2-hour sessions. A diabetic nurse and a dietician give information. It is very important that the personal GP and the patient agree on the goals and the education program. The GP knows the social circumstances of the patient and can motivate the individual so that the management plan is accepted.

The elderly have various special educational problems:

- They may not understand medical terminology.
- One-third of over-65 year olds suffer from hearing loss.
- Twenty percent cannot read normal letters in the information booklets.
- The prevalence of dementia is 5–10%.
- Memory impairment may be present.

Oral Agents

If after 3 months, the patient has not succeeded in reaching the goals for blood glucose with a diet, oral hypoglycaemic agents should be prescribed. The choice of treatment depends on the local guidelines and the personal situation: overweight, renal–hepatic function, interactions with other medications, contra-indications and side-effects (also see Chapter 11). It is important to agree in the local group of doctors upon the choice for various sulfonylureas and the indications for insulin therapy.

Insulin

Insulin treatment in general practice is a good option if the GP is well informed about the diverse range of insulins and syringes, the indications, complications and use of combination therapy. But it is essential that a nurse specialized in diabetes care be available to give intensive education to the patient and caregiver before starting the therapy. The advantage of starting insulin therapy in primary care is that the GP can follow his or her own patients and can manage the complications of the therapy. Patients fear insulin therapy because they believe that their disease is not mild but serious, and they exaggerate the pain of the injections and the difficulties of monitoring their blood glucose. The aim of insulin treatment in many elderly patients should be to make them feel better, and avoid hypoglycaemia (Tattersall 1984) (also see Chapter 12).

Acute Complications

Hypoglycemia, hyperglycemic coma and intercurrent infection are examples of acute complications presented first to the GP. A selection of these patients (the tip of the iceberg) often present to the hospital. But what is under the iceberg? In a retrospective study (Reenders 1992) in a group practice, 93 diabetic patients were studied in the period 1975–85 (483 diabetic-years). Of the 26 hypoglycemic episodes presented to the GP, five were referred to the hospital. In the same period two patients were referred with hyperglycemic coma, and of the 176 infections presented to the practice, three patients were admitted to the hospital.

Especially in elderly patients, hypoglycemia is a serious side-effect of treatment with insulin or long-acting sulfonylurea tablets. Hypoglycemia is mostly a consequence of too intensive treatment and/or too little compliance by the patient. Hypoglycemia in the elderly could have serious consequences: a car accident, a fall resulting in a fracture, insult, TIA or stroke. Sometimes more non-specific symptoms (Knight and Kesson 1986) are presented and are often attributed by patient and doctor to age: seizure, drowsy, or confused. It is important to reduce these risks by avoiding sulfonylureas with a long half-life and accepting a suboptimal level of blood glucose. Quality of life is important in the elderly, and after a serious hypoglycemic episode they fear a new episode. It is the task of the primary care team to educate the patients to prevent hypoglycemia. But education in the elderly is difficult.

DATA FROM THE AUTHOR'S PRACTICE

In the author's group practice, we have reviewed diabetes care on an annual basis. At the millennium the practice consisted of 6300 patients, of whom 18% were aged over 65 years; and of them, 3.7% were known to have diabetes. Of the over-65s, 83% were under the care of a GP (Table 17.9).

Nineteen patients were housebound and typically their care appeared to be unstructured. We decided to take the following actions:

- Create a treatment plan for each patient, including education and annual review. The treatment plan is to be kept in their medical file and the patient or his/her caregiver receives a copy.

Table 17.9 Diabetic patients in a group practice

	Age			
	<65	65–74	>75	Totals
GP	58 (63%)	64 (85%)	55 (82%)	177 (76%)
Hospital	34 (37%)	11 (15%)	12 (18%)	57 (24%)
Totals	92 (100%)	75 (100%)	67 (100%)	234 (100%)

- At the present time, the GP is in charge of these patients. Soon, we hope to have a practice nurse who can become involved in more direct care of diabetic patients. Communication with the patient and his/her caregiver will be of great importance.

CONCLUSION

In general, a primary care approach is preferred when dealing with elderly patients with diabetes. The trusting relationship between the patient and the practice GP increases the individual's ability to communicate, and allows their coexisting diseases to be actively considered. Quality care will be possible only when it is structured by means of a protocol, of which the results need to be evaluated regularly. It is important to work together within the practice as well as with the regional hospital.

In order to deliver good-quality diabetes care in a general practice, a GP needs to be motivated and responsible for this care. Besides this, extra time and manpower will be required. Governments can assess the quality of diabetes care if general practices record outcome data and make this available for inspection.

Primary care approaches can provide high-quality diabetes care in close partnership with hospital teams, but it does not happen by itself.

REFERENCES

Berger M, Jorgens V, Flatten G (1996) Health care for persons with non-insulin-dependent diabetes mellitus. *Annals of Internal Medicine*, **124**, 153–155.

Burrows PJ, Gray PJ, Kinmonth A-L, Payton DJ, Walpole GA, Walton RJ, Wilson D, Woodbine G (1987) Who cares for the patient with diabetes? Presentation and follow-up in seven Southampton practices. *Journal of the Royal College of General Practitioners*, **37**, 65–69.

Butler C, Smithers M, Stott N, Peters J (1997) Audit-enhanced, district-wide primary care for people with diabetes mellitus. *European Journal of General Practice*, **3**, 23–27.

Cahill M, Halley A, Codd M, O'Meara N, Firth R, Momey D, Acheson RW (1997) Prevalence of diabetic retinopathy in patients with diabetes mellitus diagnosed after the age of 70 years. *British Journal of Ophthalmology*, **81**, 218–222.

Chesover D, Tudor-Miles P, Hilton S (1991) Survey and audit of diabetes care in general practice in south London. *British Journal of General Practice*, **41**, 282–285.

Diabetes Integrated Care Evaluation Team (1994) Integrated care for diabetes: clinical, psychosocial, and economic evaluation. *British Medical Journal*, **308**, 1208–1212.

Dunn N, Pickering R (1998) Does good practice organization improve the outcome of care for diabetic patients? *British Journal of General Practice*, **48**, 1237–1240.

Goyder EC, McNally PG, Drucquer M, Spiers N, Botha JL (1998) Shifting of care for diabetes from secondary to primary care, 1990–5: review of general practices *British Medical Journal*, **316**, 1505–1506.

Greenhalgh PM (1994) Shared care for diabetes: a systematic review. Occasional Paper 67, Royal College of General Practitioners, London.

Griffin S (1998) Diabetes care in general practice: meta-analysis of randomized control trials. *British Medical Journal*, **317**, 390–396.

Hammersley MS, Holland MR, Walford S, Thorn PA (1985) What happens to defaulters from diabetic clinic? *British Medical Journal*, **291**, 1330–1332.

Higgs ER, Kelleher A, Simpson HCR, Reckless JPD (1992) Screening programs for microvascular complications and hypertension in a community diabetic population. *Diabetic Medicine*, **9**, 550–556.

Hill RD (1976) Community care service for diabetics in the Poole area. *British Medical Journal*, **1**, 1137–1139.

Hill RD (1994) Models of care for the elderly diabetic. *Journal of the Royal Society of Medicine*, **87**, 617–619.

Hirvela H, Laatikainen L (1997) Diabetic retinopathy in people aged 70 years or older: the Oulu eye study. *British Journal of Ophthalmology*, **81**, 214–217.

Hurwitz B, Goodman C, Yudkin J (1993) Prompting the clinical care of non-insulin dependent (Type II) diabetic patients in an inner city area: one model of community care. *British Medical Journal*, **306**, 624–630.

Jones R (2000) Self care. *British Medical Journal*, **320**, 596.

Keen H (1996) Management of non-insulin-dependent diabetes mellitus. *Annals of Internal Medicine*, **124**, 156–159.

Keen H, Hall M (1996) Saint Vincent: a new responsibility for general practitioners. *British Journal of General Practice*, **46**, 447–448.

Khunti K, Baker R, Rumsey M, Lakhani M (1999) Quality of care of patients with diabetes: collation of data from multi-practice audits of diabetes in primary care. *Family Practice*, **16**, 54–59.

Kinmonth AL, Griffin S, Wareham NJ (1999) Implications of the United Kingdom prospective diabetes study for general practice care of Type 2 diabetes. *British Journal of General Practice*, **49**, 692–694.

Knight PV, Kesson CM (1986) Educating the elderly diabetic. *Diabetic Medicine*, Education Suppl., 170–172

Koperski M (1992) How effective is systematic care of diabetic patients? A study in one general practice. *British Journal of General Practice*, **42**, 508–511.

Koperski M (2000) The state of primary care in the United States of America and lessons for primary care groups in the United Kingdom. *British Journal of General Practice*, **50**, 319–322.

Krans HR, Porta M, Keen H (1992) Diabetes care and research in Europe: The Saint Vincent Declaration. *Diabetic Medicine*, **7**, 360.

Lauritzen T (1995) Introduction to Type 2 diabetes and the primary health care team. In: Natrass M (ed) *International Symposium on Type 2 Diabetes Mellitus*. Bussum: Medicom Europe BV, 70–75.

MacKinnon M, Wilson MR, Hardisty CA, Ward JD (1989) Novel role for specialist nurses in managing diabetes in the community. *British Medical Journal*, **299**, 552–554.

McGill, Molyneaux LM, Yue DK, Turtle JR (1993) A single visit diabetes complication assessment service: a complement to diabetes management at the primary care level. *Diabetic Medicine*, **10**, 366–370.

Mooy JM, Grootenhuis PA, de Vries H (1995) Prevalence and determinants of glucose intolerance in a Caucasian population: the Hoorn study. *Diabetes Care*, **18**, 1270–1273.

Olesen F, Dickinson J, Hjortdahl P (2000) General practice: time for a new definition. *British Medical Journal*, **320**, 354–357.

Pearson P, Jones K (1994) The primary health care non-team? *British Medical Journal*, **309**, 1387–1388.

Reenders K (1992) *Complications in Non-insulin-dependent Diabetes Mellitus in General Practice*. Thesis, University of Nijmegen.

Reenders K, De Nobel E, Van den Hoogen HJM, van Weel C (1992) Screening for diabetic retinopathy by general practitioners. *Scandinavian Journal of Primary Health Care*, **10**, 306–309.

Retinopathy Working Party (1991) A protocol for screening for diabetic retinopathy in Europe. *Diabetic Medicine*, **8**, 263–267.

Sinclair AJ (1998) Diabetes mellitus. In: Pathy MST (ed) *Principles and Practice of Geriatric Medicine*. Chichester: John Wiley, 1321–1340.

Sinclair AJ, Barnett AH (1993) Special needs of elderly diabetic patients. *British Medical Journal*, **306**, 1142–1143.

Sinclair AJ, Allard I and Bayer AJ (1997a) Observations of diabetes care in long-term institutional settings with measures of cognitive function and dependency. *Diabetes Care*, **20**, 778–784.

Sinclair AJ, Turnbull CJ, Croxson SCM (1997b) Document of diabetes care for residential and nursing homes. *Postgraduate Medical Journal*, **73**, 611–612.

Sonnaville JJJ de, Bouma M, Colly LP, Devillé W, Wijkel D, Heine RJ (1997) Sustained good glycaemic control in NIDDM patients by implementation of structured care in general practice. *Diabeteologia*, **11**, 1334–1340.

Starfield B (1991) Primary care and health. *Journal of the American Medical Association*, **266**, 2268–2271.

Starfield B (1994) Is primary care essential? *Lancet*, **344**, 1129–1132.

Tattersall RB (1984) Diabetes in the elderly: a neglected area? *Diabetologia*, **27**, 167–173.

Thomson FJ, Masson EA (1992) Can elderly diabetic patients co-operate with routine foot care? *Age and Ageing*, **21**, 333–337.

Thorn PA, Russell RG (1973) Diabetic clinics today and tomorrow: mini-clinics in general practice. *British Medical Journal*, **2**, 534–536.

Van Dam HA, Crebolder HFJM, Külcü S, van Veenendaal S, van der Horst FG (1998) Non-attending diabetes patients: a literature search and enquiry of Dutch general practice diabetes experts. *Huisarts and Wetenschap*, **41**, 10–15.

Van Weel C, Tielemans W (1981) Diabetes mellitus in een huisartspraktijk. *Huisarts and Wetenschap*, **24**, 13–17.

Wagner EH (2000) The role of patient care teams in chronic disease management. *British Medical Journal*, **320**, 569–572.

Waine C (1992) The primary care team. *British Journal of General Practice*, **42**, 498–499.

Wilkes E, Lawton EE (1980) The diabetic, the hospital and primary care. *Journal of the Royal College of General Practitioners*, **30**, 199–206.

Wilks JM (1973) Diabetes: a disease for general practice. *Journal of the Royal College of General Practitioners*, **23**, 46–54.

Williams DRR, Munroe C, Hospedales CJ, Greenwood RH (1990) A three-year evaluation of the quality of diabetes care in the Norwich community care scheme. *Diabetic Medicine*, **7**, 74–79.

18

Diabetes in Care Homes

Alan J. Sinclair, Roger Gadsby

University of Birmingham, England, and Centre for Primary Healthcare Studies, University of Warwick, England

INTRODUCTION AND DEFINITIONS

Demographic changes in developed countries in the world are resulting in increasing numbers of people living well into their eighties. In the United Kingdom, a 15% increase in the 85 years and over population is expected between 1995 and 2001. This is leading to a large increase in the number of people being cared for in residential settings in many countries in the developed world. In the UK, 25% of those aged over 85 are living in residential settings (House of Commons Health Committee 1996).

In the UK the number of older frail people receiving residential care outside the National Health Service (NHS) greatly expanded in the last two decades of the twentieth century. The number living in nursing homes now are 157 000 and those in residential homes 288 750 (Royal Commission on Long Term Care 1999). Independent and charitable organizations presently provide 70% of the total provision.

In the UK there are two types of care homes:

- *Residential homes*, which provide personal and social care only. Residents within these settings are usually mobile and are often continent but require the security and provision of daily services such as meals and assistance with personal care such as bathing (Figure 18.1).
- *Nursing homes*, where the residents have much higher levels of dependency, and may have both physical and mental disabilities. These residents typically require the skills of qualified nursing staff 24 hours a day.

Dual registered homes have the facilities to offer both types of care. However, the increasing frailty of many residents makes the distinction between residential and nursing homes redundant in many ways and this chapter is applicable to diabetes care in all residential settings. The term 'care home' is often used as a generic term to cover both types of home. This chapter focuses on the special needs of residents with diabetes.

PREVALENCE OF DIABETES IN RESIDENTIAL SETTINGS

In the USA, the National Nursing Home Survey (National Center for Health Statistics 1979) estimated that 14.5% of nursing home residents had diabetes. Of these 75% were aged 74 years or over and 75% were female.

In two recent UK surveys the estimated prevalence of known diabetes in care homes was 7.2% and 9.9% (Sinclair, Allard and Bayer 1997a; Benbow, Walsh and Gill 1997). These reported prevalence figures for diabetes may, however, be underestimates. A screening program in a Canadian home reclassified 33% of residents as having diabetes during a 3-year period. (Grobin 1970). In a recent UK study of screening residential and nursing home residents for diabetes using two-point (fasting and 2-hour post-glucose challenge values) oral glucose tolerance tests, the overall prevalence was calculated to be 26% with some abnormality of glucose tolerance being present in half of the residents (Sinclair et al 2000a).

CHARACTERISTICS OF CARE IN RESIDENTIAL SETTINGS

There are relatively few reviews of diabetes care in residential settings reported in the world literature (Sinclair et al 1997b; Benbow et al 1997; Cantelon 1972; Zimmer and Franklin Williams 1978); Hamman et al 1984; Mooradian et al 1988; Coulston, Mandel-

Diabetes in Old Age. Second Edition. Edited by A. J. Sinclair and P. Finucane. © 2001 John Wiley & Sons Ltd.

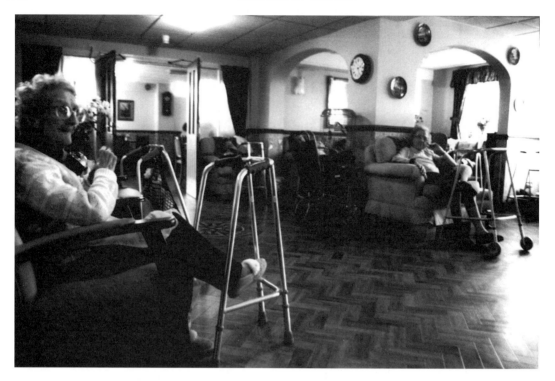

Figure 18.1   Residents within a residential care home

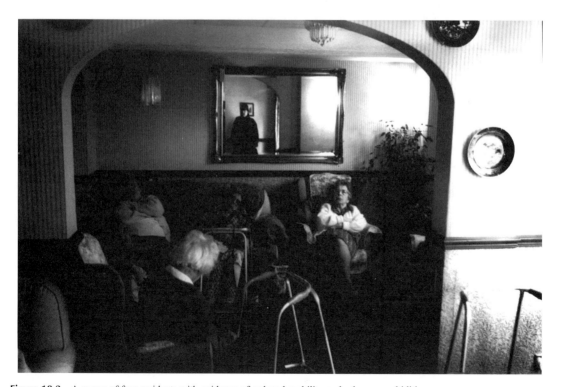

Figure 18.2   A group of four residents with evidence of reduced mobility and other comorbidities

bavum and Reaven 1990; Wolffenbuttel et al 1991; Funnel and Herman 1995). These demonstrate that residents with diabetes appear to be a highly vulnerable and neglected group, characterized by a high prevalence of macrovascular complications, marked susceptibility to infections (especially of the skin and urinary tract), increased hospitalization rates compared with ambulatory diabetic patients, and high levels of physical and cognitive disability (Figure 18.2). Such findings have been reported in studies from the USA (Zimmer and Franklin Williams 1978; Mooradian et al 1988), from Canada (Cantelon 1972), from Holland (Wolffenbuttel et al 1991), and from the UK (Sinclair, Allard and Bayer 1997a; Benbow et al 1997).

The recent UK studies also highlight problems in care delivery (Sinclair et al 1997b; Benbow et al 1997). In both of these studies it was found that health professional input was scant and fragmented and knowledge of diabetes amongst care staff was poor. In one of the studies (Benbow et al 1997), 64% of residents had no record of anyone being responsible for diabetes review and management in the proceeding year. In the UK people living in care homes will be registered with a general practitioner. However, most GPs attend residents only when called by the staff for a specific problem. Problems of transport and mobility often mean that residents cannot get to the GP's surgery or to a hospital outpatient clinic, and so routine follow-up and proactive diabetes care get neglected. In a review of a general practice diabetes clinic, the main group of those non-attending for diabetes annual reviews were those who were housebound and living in care homes (Gadsby 1994).

The UK studies emphasize the need for a reappraisal of diabetes care within institutional settings and the need for the development of agreed national standards of care. A working party of the British Diabetic Association (BDA) has been brought together to discuss these issues and its findings have been published (BDA 1997, 1999). This chapter emphasizes many of the important points highlighted in the BDA reports.

Deficiencies Identified in UK Residential Diabetes Care

The following list of deficiencies in diabetes care within care homes has been compiled from the British Diabetic Association report (1999):

1. *Lack of care plans and case management approaches for individual residents with diabetes.*

This leads to a lack of clarity in defining aims of care and metabolic targets, failure to screen for diabetes-related complications, no annual review procedures, and no allowance for age and dependency level.

2. *Inadequate dietary (nutritional) guidance policies for the anagement of residents with diabetes.*
3. *Lack of specialist health professional input, especially in relation to community dietetic services, diabetes specialist nurses and ophthalmology review.* In addition there is a lack of state registered podiatry provision for residents with diabetes of all ages; especially for those at highest risk of diabetic vascular and neuropathic damage.
4. *Indistinct medical supervision of diabetes-related problems due to lack of clarity of general practitioner and hospital specialist roles.* This leads to inadequate and unstructured follow-up practices.
5. *Inadequate treatment review and metabolic monitoring including blood glucose measurement.*
6. *Insufficient medical knowledge of diabetes and diabetes care among the staff of care homes.*
7. *No structured training and educational programmes for institutional care staff in relation to diabetes and other medical conditions which impact onto the management of diabetes.*

Deficiencies Highlighted in Reports from Other Countries

The deficiencies in care highlighted in the BDA report reflect the difficulty in providing optimum diabetes care in institutional settings. This was confirmed in a study in the United States by Funnel and Herman (1996), who examined diabetes care policies and practices in a group of 17 skilled nursing homes in Michigan. Although the American Diabetes Association (ADA) and the American Association for Diabetes Education developed guidelines for diabetes care in skilled nursing homes in 1981 (Van Nostrand 1985), the authors carried out their review using more recent but less specific criteria derived from the ADA (1995). The homes studied were generally large (mean number of beds, 137) and the number of residents with diabetes per home ranged from 1 to 46 (mean, 19). Almost all the homes reviewed had some diabetes care protocols, plans or standing orders in place, although standing orders usually consisted of guidelines relating to nutrition or some aspects of nursing care. Guidelines of care relating to parameters of metabolic control, when to call a physician, or surveillance of complications were least often present. In general the care provided did not meet local or national standards of diabetes care, but care practices were better when registered dietitians were involved in meal planning and where written institutional policies were actually present.

If these are the sort of deficiencies and difficulties in diabetes care recorded in institutional settings in both the UK and the USA, what should be the broad aims of optimal care?

AIMS OF DIABETES CARE IN INSTITUTIONAL SETTINGS

Residents with diabetes in care homes should receive a level of comprehensive diabetes care commensurate with their needs. This should be on an equitable basis with those people with diabetes who do not live in an institutional setting. The two most important objectives are:

1. To maintain the highest degree of quality of life and well-being without subjecting residents to unnecessary and inappropriate medical and therapeutic interventions.
2. To provide sufficient support and opportunity to enable residents to manage their own diabetes condition where this is a feasible and worthwhile option.

However, there are several additional processes of care which represent important goals to achieve for any resident with diabetes in a care home:

- To achieve an optimum level of metabolic control which avoids the malaise and lethargy of hyperglycaemia, substantially reduces the risk of hypoglycaemia in those residents taking sulphonylureas or insulin, and allows the greatest level of physical and cognitive function to be attained.
- To optimise footcare to preserve the integrity of the feet. This promotes the highest level of mobility possible and prevents unnecessary (and usually prolonged) hospital admissions for diabetic foot problems.
- To optimise eye care to preserve visual function.
- To screen for neurovascular complications, especially for peripheral neuropathy and peripheral vascular disease which both predispose to foot infection and ulceration.
- To manage coexisting disease in a structured way

with an emphasis on diagnosis and treatment of depressive illness, congestive cardiac failure and hypertension.

- To provide a well-balanced individualized healthy eating diet which is compatible with nutritional well-being and maintenance of bodyweight.

Effective monitoring and control of blood pressure is also an essential part of medical management within care homes.

BARRIERS TO OPTIMISING DIABETES CARE

Within any healthcare system, barriers exist which may lessen the efficiency of the organization or prevent optimal delivery of care. In care homes, lack of sufficient training, and opportunities for continuing professional development in diabetes care among all care staff may be present. This can contribute to the high staff turnover seen in many homes. This is compounded by high ratios of unqualified staff who may have little experience of looking after residents with diabetes, and lack of available resources of staff time, catering services and equipment.

In some cases, there may be a lack of clear boundaries of both medical and nursing responsibilities which may be exacerbated by poor communication channels. A basic understanding of the modern principles of dietary provision may not be known by the care staff, which may have profound implications for managing diabetes in these settings. In view of the high levels of comorbidities including neurological problems, various communication difficulties in residents with diabetes may exist which prevents needs being met. Restrictive professional boundaries which prevent healthcare professionals from having specific inputs into care homes especially within the independent sector may also be present. Quite clearly, establishing national standards of diabetes care within care homes may be an important initiative to promote care within these settings.

COMMON MANAGEMENT PROBLEMS

In view of the many barriers to care outlined above, common management problems can arise. These are listed in Table 18.1 and discussed below.

Table 18.1 Management problems in care homes

Nutritional deficiency and weight loss
Increased risk of hypoglycaemia
Infections
Urinary incontinence
Pressure sores
Leg and foot ulceration
Communication difficulties
Increased risk of adverse drug reactions

Nutritional deficiency and weight loss. This can occur through anorexic symptoms and reduced calorific intake. Other contributing factors include severe physical and cognitive impairment, as well as neurological and gastroenterological disorders associated with dysphagia, including stroke

Increased risk of hypoglycaemia. This condition may occur in residents on sulphonlyureas or insulin through several predisposing factors. These include: (a) nutritional deficiency and weight loss; (b) cognitive impairment resulting in meals being missed through poor memory and orientation; (c) anorexic conditions such as malignancy or infection; (d) lack of awareness of the symptoms and signs of hypoglycaemia by residents themselves or by care staff. The latter may be compounded by a lack of monitoring of diabetes by residents and staff.

Infections. Recurrent skin, chest and urinary infections may occur, especially if control of blood glucose is not optimal. Infections themselves predispose the resident with diabetes to marked hyperglycaemia or metabolic decompensation owing to hyperosmolar non-ketotic coma or ketosis.

Urinary incontinence. This may be secondary to hyperglycaemia, urinary infection, poor mobility or cognitive impairment.

Pressure sores and leg or foot ulceration. These can lead to rapid deterioration and need for hospital admission.

Communication difficulties. These can lead to unrecognized diabetes care needs. Predisposing factors include cognitive impairment, dysphasia and dysarthria from cerebrovascular or other neurological disease, and sensory impairments such as visual and hearing loss.

Increased risk of adverse drug reactions. These can occur because residents are often taking multiple drugs for their diabetes and other coexisting diseases. Risks can be exacerbated by infrequent review of medication and lack of monitoring of renal and hepatic function.

STRATEGIES TO IMPROVE DEFICIENCIES OF DIABETES CARE IN RESIDENTIAL SETTINGS

It is clear that there is a lack of diabetes-related experience and knowledge amongst various categories of care home staff. Unless there is appropriate education and training it is unlikely that future improvements in diabetes care will be sufficient to address the present deficiencies in care and meet any future recommended outcomes.

There are a number of difficulties in providing education and training in care homes. These include the fact that some care home managers have little or no staff training budget to pay for training and so are reliant on free advice and information. Care staff in some homes are often young and unskilled, and other older members of staff although more experienced, may often be part time and unqualified. Nursing staff in care homes work a rotating shift system which can lead to a lack of continuity of care, and which creates difficulties in attending training events. Care homes often have a high staff turnover, and poor pay and conditions can lead to low staff morale, which mitigates against effective training and education.

In spite of these difficulties some diabetes training and education events have been run in homes by local diabetes care teams, often comprising of the diabetes specialist nurse, local diabetes dietitian and podiatrist. These are usually welcomed by care home managers, and their success seems to relate to good local relationships being built up. It also requires the local diabetes team to feel a responsibility for these homes and to be allowed by their managers to go in and help.

In the United Kingdom, trade associations such as the Independent Healthcare Association—which is the largest in the independent sector, representing acute, psychiatric, and long-term care providers across the UK—can assist in improving diabetes care. By facilitating promotion and dissemination of best practice, research reports, and quality control systems within care homes, they are well placed to liaise with care home owners, managers and staff to support education and training initiatives.

Dietary Needs of Diabetic Residents

Residents are likely to have several reasons for being nutritionally at risk. These include a lack of nutritional knowledge and outdated ideas about diabetic diets held by some staff. It is vital that up-to-date information about diabetes and healthy eating be given to care home staff, especially those who have responsibility for menu planning, food purchasing and cooking.

The local community dietitian (where available) will usually be a good source of help and advice in implementing healthy eating policies. They may often be able to help in staff training on the dietary aspects of diabetes care.

Responsibility of the Physician

All residents of care homes in the UK are registered with a general practitioner. The increasing numbers of elderly people in care homes is having a significant impact on the workload of many GPs (Pell and Williams 1990; Kavanagh and Knapp 1998). Under present contractual arrangements in the NHS there is usually no recognition or encouragement to GPs to provide the appropriate levels of proactive care that those with diabetes living in residential settings need. Although some GPs make regular visits to homes to review residents, most visits to care homes are 're-active' in nature and take place only when a problem has been identified by the home staff.

Many residents of care homes have mobility problems which prevent them getting to the GP surgery for an annual review, and few GPs provide a full multidisciplinary annual review service in the care home.

The care home resident will often have been discharged from hospital outpatient review when they were admitted to the home. Those who remain under out patient review may default from follow-up because of increasing problems with mobility or transportation to the hospital clinic which may be many miles from the home.

Changes in management and clinical responsibilities of physicians in geriatric medicine have meant that in recent years they have spent more time in acute medical care, and less in continuing and community care. This is partly due to the reduction of NHS hospital long-term care beds; a withdrawal from acute admission duties by some medical specialities; and the lack of commissioning priority for the continuing healthcare needs of frail older people in the contracting process. (Bowman et al 1999a). The transfer of long-term care from hospitals to care homes has not been accompanied by any significant transfer of medical resources to the community. In consequence older people in care homes increasingly fall between primary, secondary and social care services, and all too often their needs get forgotten (Bowman et al 1999).

A number of possible solutions to the problem of developing a coherent policy to medical care in residential settings were listed in a *BMJ* editorial in 1997 (Black and Bowman 1997). These included:

1. Visiting medical officers could be appointed specifically to provide the medical management. Some have been established, but their relationships with primary and secondary care and their accountability are largely unresolved.
2. Geriatric medical and psychiatric outreach services could be set up. Hospital departments would become responsible for routine surveillance and management of people in care homes. Out-of-hours and emergency cover would be provided by co-operatives. This option would require a significant shift of resources to secondary care and become a major commitment for hospital departments.
3. Shared medical care could be established. Routine care would remain the responsibility of the GP, but hospital staff would have an increased role to support and facilitate care through visiting and advice. Though attractive in some ways, this option would not address the real problems of workload in primary care. Furthermore legal liabilities when differing opinions exist would need careful exploration.
4. Integrated medical care could be organized. Primary care would retain responsibility, with service payments for medical assessments on admission and for reviews. Geriatric services would provide structured support through the development of care management programs. This model seems to allow the strengths of primary care to be developed, defining and developing specialist responsibility, whilst providing a work-sensitive solution for remuneration of general practitioners.
5. Health maintenance organizations could be set up. Homes would then become American-style health

maintenance organizations employing their own staff on their own terms.

The fourth option has many attractions and complements the recommendations of the Burgner report for a single registration and inspection system for care homes (Burgner 1996).

No change in the medical care of residents of care homes in the UK had yet taken place three years after the publication of this editorial. At the time of writing, GPs are still responsible for medical care of individual residents registered with their practice. There is as yet no formal structure for the routine involvement of consultants in geriatric medicine nor other healthcare professionals to give the multidisciplinary diabetes care that residents need. In the absence of any formal national structure local, ad hoc arrangements occur to try to enable the best multidisciplinary care to take place.

Multidisciplinary Diabetes Care

Elements of multidisciplinary diabetes care include the following:

- An individualized diabetes care plan. Each resident with diabetes should play a part in establishing agreed objectives summarized in a care plan which should include a series of metabolic targets.
- An individualized dietary and nutritional plan as part of the overall care plan.
- An annual review assessment involving a diabetes eye check and foot check.
- Support and assistance in diabetes care from a named person who will be involved in metabolic monitoring with the resident.
- Ensuring that the residents with diabetes have their names recorded in the local district diabetes register and participate in local clinical diabetes audit.

In the locally variable arrangements that exist in the UK, these elements may (or may not) be provided by a number of healthcare professionals. These are now outlined, although some of the statements made may not be applicable outside the UK.

Diabetes specialist nurses. These nurses, who have had special training and education in diabetes, are known to be an invaluable link between primary and secondary diabetes care for older people (Sinclair, Turnbull and Croxson 1996) and can provide a high-quality service to disadvantaged people with diabetes

(Norman et al 1998). Some DSNs are employed to work in the community, and within the time constraints of their busy jobs may become involved in diabetes education and support for all home care staff, assisting in the development of the diabetes care policies for the home and individual care plans.

Primary care practice nurses. In some general practices the practice nurse who has had special training in diabetes may be empowered to visit residents of the practice who are living in care homes, to assist in the delivery of the care objectives outlined above.

District (community) nurses. District nurses can play an immense supporting role in diabetes care in residential settings, despite many receiving little if any special training in this area. The major remit of the district nurse is in the provision of nursing support to residents with diabetes and advice to care staff in residential homes. They are also involved in insulin administration (in some cases twice a day) to residents who require insulin and are unable to self-inject because of physical or cognitive disability or behavioural disturbance. In selected cases, and where a specific contract exists between the care home and the District Nursing service on behalf of the District Health Authority (UK), district nurses may be responsible for delegating specific diabetes care tasks to named members of a care home. These duties require to be closely monitored by the nurse and remain their professional responsibility for providing adequate training of the care staff member (Department of Health 1996).

Provision of Footcare

Published information from many countries of the world testifies to the high prevalence of diabetic foot disease in residents of care homes (Sinclair et al 1997b; Cantelon 1972; Mooradian et al 1988; Wolffenbuttel et al 1991). The risk of foot ulceration is increased in those with advancing age, loss of protective pain sensation due to diabetic peripheral neuropathy, peripheral vascular disease, and bony foot abnormalities (Gadsby and McInnes 1998).

The residents in some homes have access to free care from state registered podiatrists, whilst in other homes private podiatrists are employed, when residents may have to pay fees for footcare. In some care homes there is no structured plan for footcare. Where available, a local state registered podiatrist with an interest in diabetes is a very important member of the district multidisciplinary diabetes team, and his or her skills need to be utilized by care home staff in appropriate ways.

All people with diabetes should have a foot examination yearly as part of the review process, and residents in care homes are not exempt from this recommendation (BDA 1997). This examination is to detect feet at risk of ulceration. At its simplest this involves a brief history to discover any previous episodes of ulceration, inspection of the feet to check for bony abnormalities, palpation of the dorsalis pedis and posterior tibial pulses to detect ischaemia, and use of the 5.07 g nylon monofilament to detect loss of protective pain sensation. This foot examination can be done by any member of the community diabetes team who has the relevant skills and experience. If the foot is deemed to be at risk it should be checked every 3 months by a podiatrist, and extra foot education given (Gadsby and McInnes 1998).

It is also important to train care home staff to understand the importance of preventive footcare, and to alert them to the importance of detecting early signs of foot ulceration and/or infection so that urgent prompt referral and action can be taken. The local state registered podiatrist with an interest in diabetes will usually be the best person to provide this help.

Provision of Eye Care

Lack of specialist eye care and regular ophthalmology review of residents with diabetes has been demonstrated in UK care homes (Sinclair et al 1997b; Benbow et al 1997). In a recent large community-based study of older people with diabetes, some of whom were residents of care homes, a large proportion of subjects had evidence of major undetected refractive error. (Sinclair et al 2000b).

Screening programs for detecting diabetes-related eye problems are being set up in many districts of the UK. Many are based on examinations being carried out by experienced and specially trained optometrists who are able to check for refractive error, glaucoma and cataract whilst also checking for diabetic retinopathy using the technique of indirect opthalmoscopy through dilated pupils. In other districts, diabetes eye screening is based on taking photographs of the retina using a special camera. The evidence is at present insufficient to make specific recommendation on which is the best method of screening (Department of Health 1999).

However, both of these screening techniques require the use of expensive equipment which is not easily portable, and so may be difficult to use in care homes.

There may also be other organizational and professional barriers to the involvement of optometrists in care homes. These include a lack of locally agreed protocols and funding arrangements to make optometric examination in care homes a financially viable option for the self-employed optometrist.

Optometric assessment for residents of care homes could be improved by several measures as follows:

- Adequate funding of optometric assessment by contractual arrangements with the local health authority and social services, to allow (a) improved and regular access of optometrists into care homes, and (b) visual screening of all new admissions who have diabetes.
- Improved accommodation and facilities at each care home to allow full optometric assessment to be carried out.
- Education of care staff about the importance of maintaining visual health in residents.
- Identifying a member of the care home staff to take responsibility for organizing visits by the optometrist and prior instilling (where appropriate) of eye-drops for retinal examination through dilated pupils
- An improved referral system for residents in care homes who have eye problems identified requiring specialist secondary care.

ASSESSING THE EFFICACY AND EFFICIENCY OF DIABETES CARE

Outcome measurement of *hospital-based* care, and of acute inpatient and outpatient services, is fairly well developed in the UK (Higginson 1994). A uniform, comprehensive, standardized assessment for routine long-term care of older people, the minimum dataset–resident assessment instrument (MDS-RAI), has been introduced into all nursing homes in the United States, Iceland, and three provinces in Canada. A US research group has combined data from the MDS-RAI instrument, including detailed drug use information, with data from Medicare enrolment and hospital discharge claims files, enabling the study of drug treatment effects using valid measures of outcome in this frail population (Carpenter 2000).

Outcome measures for older adults with diabetes have been published (Sinclair et al 1996), but they have not been tested in care home settings. Outcomes chosen need to be sensitive to an intervention; but care delivered within residential settings consists of multiple interventions, making the correct choice of suitable outcomes to measure complex and difficult. In addition, resident-centred outcomes which require self-assessment forms to be completed may not be appropriate for many frail residents of care homes.

The purpose of outcome measures in care homes is:

- to assess the quality of care delivered to each resident with diabetes
- to assess the impact of diabetes on each resident in terms of personal well-being, functional disability, and rate of diabetes complications
- to determine the impact of use of care home resources for residents with diabetes in terms of use of care staff time, dietary planning, monitoring equipment, and educational initiatives.

Potential outcome measures are summarized in Table 18.2.

Data collection needs to be done by care staff and visiting healthcare professionals and must represent common objectives of diabetes care for all parties.

SUSTAINING EFFECTIVE DIABETES CARE

A summary of recommendations relating to diabetes care of older residents in residential settings has been published (Sinclair et al 1997b). Further more detailed recommendations are contained the recent BDA report (1999), outlining what must be provided at a care home

Table 18.2 Outcome measures for use in residential diabetes care

1. The percentage of residents achieving agreed metabolic targets of HBA_{1c}, blood pressure, and weight during previous 12 months
2. Frequency and severity of hypoglycaemic episodes in previous 12 months
3. Frequency of hospital admissions for diabetes-related problems in previous 12 months
4. Complication rates of visual loss, foot ulceration, renal impairment, and angina
5. Changes in level of dependency and physical and mental functions using the Barthel ADL or extended ADL measures during previous 12 months
6. Quality of life and well-being of each resident with diabetes using the SF 36 or sickness impact profile measures; changes from admission to now, or changes within previous 12 months
7. The percentage of patients with completed diabetes care plans and annual reviews in past 12 months
8. Number of staff who have received education in diabetes care

and in the locality to sustain effective diabetes care. These are outlined below.

What the Care Home Needs to Provide

In order to sustain effective diabetes care, homes need to provide a suitable care environment in terms of staff, resources, equipment and facilities. These should include: (a) one or more staff members who have received appropriate training and education in the basic management of residents with diabetes in care home settings; (b) facilities to carry out blood glucose monitoring, and staff trained in the use of the equipment; (c) provision of a room suitable for annual review examination of residents, and podiatric footcare; (d) a member of catering staff familiar with dietary planning for residents with diabetes who is able to provide suitable meals; (e) a protocol of diabetes care agreed by the staff of the home, visiting diabetes healthcare professionals and the GP; (f) a method of collecting agreed diabetes outcome indicator data; (g) one or more members of staff trained to administer insulin; (h) educational resources on diabetes for residents and their families; (i) access to transport to enable residents to receive specialist treatment outside the home; and (j) an admission policy that highlights those with known diabetes and screens for diabetes in those not known to have it.

What Needs to be Provided at the Local Level

Local diabetes care services must encompass the special needs of residents with diabetes in care homes and must provide support and guidance for the homes. This could include the following recommendations:

1. Health and social service contracts should be agreed which provide adequate funding to enable high-quality diabetes care to be delivered. This will require local negotiation within nationally agreed guidelines. Such guidelines are not yet in place, and the funding of care in care homes is still the subject of government debate in the UK. The process of local negotiation may be helped in the UK through the emergence of Primary Care Groups (PCGs) many of whom will develop into Primary Care Trusts (PCTs) within a few years. PCGs aim to bring together both primary care medical services and social services to develop

common policies and budgets, which ought to be a help to care home residents.

2. Optometric services should be supported and funded to provide both on-site and clinic-based eye services for residents with diabetes in care homes.

3. Podiatry services should be supported and funded to provide services for care home residents.

4. Criteria for referral to secondary care specialist services should be agreed by all relevant parties including GPs and secondary care staff.

5. At least one diabetes specialist nurse with specific remit for older people with diabetes should be appointed in each district. His or her remit would encompass the requirements of residents within care homes. They would play a prominent role in the effective organization of diabetes care for care homes in their area, and provide momentum for developing diabetes educational initiatives in care homes.

6. At least one community dietitian should be identified in each locality, whose responsibility would be the dietary and nutritional support for residents in care homes.

7. Residents in care homes should be on the locality diabetes register to ensure that they are involved in diabetes clinical audit projects.

8. Diabetes educational and training programs for care home staff need to be established at either a local, regional or national level to ensure that staff are kept up to date with developments in diabetes care.

CONCLUSIONS

Diabetes care in residential settings has not previously attracted a great deal of scientific clinical enquiry, and so little has been known about the quality of diabetes care delivered, or the outcomes of care in residential settings. Thus there are many important topics for future clinical research as the number of people with diabetes resident in care homes across the world continues to grow rapidly.

The tremendous morbidity and disability of residents with diabetes within long-term care poses many complex and challenging problems for all healthcare professionals involved in delivering diabetes care. This chapter has outlined these and offered a number of practical strategies to improve care. Our hope is that these will be taken up and acted upon by all who can influence diabetes care delivery in residential settings in other countries.

REFERENCES

ADA (American Diabetes Association) (1995) Clinical practice recommendations. *Diabetes Care*, **18** (Suppl. 1), 1–96.

BDA (British Diabetic Association) (1997) *Recommendations for the Management of Diabetes in Primary Care*. London: BDA.

BDA (British Diabetic Association) (1999) *Guidelines of Practice for Residents with Diabetes in Care Homes*. London: BDA.

Benbow SJ, Walsh A, Gill GV (1997) Diabetes in institutionalised elderly people: a forgotten population. *British Medical Journal*, **314**, 1868–1869.

Black D, Bowman C (1997) Community institutional care for frail elderly people: time to structure professional responsibility. *British Medical Journal*, **315**, 441–442.

Bowman C, Johnson M, Venebles D, Foote C, Kane RL (1999) Geriatric care in the UK: aligning services to needs. *British Medical Journal*, **319**, 1119–1122.

Burgner T (1996) *The Regulation and Inspection of Social Services*. London: Department of Health.

Cantelon JFD (1972) Diabetic residents of homes for the aged: observations for an eleven year period. *Journal of the American Geriatrics Society*, **26**, 17–21.

Carpenter GI, Bernabei R, Hirdes JP, Mor V, Steel K (2000) Building evidence on chronic disease in old age. *British Medical Journal*, **320**, 528–529.

Coulston AM, Mandelbaum D, Reaven GM (1990) Dietary management of nursing home residents with non insulin dependent diabetes mellitus. *American Journal of Clinical Nutrition*, **51**, 67–71.

Department of Health (1996) *NHS Continuing Care Guidance*. London: DOH.

Department of Health (1999) *Effective Health Care Bulletin*, **5**(4), 1–6.

Funnel MM, Herman WH (1995) Diabetes care policies and practices in Michigan nursing homes, 1991. *Diabetes Care*, 1995; **18**, 862–866.

Gadsby R (1994) Care of people with diabetes who are housebound or in nursing and residential homes. *Diabetes in General Practice*, **4**(3), 30–31

Gadsby R, McInnes A (1998) The at-risk foot: the role of the primary care team in achieving St Vincent targets for reducing amputation. *Diabetic Medicine*, 1998 **15** (Suppl. 3), S61–S64.

Grobin W (1970) Diabetes in the aged: underdiagnosis and over-treatment. *CMA Journal*, **103**, 915–923.

Hamman RF, Michael SL, Keefer SM, Young WF (1984) Impact of policy and procedure changes on hospital days among diabetic nursing home residents—Colorado. *Morbidity and Mortality Weekly Report* **33**, 621–629.

Higginson I (1994) Clinical teams, general practice, audit and outcomes. In: Delamothe T (ed.) *Outcomes in Clinical Practice*. London: BMJ Publishing Group, 28–39.

House of Commons Health Committee (1996) *Review of Long-term Care*. London: HMSO.

Kavanagh S, Knapp M (1998) The impact on general practitioners of the changing balance of care for elderly people living in institutions. *British Medical Journal* **317**, 322–327.

Mooradian AD, Osterweil D, Petrasek D Morley JE (1998) Diabetes mellitus in elderly nursing home patients: a survey of clinical characteristics and management. *Journal of the American Geriatrics Society* **36**, 391–396.

National Center for Health Statistics (1979) *The National Nursing Home Survey 1977. Summary for the United States*. Hyattsville, MD: US Government Printing Office.

Norman A, French M, Hyam V, Hicks D (1998) Development and audit of a home clinic service. *Journal of Diabetes Nursing*, **2**(2), 51–54.

Pell J, Williams S (1999) Do nursing home residents make greater demands on GPs? A prospective comparative study. *British Journal of General Practice*, **49**, 527–530.

Royal Commission on Long Term Care (1999) *With Respect to Old Age*. London: Stationary Office.

Sinclair AJ, Turnbull CJ, Croxson SCM (1996) Document of care for older people with diabetes: Clinical guidelines. *Postgraduate Medical Journal*, **72**, 334–338.

Sinclair AJ, Allard I, Bayer AJ (1997a) Observations of diabetes care in long-term institutional settings with measures of cognitive function and dependency. *Diabetes Care*, **20**, 778–784.

Sinclair AJ, Turnbull CJ, Croxson SCM (1997b) Document of diabetes care for residential and nusing homes. *Postgraduate Medical Journal*, **73**, 611–612.

Sinclair AJ, Gadsby R, Penfold S, Croxson S (2000a) Diabetes mellitus in care homes: underdetected and untreated. *Age and Ageing* Abstract (in press).

Sinclair AJ, Bayer AJ, Girling AJ and Woodhouse KW (2000b) Older adults, diabetes mellitus and visual acuity: a community-based case-control study. *Age and Ageing* **29**, 335–339.

Van Nostrand JF (1985) Nursing home care for diabetics. In: *Diabetes in America: Diabetes Data Compiled by National Diabetes Data Group*. Washington, DC: US Govt Printing Office (NIH publ. 85–1468).

Wolffenbuttel BHR, van Vliet S, Knols AJF, Slits WLH, Sels J-PJE, Nieuwenhuijzen Kruseman ACN (1991) Clinical characteristics and management of diabetic patients residing in a nursing home. *Diabetes Research and Clinical Practice*, **13**, 199–206.

Zimmer JG, Franklin Williams T (1978) Spectrum of severity and control of diabetes mellitus in skilled nursing facilities. *Journal of the American Geriatrics Society*, **26**, 443–452.

19

Modern Perspectives and Recent Advances

Christopher J. Turnbull, Alan J. Sinclair

Arrowe Park Hospital and University of Birmingham

INTRODUCTION

Diabetes in old age is not to be taken lightly. Not only are the numbers of older people increasing, but also obesity which is a major risk factor for Type 2 diabetes is more prevalent in the Western world and levels of physical activity are reduced. This creates the potential for a large increase in the prevalence of this metabolic disorder. We know that complications are common at the onset of diabetes, so early detection would appear to be justified. In the last few years there is increasing evidence of the value of improved glucose control in reducing the frequency of complications. Regrettably these studies have not yet included the very old. However, we know that diabetes in old age is associated with an increased mortality and morbidity (Bourdel-Marchanon et al 1998; Sinclair, Robert and Croxson 1997). It would seem particularly important to take diabetes in old age seriously.

There is considerable evidence of the poor organization of diabetes care especially for older people. Good organization with structured care does lead to better outcomes. Many European countries have been attempting to implement the St Vincent Declaration whose aims are to improve management of diabetes and reduce complications (World Health Organization 1989). One important way to improve care within a district or specific region is to recognize all those with diabetes by construction of a register. This can be used to target structured care.

In the last few years a lot of research on diabetes in old age has taken place. The value of screening for diabetes has been investigated and a change in the standards for diagnosis has been implemented in many countries. Research has shown us more of the specific effects of age on glucose tolerance and in management of diabetes and recognition of hypoglycaemia. In older people, good footcare is especially important as is prevention of cardiovascular disease and management of hypertension and hyperlipidaemia. The effect of diabetes on cognitive function has received increasing attention. We know more about the effective prevention of retinopathy and the organization of schemes for early detection is under way. More work is being done on prevention and management of neuropathy. Finally, there is a lot of research on new drugs for Type 2 diabetes which is finally bearing fruit, giving more options for treatment. Also the role, safety and method of insulin administration in older people are now being actively researched. These areas will be considered in more detail.

SCREENING

Regrettably no study has been done to show that early diagnosis of Type 2 diabetes improves outcome. In the past it has been argued that the new onset of diabetes in old age does not affect overall life expectancy. Recent research shows that this is not the case (Sinclair et al 1997). In addition, the United Kingdom Prospective Diabetes Study (UKPDS) has shown that tighter control of Type 2 diabetes improves outcome (UKPDS 1998a). If treatment does make a difference, and untreated the outcome is adverse, it seems quite likely that early diagnosis would be beneficial. It is possible to reduce the late microvascular and macrovascular complications of diabetes by effective management of glucose control, hypertension and hyperlipidaemia. This should take into account the fact that patients with diabetes have on average probably had an impairment of glucose tolerance for about 12 years prior to diagnosis (Adler et al 1999).

Diabetes in Old Age. Second Edition. Edited by A. J. Sinclair and P. Finucane. © 2001 John Wiley & Sons Ltd.

Which Screening Test?

If we consider that screening for diabetes in older people is worthwhile, how should it be done? In screening studies the most appropriate tests depend on the prevalence of diabetes in the tested population. A different test is required in Pima Indians, where the prevalence of diabetes is 45%, to that required for residents of Melton Mowbray in Leicestershire where it is 6% (Croxson et al 1991). Thus testing in an area with a high Asian population in whom the prevalence of diabetes is high may require different tests compared with a Caucasian population. One method commonly employed is to check a fasting urine sample for glucose. However, this test is too insensitive, detecting < 20% of cases even though > 95% of positive cases have diabetes. These figures would apply to a typical British population. Some tests are too difficult to carry out for screening large populations with a low prevalence of diabetes; e.g. the oral glucose tolerance test (OGTT). Probably the simplest tests are a post-prandial blood glucose with a sensitivity of 80% and a positive predictive value of 5–10%, or 1-hour post-prandial glycosuria with a sensitivity of about 70% and positive predictive value of 20–30%. Testing for glycosylated hemoglobin (HbA_{1c}) is sensitive (90%)—a result outside the normal range is considered positive but the positive predictive value is low (14–33%). It is also expensive, and for this reason another test of longer-term glucose control which is used is fructosamine. There are those who argue that a fasting blood glucose is useful because a low threshold (e.g. > 5.5 mM) gives reasonable sensitivity of 70–90% and a positive predictive value of 20–45% (Paterson 1994) (Table 19.1).

Only about 25% of new patients with diabetes diagnosed by screening have symptoms of polyuria and polydipsia, so 75% are asymptomatic (Croxson and Burden 1998).

How Should Screening be Carried Out?

Carrying out screening is difficult on a population basis in older people as many are not keen to attend screening; but opportunistic screening, such as at the over-75 year old annual check by general practitioners in the UK, may be worthwhile. In fact the test probably does not need to be done every year. With the average deterioration in glucose tolerance with age that is expected, a frequency of testing every 3–5 years would be satisfactory.

Offering screening in the open (e.g. at outdoor meetings or in a pharmacy) is advocated by some but can be difficult to organize and carry out effectively. For example, the policy should state clearly what should be done when a positive test is found. Techniques used by the screeners should be safe and eliminate the risk of cross-infection when using fingerprick lancets or automated fingerpricking devices. It may be more valuable to use a screening questionnaire to detect diabetes (Ruige et al 1997).

In hospitals blood glucose is often measured on admission. This could be a good way of early detection of diabetes; but owing to organizational difficulties in hospitals, such an opportunity is often missed (Levetan et al 1998).

ORGANIZATION OF DIABETES SERVICES

In the wake of the St Vincent Declaration, there has been increasing evidence of the value of regular review of people with diabetes and sustained efforts made to improve the organization of services for people with diabetes (World Health Organization 1989). In the UK, for example, many health districts have established a register of people with diabetes which can be used to arrange regular recall for review. Some people have, however, questioned the value of these registers (Elwyn et al 1998). Structured care is particularly important for older people with diabetes who are often missing out at present (Sinclair and Barnett 1993). Care can improve as a result of proper organization (Griffin 1998). In the UK one important factor is the shift of care from secondary (hospital) to primary care, so it is particularly important that general practitioners are well organized (Goyder et al 1998). Using nursing staff provided with protocols can improve care within a

Table 19.1 The sensitivity and positive predictive value of different screening tests for diabetes

Test	Sensitivity (%)	Positive predictive value (%)
Fasting urine	<20%	>95%
Post-prandial blood glucose >11.1 mM	80%	5–10%
Post-prandial glycosuria	70%	20–30%
Glycosylated haemoglobin	90%	14–33%
Fasting blood glucose >5.5 mM	70–90%	20–45%

Source: Paterson (1994).

structured program (Peters and Davidson 1998). Diabetes specialist nurses (DSNs) have an especially important role in diabetes care of older people. They should be available not only to manage individual patients but also to provide advice and support to the many general practice (primary healthcare) nurses who provide much of the routine care. Audits have demonstrated that many housebound and institutionalized people with diabetes have been missing out on routine preventative care (Gadsby 1994). One useful response to this has been the appointment of community-based diabetes nurses who visit these patients in their own homes.

Geriatricians manage many older people with diabetes in hospital, but a few only provide structured outpatient care. As many of these frail older patients do not receive diabetes care elsewhere, it would seem important for geriatricians to provide it (Hendra and Sinclair 1997). More recently, new developments in providing diabetes care within the secondary sector have been proposed and include fast-tract vascular work-up, functional assessment and active screening for complications, and establishing specific diabetic rehabilitation programs (Sinclair 2000). Another feature is the emergence of critical-event monitoring, which is a system of monitoring those critical periods or episodes of major health or social care need when patient vulnerability is highest and when a suitable intervention is likely to be present. Examples include foot ulceration or admission to hospital for metabolic coma.

A favoured model of care in the UK is joint shared care between a hospital team and primary (general practice) care. This needs to be structured to be effective so that everyone understands exactly what their own role is in this joint care program. The hospital can provide technical aspects of care not readily available in the community; e.g. eye screening if not available in the community, and access to a mutidisciplinary rehabilitation team where disability is an issue.

THE ANNUAL REVIEW

In the last few years research has refined some aspects of the annual review. Eye screening is now known to be better provided using a camera to photograph the fundus, either with a Polaroid multiple field view approach or by newly developing digital photography (Ryder 1995; Taylor et al 1999). However, many ophthalmologists feel that direct stereoscopic slit lamp examination is the best method of examination. Increasingly, optometrists are being trained to provide this technique so that effective eye screening is now available outside hospital. Where careful training of optometrists and audit of the service is inbuilt, this can be an effective technique.

Amputation remains a major complication of older people with diabetes, and so good footcare is essential as is a properly organized preventative care program. A 10 g nylon monofilament is a simple way to test for evidence of neuropathy in diabetes. Patients can be taught to use this simple device for themselves (Birke and Rolfsen 1998). Good education and adequate literature are important (Connor 1997). Diabetic patients need to be especially careful about footwear, which needs to be properly measured (Litzelman and Marriott 1997; Uccioli et al 1995). Early intervention is needed when problems are detected, to avoid amputation. This would include good vascular surgical support (Levin 1995). Many older people cannot manage to reach or inspect their own feet, so it is important that caregivers are also taught the appropriate techniques (Thomson and Masson 1996).

The annual review is not only about detection and management of complications. Education and verifying comprehension of and concordance with dietary guidelines are important. Patients must be made aware about driving regulations which, in Europe, are now internationally based (Sheppard 1998). Patients also need to know how to obtain adequate life insurance, health insurance, motor insurance etc. Crash rates are said not to be increased in the diabetic elderly (McGwin et al 1999). Where the patient has any form of disability, it is necessary to check how the patient is coping and whether any therapeutic or rehabilitative management is appropriate. Home adaptations may be required and the patient may be eligible for additional welfare support (e.g. in the UK, attendance allowance). For some patients, blind registration may be appropriate to ensure adequate social support. The annual review gives the opportunity to find out how caregivers are coping and arrange caregiver support if it is available, such as through home care, day care or respite care if required.

SELF-MONITORING

Setting targets for diabetic control can improve blood glucose control (Martin, Young and Kesson 1986) but increases treatment burden (van der Does et al 1998) and does not necessarily increase well-being. However, the effect on reducing complications is still uncertain (Faas, Schellevis and Van Eijk 1997). It is argued, therefore, that only patients with poor glycemic control are likely to benefit from self monitoring, but these may be the very patients who are least able to carry it out. In order to implement changes in management arising from varying glucose levels, good patient comprehension and compliance are essential. Patients using insulin should be instructed on self-monitoring where they are capable of understanding it (American Diabetes Association 1990). This is particularly important if the patient is subject to hypoglycaemia and when it is necessary to implement 'sick day rules' (Diabetes UK, 10 Queen Anne St, London W1M OBD). When the basis of blood glucose monitoring is understood by the patient, increased accuracy of monitoring may be superior to urine monitoring. Urine monitoring is thought by some to be adequate for non-insulin treated patients (Gatling 1989).

PRIMARY CARE

There has been a shift towards providing care of diabetes in the primary care setting in the UK (Goyder et al 1998). Primary care clinics have been developed. These are frequently managed almost entirely by nursing staff with little medical input except in the design of protocols of care. In many cases, practice nurses who supervise these clinics have received some special training. They need to be aware of issues such as driving and diabetes, coping with insurance problems, optimum use of oral medications taking into account the physiology and pathology of the patient, techniques of self-monitoring and their results, correct dietary recommendations, the role of patient associations (e.g. Diabetes UK), travel and management of diabetes, management of hypoglycaemia, and the application of the 'sick day rules'. If they are responsible for patients using insulin they will need to know about the action of various types of insulin, methods of administration, storage, inspection of insulin sites, detection and management of ketonuria, education about the various methods of management of hypoglycaemia, education of caregivers, as well as how to carry out a comprehensive annual review.

Some patients are unable to travel to their family doctor or primary health care centre and have been missing out on structured care (Gadsby 1994). However, in Britain for example, community diabetes nurses (CDNs) have been appointed to visit the diabetic housebound and those in residential and nursing homes. These specialist nurses can be a valuable addition to the primary healthcare team.

COGNITIVE FUNCTION AND DEPRESSION

There is increasing evidence to link Type 2 diabetes with cognitive dysfunction. In some studies, hypoglycaemia has not been thought to play a major causal role (Austin and Deary 1999), though other studies have shown cognitive impairment with recurrent hypoglycaemia (Lincoln et al 1996). However, even impaired glucose tolerance can cause cognitive dysfunction (Vanhanen et al 1998), possibly due to hyperinsulinaemia as this can impair cognitive function even in non-diabetic persons (Stolk et al 1997). In diabetic elderly patients, impaired learning processes have been found (Croxson and Jagger 1995). Community-based studies have also shown impaired cognitive function on simple mental tests (Croxson and Jagger 1995; Dornan et al 1992; Sinclair and Bayer 1998). A recent review has suggested that many of the deficits seen in the metabolic syndrome (hypertension, hyperglycaemia, dyslipidemia) may each play a role in memory disturbance in Type 2 diabetes (Kumari, Brunner and Fuhrer 2000).

Older people with diabetes who are subject to major lifestyle changes, vascular complications and chronic ill-health may well have symptoms of clinical depression. It is important to exclude depression as a cause of cognitive impairment, as people with diabetes are more likely to be depressed (Sinclair and Croxson 1998). Indeed, the presence of depression appears to increase the risk of diabetes two-fold (Eaton et al 1996). In the presence of depressed mood, anxiety symptoms, withdrawal phenomena, and anorexia, depression must be excluded. Simple screening tests such as the Geriatric Depression Score can be used. Other explanations of cognitive impairment in diabetes can include cerebral atrophy and cerebrovascular disease (Tarcot et al 1999). Poor glucose control can cause cognitive impairment which recovers following improvement in control of diabetes (Gradman et al 1993; Jagust et al 1987). Hypertension which is commonly associated with Type 2 diabetes is also a risk factor for impaired cognitive function (Elias et al 1997).

METABOLIC CONTROL OF DIABETES

Evidence of the adverse effects of poor glucose control comes from a number of studies. For example a study has shown that mortality in patients with Type 2 diabetes increases with poor control (Anderson and Svardsudd 1995). Likewise, the worse the control the more progressive is retinopathy in NIDDM (Nakagami et al 1997).

Traditionally, diabetes management in older people was aimed just at reducing symptoms of hyper- and hypoglycaemia. It has become apparent that mortality is increased in older people with diabetes, and that poor control leads to a poor outcome in other ways, so it has become important to evaluate the effect of more intensive management of glucose and other metabolic abnormalities.

A number of studies now suggest that improving diabetic control can lead to an improved outcome. The most relevant of these is the United Kingdom Prospective Diabetes Study (UKPDS) which included patients with Type 2 diabetes diagnosed before the age of 65 years. In the intensive-glucose-reduction arm of the study (UKPDS 1998a), an 11% reduction in glycosylated haemoglobin was associated with significant risk reductions in any diabetes-related endpoint, and, in particular, microvascular endpoints. The risk of having a macrovascular endpoint was not reduced. In the blood-pressure-reduction arm (UKPDS 1998b), the principal benefits of the 10 and 5 mmHg reductions in systolic and diastolic pressures in the intensively treated group related to significant reductions in risk of both microvascular and macrovascular disease endpoints. The 44% risk reduction in stroke was particularly relevant in older populations. For every 10 mmHg reduction in systolic blood pressure, a 12% risk reduction in diabetes-related endpoints were seen.

Because this trial did not include newly diagnosed patients over 65 years of age, it is possible only to speculate that these findings relate to older patients. In particular, it is important not to extend the findings without confirmation to the frail elderly, who will have additional risk factors such as complications, or may be taking treatment for other conditions. This will result from their multiple pathology and altered physiology. In addition the lack of proof of an effect of reduced glycaemia on cardiovascular disease is disappointing when these problems are so common in older patients. However, reducing cardiovascular risk in people with diabetes involves active management of hypertension as confirmed in the UKPDS, control of hyperlipidaemia and stopping smoking as well as effective management of glucose levels (UKPDS 1998b; Sinclair and Meneilly 2000).

It has now been shown that improved glucose control is also important following myocardial infarction in patients with hyperglycaemia (Diabetes Mellitus, Insulin Glucose Infusion in Acute Myocardial Infarction Study; Malmberg 1997). Though this study was restricted to patients immediately following a myocardial infarction, it does demonstrate that more intensive treatment can improve outcome. New evidence suggests that this may also apply to patients with hyperglycaemia and acute stroke (Scott et al 1999). In the DIGAMI study, 620 patients with a blood glucose of >11 mM on admission to hospital were randomized to an immediate insulin infusion followed by four times daily insulin for at least 3 months (three times daily soluble insulin and an evening medium long-acting insulin) or conventional therapy. Glycosylated haemoglobin 3 months after entry into the study was 7.0% ($\pm$1.6%) in the infusion group and 7.5% ($\pm$1.8%) in the control group. At 3 months, 80% of those in the intensive group and 45% in the control group (much higher than one might expect) were being treated with insulin. The mortality reduction at 12 months in the more intensively treated group was 26.1% but with wide confidence limits. Surprisingly the benefit was greatest in those with a lower cardiovascular risk profile. The precise reason for this last finding is unexplained. It is worrying that insulin appears to have a less beneficial effect in those with established atherosclerosis. An important feature of this study is that older people were not excluded and the mean age was 68 years. Of course this study included patients with any type of diabetes, though 83% had Type 2.

BLOOD PRESSURE CONTROL

In the last few years research has shown the importance of good blood pressure control, especially for people with diabetes for whom much lower target blood pressures are recommended. Indeed for people with diabetes who have microalbuminuria, proteinuria or renal impairment, it is even worth lowering blood pressure in those who conventionally would be regarded as having normal levels. Angiotensin-converting enzyme (ACE) inhibitors are particularly recommended for treatment as they appear to protect renal function in the long term (Sano et al 1996; Leitz and Vora 1998).

In the UKPDS, atenolol and captopril were compared for their effects and were equally beneficial—an important finding as there has been concern about the effects of beta-blockers on lipid and glucose levels (UKPDS 1998c).

The HOT study confirmed the importance of good blood pressure control especially in people with diabetes (Hansson et al 1998). Some concern has been expressed about calcium antagonists which have been suggested to increase the risk of gastrointestinal haemorrhage and possibly also myocardial infarction, as found in the ABCD study (Estacio et al 1998). The FACET study found similar results (Tatti et al 1998). However, the HOT study and the SYST-EUR study (Fagard and Staessen 1999) are more reassuring with regard to the safety of calcium antagonists. Despite concerns expressed about thiazides increasing glucose intolerance and other adverse metabolic effects, and beta-blockers increasing the risk of hypoglycaemia, studies including patients with diabetes such as the SHEP study (Curb et al 1996) and UKPDS are reassuring.

WHAT ABOUT LIPIDS?

Diabetes is well known to be associated with hyperlipidaemia, often as a part of the metabolic (Reaven's) syndrome. A lot of research has quantified the risks and benefits of lowering lipid levels. The benefits in Type 2 diabetes are relatively well recognized (Tikkanen et al 1998; Pyorala, Olsson and Pedersen 1997). These studies have used or compared statins and fibrates (Jeck et al 1997). Unfortunately these studies have not included many very elderly patients, though the 4S study, which reported on a subset of diabetic patients, did include patients up to the age of 70 years. The VA-HIT study included male patients up to the age of 74 years (Veterans Affairs High-Density Lipoprotein Cholesterol Intervention Trial Study Group 1999). Some attempts to set metabolic thresholds for older people with diabetes have been made and these have included data on lipid levels (Sinclair 2000). There is concern in extending the findings in younger patients to the old as the relative risk of hyperlipidaemia falls with age, though the absolute risk rises. The risk/benefit ratio might therefore be very different in the very old. In the very elderly non-diabetic person, for example, there is an inverse association of cholesterol with mortality, possibly owing to the association of a

low cholesterol with serious terminal diseases such as cancer.

Treatments other than statins and fibrates, such as hormone replacement therapy in women (Robinson et al 1996) or fish oils (Friedberg et al 1998), have beneficial effects on lipids and therefore may reduce cardiovascular risk. Fish oils also have a beneficial effect on glycaemic control.

As evidence for treatment of the over-75 year olds is lacking, trials in this age group are justified. It would appear reasonable to treat older patients with hyperlipidaemia who have established vascular disease. Cost-effectiveness must be taken into account as the extension to life is likely to be reduced in the very elderly.

QUALITY OF LIFE

Diabetes mellitus, like many chronic diseases, imposes life-long stresses on achieving optimal quality of life and well-being, and this goal may be strongly influenced by how well an individual views their own health (Linn et al 1980). By virtue of high levels of comorbidities and marked disability from long-term vascular complications (Morley et al 1987), diabetes mellitus in older adults presents significant challenges in delivering healthcare, making the attainment of a satisfactory quality of life essential (Sinclair and Barnett 1993).

The effect of diabetes on health-related quality of life in older people has been reported from a varying number of perspectives and use of disease-specific and generic outcome measures. Poorer quality of life in older people with diabetes was observed in a large French community study (PAQUID Epidemiological Survey; Bourdel-Marchasson et al 1997), but demented subjects were excluded and a subjective health questionnaire based on four questions only was used. A recent British postal questionnaire study employing two diabetes-specific scales (Well-Being Questionnaire; Diabetes Treatment Satisfaction Questionnaire) examined quality of life in a random selection of inner-city patients with diabetes in Salford, UK (Petterson et al 1998). No significant relationship between glycaemic control and either quality of life measure was observed, but treatment with insulin was associated with significantly lower well-being scores. However, this finding is not universal since an improved quality of life of poorly controlled patients with diabetes being switched over to insulin has been reported (Reza et al 1999).

CHANGING OVER TO INSULIN

Early insulin transfer is now being advocated (Glaser 1998). It should not be forgotten that some older patients with diabetes require insulin within a few years of diagnosis. Studies have suggested that glutamic acid decarboxylase (GAD) and islet cell antibodies and insulin sensitivity predict early need for insulin (Turner et al 1997). Diabetes in elderly people can also present with insulin dependence (Sturrock et al 1995; Sinclair 2000). Insulin in general has been shown to be safe for older people with diabetes, a twice-daily regimen being cost-effective (Wolfenbuttel et al 1996).

CONCLUSION

There has been a huge increase in knowledge about diabetes in old age, but much work remains to be done. Knowledge has advanced particularly in the management of risk factors for the complications of diabetes, such as hypertension, hyperlipidaemia and diabetes control. There has also been some advance in service organization of diabetes care in old age. In the UK, we have seen improvements with the development of shared-care guidelines between primary healthcare (general practice) and secondary healthcare (hospital practice). The implementation of disease registers which are often computerized, and their use to ensure structured care for older people with diabetes, is noteworthy since previously older patients were left out from provision of structured care. There is an increasing array of new drug therapies with many more being actively developed. More work needs to be done on evaluation of the real benefits of these new therapies. The availability of better insulin administration devices has enhanced the care of older people with diabetes, making the use of insulin easier and safer. Likewise, better equipment for the home monitoring of diabetes has improved control.

Diabetes in old age presents many research and clinical questions, such as the management of the patient with cognitive dysfunction and its relationship to diabetes. There needs to be research to determine the easiest ways of improving glucose control, especially in patients with myocardial infarction and stroke. Hopefully there will be more knowledge of how to prevent the neurological complications of diabetes—

such as peripheral neuropathy, amyotrophy and neuropathic cachexia—that are more common in old age. Strategies for avoiding hypoglycaemia need to be researched to find out which management regimes are most effective. We need to know more about the most effective ways of screening and early diagnosis.

In short, for those interested in the unique and fascinating area of geriatric diabetes, a lifetime of challenges is available.

REFERENCES

Adler AI, Neil HA, Manley SE, Holman RR, Turner RC (1999) Hyperglycemia and hyperinsulinemia at diagnosis of diabetes: association with subsequent cardiovascular disease in the United Kingdom prospective diabetes study (UKPDS 47). *American Heart Journal*, **138**, 353–9).

American Diabetes Association (1990) Clinical practice recommendations. *Diabetes Care*, **13** (Suppl.), 41–46.

Andersson DK, Svardsudd K (1995) Long-term glycemic control relates to mortality in Type II diabetes. *Diabetes Care*, **18**, 1534–1543.

Austin EJ, Deary IJ (1999) Effects of repeated hypoglycemia on cognitive function: a psychometrically validated reanalysis of the Diabetes Control and Complications Trial data. *Diabetes Care*, **22**, 1273–1277.

Birke JA, Rolfsen RJ (1998) Evaluation of a self administered sensory testing tool to identify patients at risk of diabetes related foot problems. *Diabetes Care*, **21**, 23–25.

Bourdel-Marchasson I, Dubroca B, Manciet G, Decamps A, Emeriau J-P, Dartigues J-F (1997) Prevalence of diabetes and effect on quality of life in older French living in the community; the PAQUID Epidemiological Survey. *Journal of the American Geriatrics Society*, **45**, 295–301.

Bourdel-Marchasson I, Dubroca B, Decamps A, Richard-Hanton S, Emeriau J-P, Dartigues JF (1998) Five year mortality in elderly French subjects from the PAQUID Epidemiological survey. *Diabetic Medicine*, **15**, 830–835.

Connor H (1997) Footcare advice: what do we tell out patients and what should we tell them? *Practical Diabetes International*, **14**, 75–77.

Croxson SCM, Burden AC (1998) Polyuria and polydipsia in an elderly population: its relationship to previously undiagnosed diabetes. *Practical Diabetes*, **15**, 170–172.

Croxson SCM, Burden AC, Bodlington M and Botha JL (1991) The prevalence of diabetes in elderly people. *Diabetic Medicine*, **8**, 28–31.

Croxson S, Jagger C (1995) Diabetes and cognitive impairment: a community based study of elderly subjects. *Age and aging*, **24**, 421–424.

Curb JD, Pressel SL, Cutler JA, Savage PJ, Applegate WB, Black H, Camel G, Davies BR, Frost PH, Gonzalez N, Guthrie G, Oberman A, Rutan GH, Stamler J (1996) Effect of diuretic-based antihypertensive treatment on cardiovascular disease risk in older diabetic patients with isolated systolic hypertension. Systolic Hypertension in the Elderly Program Cooperative Research Group. *JAMA*, **276**, 1886–1892.

Dornan TL, Peck GM, Dow JD, Tattersall RB (1992) A community survey of diabetes in the elderly. *Diabetic Medicine*, **9**, 860–865.

Eaton WW, Armenian H, Gallo J, Pratt L, Ford DE (1996) Depression and risk for onset of Type II diabetes: a prospective population based study. *Diabetes Care*, **19**, 1097–1102.

Elias PK, Wilson PW, Elias ME, Silbershatz H, D'Agostino RB, Wolf PA, Cupples LA (1997) NIDDM and blood pressure as risk factors for poor cognitive performance: the Framingham Study. *Diabetes Care*, **20**, 1388–1395.

Elwyn GJ, Vaughan NJA, Stott NCH (1998) District diabetes registers: more trouble than they're worth? *Diabetic Medicine*, **15** (Suppl. 3), S44–48.

Estacio RO, Jeffers BW, Hiatt WR, Biggerstaff SL, Gifford N, Schrier RW (1998) The effect of nisoldipine as compared with enalapril on cardiovascular outcomes in patients with non-insulin-dependent diabetes and hypertension. *New England Journal of Medicine*, **338**, 645–652.

Faas A, Schellevis FG, Van Eijk JT (1997) The efficacy of self-monitoring of blood glucose in NIDDM subjects. a criteria-based literature review. *Diabetes Care*, **20**, 1482–1486.

Fagard RH, Staessen JA (1999) Treatment of isolated systolic hypertension in the elderly: the Syst-Eur Trial. Systolic Hypertension in Europe (Syst-Eur) Trial Investigators. *Clinical and Experimental Hypertension*, **21**, 491–497.

Friedberg CE, Janssen MJ, Heine RJ, Grobbee DE (1998) Fish oil and glycemic control in diabetes: a meta-analysis. *Diabetes Care*, **21**, 494–500.

Gadsby R (1994) Care of people with diabetes who are housebound or in nursing and residential homes. *Diabetes in General Practice*, **4**, 30–31.

Gatling W (1989) Home monitoring of diabetes. *Practical Diabetes*, **6**, 100–101.

Glaser B (1998) Insulin treatment of Type 2 diabetes mellitus. *Diabetes Reviews International*, **7**, 5–8.

Goyder EC, McNally PG, Drucquer M, Spiers N, Botha JL (1998) Shifting of care for diabetes from secondary to primary care, 1990–5: review of general practices. *British Medical Journal*, **316**, 1505–1506.

Gradman TJ, Laws A, Thompson LW, Reaven GM (1993) Verbal learning and/or memory improves with glycemic control in older subjects with non-insulin-dependent diabetes mellitus. *Journal of the American Geriatrics Society*, **41**, 1305–1312.

Griffin S (1998) Diabetes care in general practice: meta-analysis of randomised controlled trials. *British Medical Journal*, **317**, 390–396.

Hansson L, Zanchetti A, Carruthers SG, Dahlof B, Elmfeldt D, Julius S, Menard J, Wedel H, Westerling S (1998) Effects of intensive blood-pressure lowering and low-dose aspirin in patients with hypertension: principal results of the Hypertension Optimal Treatment (HOT) randomised trial. *Lancet*, **351**, 1755–1762.

Helkala EL, Niskanen L, Viinamaki H, Partanen J, Uusitupa M (1995) Short-term and long-term memory in elderly patients with NIDDM. *Diabetes Care*, **18**, 681–685.

Hendra TJ, Sinclair AJ (1997) Improving the care of elderly diabetic patients: the final report of the St Vincent Joint Task Force for Diabetes. *Age and Ageing*, **26**, 3–6.

Jagust W, Cramon DY, Renner R, Hepp KD (1987) Tight metabolic control improves cerebral function in older Type 2 diabetic patients. *Diabetologia*, **30**: 535A (abstract).

Jeck T, Riesen WF, Keller U (1997) Comparison of bezafibrate and simvastatin in the treatment of dyslipidaemia in patients with NIDDM. *Diabetic Medicine*, **14**, 564–570.

Kumari M, Brunner E, Fuhrer R (2000) Minireview: mechanisms by which the metabolic syndrome and diabetes impair memory. *Journal of Gerontology (Biological Sciences)*, **55A**, B228–232.

Leitz G, Vora JP (1996) The management of hypertension in diabetes with special reference to diabetic kidney disease. *Diabetic Medicine*, **13**, 401–410.

Levetan CS, Passaro M, Jablonski K, Kass M, Ratne RE (1998) Unrecognized diabetes among hospital patients. *Diabetes Care*, **21**, 246–249.

Levin ME (1995) Preventing amputation in the patient with diabetes. *Diabetes Care*, **18**, 1383–1394.

Lincoln NB, Faleiro RM, Kelly C, Kirk BA, Jeffcoate WJ (1996) Effect of long-term glycemic control on cognitive function. *Diabetes Care*, **19**, 656–658.

Linn MW, Linn BS, Skyler JS, Harris R (1980) The importance of self-assessed health in patients with diabetes. *Diabetes Care*, **3**, 599–606.

Litzelman DK, Marriott DJ (1997) The role of footwear in the prevention of foot lesions in patients with NIDDM: conventional wisdom or evidenced-based practice? *Diabetes Care*, **20**, 856–862.

Malmberg K for the DIGAMI Study Group (1997) Prospective randomised study of intensive insulin treatment on long term survival after acute myocardial infarction in patients with diabetes mellitus. *British Medical Journal*, **314**, 1512–1515.

Martin BJ, Young RE, Kesson KM (1986) Home monitoring of blood glucose in elderly non-insulin-dependent diabetics. *Practical Diabetes*, **3**, 37.

McGwin G Jr, Sims RV, Pulley L, Roseman M (1999) Diabetes and automobile crashes in the elderly: a population-based case-control study. *Diabetes Care*, **22**, 20–27.

Morley JE, Mooradian AD, Rosenthal MJ, Kaiser FE (1987) Diabetes mellitus in elderly patients: is it different? *American Journal of Medicine*, **83**, 533–544.

Nakagami T, Kawahara R, Hori S, Omori Y (1997) Glycemic control and prevention of retinopathy in Japanese NIDDM patients: a 10-year follow-up study. *Diabetes Care*, **20**, 621–626.

Paterson KR (1994) Population screening for diabetes mellitus. Professional Advisory Committee of the British Diabetic Association. *Diabetic Medicine*, **11**, 517–518.

Peters AL, Davidson MB (1998) Application of a diabetic managed care program: the feasability of using nurses and a computer system to provide effective care. *Diabetes Care*, **21**, 1037–1043.

Petterson T, Lee P, Hollis S, Young B, Newton P, Dornan T (1998) Well-being and treatment satisfaction in older people with diabetes. *Diabetes Care*, **21**, 930–935.

Pyorala K, Olsson AG, Pedersen TR, Thorgeirsson G, Kjekshus J, Faergeman O (1997) Cholesterol lowering with simvastatin improves prognosis of diabetic patients with coronary heart disease: a subgroup analysis of the Scandinavian Simvastatin Survival Study (4S). *Diabetes Care*, **20**, 614–620.

Reza M, Taylor C, Towse K, Ward JD, Hendra TJ (1999) Impact of insulin treatment in elderly subjects with non insulin dependent diabetes mellitus on quality of life, satisfaction with treatment and carer strain. *Age and Ageing*, **28** (Suppl. 1), 30.

Robinson JG, Folsom AR, Nabulsi AA, Watson R, Brancati FL, Cai J (1996) Can postmenopausal hormone replacement improve plasma lipids in women with diabetes? The Atherosclerosis Risk in Communities Study Investigators. *Diabetes Care*, **19**, 480–485.

Ruige JR, Bouter LM, de Neiling JND, Heine RJ, Kostenue PJ (1997) Performance of an NIDDM screening questionnaire based on symptoms and risk factors. *Diabetes Care*, **20**, 491–496.

Ryder B (1995) Screening for diabetic retinopathy. *British Medical Journal*, **311**, 207–208.

Sano T, Hotta N, Kawamura T, Matsuna H, Chaya S, Sasaki H, Nakayama M, Hara T, Matsui S, Skamito N (1996) Effects of long-term enalapril on persistent microalbuminuria in normotensive Type 2 diabetic patients: results of a 4 year, prospective, randomised study. *Diabetic Medicine*, **13**, 220–224.

Scott JF, Robinson G, French JM, O'Connell JE, Alberti KGMM, Gray CS (1999) Glucose potassium insulin (GKI) infusions in the treatment of acute stroke patients with mild to moderate hyperglycaemia (the GIST trial). *Age and aging*, **28** (Suppl. 1), 46.

Sheppard DA (1998) Driving regulations and diabetes: recent changes. *Practical Diabetes International*, **15**, 69.

Sinclair AJ (2000) Diabetes in old age: changing concepts in the secondary care arena. *Journal of the Royal College of Physicians of London*, **34**, 240–244.

Sinclair AJ, Barnett AH (1993) Special needs of elderly diabetic patients. *British Medical Journal*, **306**, 1142–1143.

Sinclair AJ, Bayer AJ (1998) *All Wales Research in Elderly (AWARE) Diabetes Study*. Department of Health Report 121/3040. London: UK government.

Sinclair AJ, Croxson SCM (1998) Diabetes mellitus in the older adult. In: Tallis R, Fillit H, Brocklehurst JC (eds) *Textbook of Geriatric Medicine and Gerontology, 5th edn*. London: Churchill-Livingstone, 1051–1072.

Sinclair AJ, Meneilly GS (2000) Re-thinking metabolic strategies for older people with Type 2 diabetes mellitus: implications of the UKPDS and other recent studies. *Age and aging*, (in press).

Sinclair AJ, Robert IE, Croxson SCM (1997) Mortality in older people with diabetes mellitus. *Diabetic Medicine*, **14**, 639–647.

Stolk RP, Breteler MM, Ott A, Pols HA, Lamberts SW, Grobbee DE, Hofman A (1997) Insulin and cognitive function in an elderly population: the Rotterdam Study. *Diabetes Care*, **20**, 792–795.

Sturrock NBC, Page SR, Clarke P, Tattersall RB (1995) Insulin dependent diabetes in nonagenarians. *British Medical Journal*, **310**, 1117–1118.

Tarcot PN, Ogden MA, Cox C, Williams TF (1999) Diabetes and dementia in long-term care. *Journal of the American Geriatrics Society*, **47**, 423–429.

Tatti P, Pahor M, Byington RP, Di Mauro P, Guaresco R, Strollo G, Strollo F (1998) Outcome results of the Fosinopril versus Amlodipine Cardiovascular Events Randomized Trial (FACET) in patients with NIDDM. *Diabetes Care*, **21**, 597–603.

Taylor DJ, Fisher J, Jacob J, Tooke JE (1999) The use of digital cameras in a mobile retinal screening environment. *Diabetic Medicine*, **16**, 680–686.

Thomson FJ, Masson EA (1996). Can elderly persons co-operate with routine footcare. *Age and Ageing*, **21**, 333–337.

Tikkanen MJ, Laakso M, Ilmonen M, Helve E, Kaarsalo E, Kilkki E, Saltevo J (1998) Treatment of hypercholesterolaemia and combined hyperlipidaemia with simvastatin and gemfibrozil in patients with NIDDM: a multicenter comparison study. *Diabetes Care*, **21**, 477–481.

Turner R, Stratton I, Horton V, Manley S, Zimmet P, Mckay IR, Shattock M, Bottazu GF, Holman R (1997) UKPDS 25: autoantibodies to islet-cell cytoplasm and glutamic acid decarboxylase for prediction of insulin requirement in Type 2 diabetes. *Lancet*, **350**, 1288–1293.

Uccioli L, Faglia E, Monticone E, Favales F, Durola L, Aldeghi A, Quarantillo A, Calia P, Menzinger G (1995) Manufactured shoes in the prevention of diabetic ulcers. *Diabetes Care*, **18**, 1376–1378.

UK Prospective Diabetes Study (UKPDS) Group (1998a) Intensive blood-glucose control with sulphonylureas or insulin compared with conventional treatment and risk of complications in patients with Type 2 diabetes. *Lancet*, **352**, 837–853.

UK Prospective Diabetes Study Group (1998b) Tight blood pressure control and risk of microvascular and macrovascular complications in Type 2 diabetes. *British Medical Journal*, **317**, 703–713.

UK Prospective Diabetes Study Group (1998c) Efficacy of atenolol and captopril in reducing risk of macrovascular and microvascular complications in Type 2 diabetes. *British Medical Journal*, **317**, 713–720.

van der Does FE, de Neeling JN, Snoek FJ, Grootenhuis PA, Kostense PJ, Bouter LM, Heine RJ (1998) Randomized study of two different target levels of glycemic control within the acceptable range in Type 2 diabetes: effects on well-being at 1 year. *Diabetes Care*, **21**, 2085–2093.

Vanhanen M, Koivisto K, Kuusisto J, Mykkanen L, Helkala EL, Hanninen T, Riekkinen P Sr, Soininen H, Laakso M (1998) Cognitive function in an elderly population with persistent impaired glucose tolerance. *Diabetes Care*, **21**, 398–402.

Veterans Affairs High-Density Lipoprotein Cholesterol Intervention Trial Study Group (1999) Gemfibrozil for the secondary prevention of coronary heart disease in men with low levels of high-density lipoprotein cholesterol. *New England Journal of Medicine*, **341**, 410–418.

Wolffenbuttel BHR, Sels JP, Rondas-Colbers GJ, Menheere PP, Kruseman AC (1996) Comparison of different insulin regimens in elderly patients with NIDDM. *Diabetes Care*, **19**, 1326–1634.

World Health Organization Europe and European Region of International Diabetes Federation (1989) *The St Vincent Declaration*. Copenhagen: WHO Europe and the European Region of IDF.

Index

Index compiled by Liza Furnival